Acta Neurochirurgica Supplement 136

Series Editor
Hans-Jakob Steiger
Department of Neurosurgery
Heinrich Heine University
Düsseldorf, Germany

ACTA NEUROCHIRURGICA's Supplement Volumes provide a unique opportunity to publish the content of special meetings in the form of a Proceedings Volume. Proceedings of international meetings concerning a special topic of interest to a large group of the neuroscience community are suitable for publication in ACTA NEUROCHIRURGICA. Links to ACTA NEUROCHIRURGICA's distribution network guarantee wide dissemination at a comparably low cost. The individual volumes should comprise between 120 and max. 250 printed pages, corresponding to 20-50 papers. It is recommended that you get in contact with us as early as possible during the preparatory stage of a meeting. Please supply a preliminary program for the planned meeting. The papers of the volumes represent original publications. They pass a peer review process and are listed in PubMed and other scientific databases. Publication can be effected within 6 months. Hans-Jakob Steiger is the Editor of ACTA NEUROCHIRURGICA's Supplement Volumes. Springer Verlag International is responsible for the technical aspects and calculation of the costs. If you decide to publish your proceedings in the Supplements of ACTA NEUROCHIRURGICA, you can expect the following: • An editing process with editors both from the neurosurgical community and professional language editing. After your book is accepted, you will be assigned a developmental editor who will work with you as well as with the entire editing group to bring your book to the highest quality possible. • Effective text and illustration layout for your book. • Worldwide distribution through Springer-Verlag International's distribution channels.

Giuseppe Esposito · Yasuhiko Kaku
Martina Sebök · Luca Regli
Tetsuya Tsukahara
Editors

Trends in the Treatment of Cerebrovascular Diseases

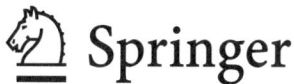

Editors
Giuseppe Esposito
Department of Neurosurgery
University Hospital Zurich
Zurich, Switzerland

Martina Sebök
Department of Neurosurgery
University Hospital Zurich
Zurich, Switzerland

Tetsuya Tsukahara
Department of Neurosurgery
Kyoto Medical Center
Kyoto, Japan

Yasuhiko Kaku
Department of Neurosurgery
Asahi University Hospital
Gifu, Japan

Luca Regli
Department of Neurosurgery
University Hospital Zurich
Zurich, Switzerland

European – Japanese Cerebrovascular Congress
ejcvc, ejcvc2022, EJCVC, Kyoto, Japan, 2022, 11, 13, 2022, 11, 16
https://site.convention.co.jp/ejcvc2020/

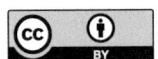

ISSN 0065-1419   ISSN 2197-8395 (electronic)
Acta Neurochirurgica Supplement 136
ISBN 978-3-031-89843-3   ISBN 978-3-031-89844-0 (eBook)
https://doi.org/10.1007/978-3-031-89844-0

This work was supported by Kyoto University.

© The Editor(s) (if applicable) and The Author(s) 2025. This book is an open access publication.

Open Access This book is licensed under the terms of the Creative Commons Attribution 4.0 International License (http://creativecommons.org/licenses/by/4.0/), which permits use, sharing, adaptation, distribution and reproduction in any medium or format, as long as you give appropriate credit to the original author(s) and the source, provide a link to the Creative Commons license and indicate if changes were made.

The images or other third party material in this book are included in the book's Creative Commons license, unless indicated otherwise in a credit line to the material. If material is not included in the book's Creative Commons license and your intended use is not permitted by statutory regulation or exceeds the permitted use, you will need to obtain permission directly from the copyright holder.

The use of general descriptive names, registered names, trademarks, service marks, etc. in this publication does not imply, even in the absence of a specific statement, that such names are exempt from the relevant protective laws and regulations and therefore free for general use.

The publisher, the authors and the editors are safe to assume that the advice and information in this book are believed to be true and accurate at the date of publication. Neither the publisher nor the authors or the editors give a warranty, expressed or implied, with respect to the material contained herein or for any errors or omissions that may have been made. The publisher remains neutral with regard to jurisdictional claims in published maps and institutional affiliations.

This Springer imprint is published by the registered company Springer Nature Switzerland AG
The registered company address is: Gewerbestrasse 11, 6330 Cham, Switzerland

If disposing of this product, please recycle the paper.

Preface

The 10th European–Japanese Cerebrovascular Congress (EJCVC), held in Kyoto from November 13 to 16, 2022, marked a pivotal moment in the history of this esteemed series of meetings. For the 10th anniversary edition and for the first time, the congress took place in Japan, representing a significant step toward strengthening international collaboration in the treatment of cerebrovascular diseases. Originally scheduled for an earlier date, the meeting experienced delays due to the global COVID-19 pandemic, with Japan's strict travel restrictions causing two postponements. The decision to proceed with the congress, made during the summer of 2022, despite ongoing travel limitations, highlighted the organizers' resilience and their commitment to advancing the field.

The lifting of Japan's travel restrictions just 1 month before the congress enabled an in-person gathering that highlighted the profound value of face-to-face scientific exchange. After 2 years of virtual meetings, the return to a live format revitalized the community, emphasizing the irreplaceable role of direct engagement in fostering innovation and collaboration. The palpable energy of the attendees, coupled with the historic setting of Kyoto, created an environment that nurtured both scientific rigor and cross-cultural exchange.

The scientific program of the 10th EJCVC showcased an impressive array of technical progress and clinical advancements. Experts from Japan and Europe presented cutting-edge research and engaged in robust discussions on the most pressing challenges in the field of cerebrovascular disease. These exchanges not only advanced understanding but also inspired new lines of inquiry and collaboration, reinforcing the congress's role as a cornerstone of progress in cerebrovascular research and treatment.

This volume, part of the ongoing series *Trends in Cerebrovascular Disease*, the proceedings of the European–Japanese Cerebrovascular Congresses, encapsulates the high-level presentations and discussions that took place during this memorable event. The chapters provide a comprehensive overview of the current state of the field, covering topics from novel surgical techniques and interventional approaches to advancements in imaging, pharmacology, and patient management. Together, these contributions highlight the dynamic nature of cerebrovascular research and the critical role of multidisciplinary collaboration in driving innovation.

We extend our deepest gratitude to all the contributors, whose dedication and expertise have made this volume possible. Special thanks are due to the organizing committee, whose unwavering efforts ensured the success of the 10th EJCVC despite unprecedented challenges. We are also grateful to the city of Kyoto for offering a setting that enriched the congress experience, seamlessly blending tradition and modernity in a way that reflects the spirit of progress in our field.

As you explore the contents of this volume, we hope you will find inspiration in the remarkable advancements presented and a renewed sense of purpose in addressing the complex challenges of cerebrovascular disease. May this compilation serve not only as a record of a historic meeting but also as a catalyst for future discoveries and innovations.

Sincerely,

Zurich, Switzerland	Giuseppe Esposito
Gifu, Japan	Yasuhiko Kaku
Zurich, Switzerland	Martina Sebök
Zurich, Switzerland	Luca Regli
Kyoto, Japan	Tetsuya Tsukahara

Contents

Part I Aneurysms and SAH

Clinical Evidence for Intravenous Milrinone to Treat Secondary Cerebral Ischemia After Aneurysmal Subarachnoid Hemorrhage—A Narrative Review.................................... 3
Hans-Jakob Steiger, Lukas Andereggen, and Serge Marbacher

Tenascin-C as a Target for Intervention in Delayed Cerebral Ischemia After Subarachnoid Hemorrhage............................ 11
Hidenori Suzuki, Fumihiro Kawakita, Hideki Nakajima, Hiroki Oinaka, Mai Nampei, and Yume Suzuki

Introducing Bayesian Analysis for Clinicians: Sex-Associated Risk Assessment of Intracranial Aneurysms............................ 19
Philippe Bijlenga, Georg Ralph Spinner, Marco Scutari, Matteo Delucchi, and Sven Hirsch

Challenges of the Endovascular Approach for Difficult Cerebral Aneurysms... 27
Shigeru Miyachi

Part II AVM and dAVF

An Evaluation of Motor Function in Surgery for Cerebral Arteriovenous Malformations via 3-Tesla Magnetic Resonance Tractography.. 37
Ayumi Akazawa, Yoshifumi Higashino, Makoto Isozaki, Takahiro Yamauchi, Satoshi Kawajiri, Munetaka Yomo, Ken Matsuda, Hidetaka Arishima, Shintaro Yamada, Miduki Oiwa, Tsutomu Okada, Yasutaka Fushimi, Nobuyuki Miki, Yoshiki Arakawa, and Kenichiro Kikuta

The Forefront of Gamma Knife Radiosurgery for Brain Arteriovenous Malformations: Our History of Treatment Optimisation Over 30 Years and the Modern Outcomes................ 47
Yuki Shinya, Hirotaka Hasegawa, Motoyuki Umekawa, Masahiro Shin, Mariko Kawashima, Satoshi Koizumi, Atsuto Katano, Yuichi Suzuki, Taichi Kin, and Nobuhito Saito

Role and Efficacy of Direct Surgery in the Management of Intracranial Dural Arteriovenous Fistulas........................... 61
Taku Sugiyama, Toshiya Osanai, Masaki Ito, Haruto Uchino, and Miki Fujimura

Paraspinal Arteriovenous Shunt Associated with PTEN Hamartoma Tumor Syndrome: A Case Report and Literature Review................ 69
Sayaka Ito and Naoki Hatsuda

Efficacy of High-Resolution Cone-Beam CT for the Endovascular Treatment of Dural Arteriovenous Fistulas............................ 73
Michihiro Tanaka, Keisuke Kadooka, Takafumi Mitsutake, Shimpei Tsuboki, and Kotaro Ueda

Part III Bypass and Moyamoya

Cerebral Ischemic Complications of Surgical Treatment in Patients with Moyamoya Disease.. 85
Anna A. Shulgina, Vasily A. Lukshin, Anton A. Korshunov, and Dmitry Yu. Usachev

Long-Term Outcome of Moyamoya Disease.......................... 93
Peter Birkeland, Victoria Hansen, Vinosha Tharmabalan, Jens Lauritsen, Troels Nielsen, Thomas Truelsen, Sverre Rosenbaum, and Paul von Weitzel-Mudersbach

Efficacy and Safety of Combined Revascularization Surgery for Moyamoya Disease: Standard Procedure and Perioperative Management... 99
Miki Fujimura, Masaki Ito, Haruto Uchino, Masahito Kawabori, and Taku Sugiyama

Comparison of Exoscopic and Microscopic Superficial Temporal Artery to Middle Cerebral Artery Bypass............................ 105
Takuma Maeda, Hidetoshi Ooigawa, Koki Onodera, Yushiro Take, Hiroki Sato, Kaima Suzuki, and Hiroki Kurita

Flow-Augmentation Bypass Surgery: Indications and Decision-Making... 113
Giuseppe Esposito, Martina Sebök, Jorn Fierstra, and Luca Regli

Part IV Neuroimaging

New Classification of the Degree of Cerebrovascular Insufficiency in Patients with Moyamoya Disease Measured According to ASL-MRI Perfusion... 121
Anna A. Shulgina, Vasily A. Lukshin, Anton A. Korshunov, Dmitry Yu Usachev, and Igor N. Pronin

ADC Threshold Indicating the Ischemic Region for Predicting Efficacy in Thrombectomy.. 129
Hideyuki Ishihara, Fumiaki Oka, Takuma Nishimoto, Masatoshi Yamane, Kazutaka Sugimoto, and Hirokazu Sadahiro

Novel Hemodynamic Parameters for Cerebral Ischemia in Patients with Occlusive Cerebrovascular Disease Using Dual ASL Perfusion Imaging.. 135
Jyoji Nakagawara

Part V Cavernoma and Others

Epidemiology and Aetiology of Cerebral Cavernous Malformations ... 143
Hiroki Hongo, Satoru Miyawaki, and Nobuhito Saito

Part VI Innovations

Experiences with and Practical Implications of Using a Hybrid Operating Room ... 153
Matthias Gmeiner, Vanessa Mazanec, Michael Sonnberger, and Andreas Gruber

Artificial Intelligence and Augmented Reality in Vascular Neurosurgery ... 157
Tristan van Doormaal, Elisa Colombo, Tim Fick, Jesse A. M. van Doormaal, Tessa M. Kos, Mathijs de Boer, Pierre Robe, Eelco Hoving, Lambertus W. Bartels, and Luca Regli

Educational Impact of an Annotation System Integrated with an Exoscope for Cerebral Aneurysm Surgery: Case Description ... 165
Yoji Tanaka, Motoki Inaji, Daisu Abe, Kazuhide Shimizu, and Taketoshi Maehara

Part VII Editorials

Microneurosurgical Training on Simulators: The Zurich Microsurgery Lab Experience ... 173
Elisa Colombo, Lara Höbner, Martina Sebök, Tristan van Doormaal, Luca Regli, and Giuseppe Esposito

Index ... 177

Part I
Aneurysms and SAH

Clinical Evidence for Intravenous Milrinone to Treat Secondary Cerebral Ischemia After Aneurysmal Subarachnoid Hemorrhage—A Narrative Review

Hans-Jakob Steiger, Lukas Andereggen, and Serge Marbacher

Introduction

For almost half a century, induced normovolemic or hypervolemic arterial hypertension has been the mainstay of treatment for delayed cerebral ischemia (DCI) after aneurysmal subarachnoid hemorrhage (SAH) [8, 18, 20, 26]. Within the frame of induced hypertension, hypervolemia, and hemodilution (triple-H therapy), more-detailed studies have suggested that induced hypertension is the principal effector [18]. Induced hypervolemia and hemodilution have subsequently been seen more critically. In the most recent version of the guidelines of the American Stroke Association, dating from 2012, euvolemia is recommended, and hemodilution is no longer an issue, partially influenced by the negative effects of albumin in traumatic brain injury [8, 9]. In addition to systemic therapy, the mentioned guidelines have recommended cerebral angioplasty and/or selective intra-arterial vasodilator therapy in patients with symptomatic cerebral vasospasm, particularly those who are not rapidly responding to hypertensive therapy [8].

The intra-arterial and intravenous administration of milrinone has become popular over the past 20 years, and many clinical series have been published. Milrinone is promising as an inotropic vasodilator to increase perfusion and eliminate arterial constriction [5–7, 12]. Milrinone belongs to the group of phosphdiesterase-3 inhibitors (see Table 1).

In 2016, hyperdynamic therapy with the intravenous administration of milrinone and norepinephrine was introduced as the standard treatment for symptomatic cerebral vasospasm or DCI after SAH at the Kantonsspital Aarau [25]. Because milrinone can cause arterial hypotension or at least lower the blood pressure below levels recommended by current international guidelines [8], therapy requires the additional use of vasopressors, in our case norepinephrine. Our treatment protocol included a strict schedule of computed tomography (CT) perfusion studies to monitor cerebral perfusion. The scheme also included the possibility of additional intra-arterial infusion of nimodipine in case of the ineffectiveness of systemic therapy. A retrospective analysis of the treatment results showed and immediate improvement in ischemic symptoms and in brain perfusion following the induction of the rescue therapy.

The aim of the current analysis is to contextualize our results with the published clinical studies on the use of milrinone as a rescue strategy for DCI following SAH. For this purpose, PubMed was searched for subarachnoid hemorrhage and milrinone, with the filter *clinical trial*.

Table 1 Main phosphodiesterase-3 inhibitors, including effects and side effects [17]

PDE-3 inhibitor	Main indications	Effects	Common side effects
Cilostazol	Peripheral artery disease, intermittent claudication	Antiplatelet, vasodilation, increased walking distance	Headache, diarrhea, palpitations, dizziness, abdominal pain
Milrinone	Acute decompensated heart failure, short-term treatment of heart failure	Positive inotropic effect, vasodilation	Hypotension, arrhythmias, thrombocytopenia, tremor
Amrinone	Short-term treatment of heart failure	Positive inotropic effect, vasodilation	Thrombocytopenia, arrhythmias, hypotension, nausea, vomiting
Enoximone	Short-term treatment of heart failure	Positive inotropic effect, vasodilation	Hypotension, arrhythmias, nausea, vomiting, headache

Note: *PDE* phosphodiesterase

Results

Summary of Our Results

In our analysis, we retrospectively analyzed 176 patients with aneurysmal SAH treated at the Kantonsspital Aarau between April 2016 and March 2021 [25]. Ninety-eight of these suffered from DCI and were submitted to rescue therapy with intravenous milrinone and norepinephrine and to additional intra-arterial spasmolysis with nimodipine in the case of the insufficient effect of systemic therapy. For the numeric analysis of the treatment results, characteristics of patients and clinical responses to rescue therapy were correlated with hemodynamic parameters, as assessed via CT angiography (CTA) and perfusion CT. Time-to-peak (TTP) delay in the ischemic focus and the volume with a TTP delay of more than 4 s (T4 volume) were used as hemodynamic parameters.

The median delay to neurological deterioration following SAH was 5 days. Perfusion CT at that time showed median T4 volumes of 40 cc and mean focal TTP delays of 2.5 ± 2.1 s in these patients. Following rescue therapy, median T4 volume decreased to 10 cc and mean focal TTP delay to 1.7 ± 1.9 s. Seventeen patients (17% of patients with DCI) underwent additional intra-arterial spasmolysis using nimodipine. The visible resolution of macroscopic vasospasm on CTA was observed in 43% of the patients with DCI and verified vasospasm on CTA, including those managed with additional intra-arterial spasmolysis. Initial World Federation of Neurological Surgeons (WFNS) grade, the occurrence of secondary infarction, age, ischemic volumes and TTP delays at the time of decline, the time to clinical decline, and the necessity for additional intra-arterial spasmolysis were identified as the most important features determining neurological outcome at 6 months (Table 2). The more severe the initial SAH, the older the patients, and the earlier that DCI occurred, the worse the outcome.

In conclusion, our analysis showed that cerebral perfusion in the setting of secondary cerebral ischemia following SAH is measurably improved through milrinone and norepinephrine-based hyperdynamic therapy. A long-term clinical benefit from the addition of milrinone appears likely. The separation of the direct effect of milrinone from the effect of induced hypertension is not possible according to the present dataset.

Table 2 Importance of features governing dichotomized outcome (mRS 0–2 vs. mRS $\geq$ 3) in our patients suffering delayed ischemic decline according to Random Forest Classifier [25]

Feature	Relative importance (%)
Initial WFNS grade	23.12
Post-aneurysm occlusion T4 volume	10.35
Day of DCI onset	09.55
Age	07.67
Post-aneurysm occlusion TTP delay	07.62
Pre-existing hypertension	06.30
Additional intra-arterial spasmolysis	06.28
TTP delay at DCI onset	05.16
Secondary infarction at discharge	05.07
T4 volume at DCI onset	04.81
Fisher grade	03.91
Resolution of vasospasm on CTA after rescue therapy	03.85
Vasospasm on CTA at DCI onset	03.17
Gender	02.69
Pre-existing diabetes	00.46

Summary of Published Controlled Trials Using Intravenous Milrinone

The published controlled studies on the intravenous use of milrinone are summarized in Table 3.

Soliman and Zohry published the results of a randomized trial to compare the effect of prophylactic magnesium sulfate and milrinone on the incidence of cerebral vasospasm after

Table 3 Comparative clinical studies using intravenous milrinone for vasospasm and DCI following aneurysmal subarachnoid hemorrhage

Author, year	Type of study	Total number of patients	Additional measures in milrinone group	Measures in control group	Primary outcome	Result
Soliman, 2019 [24]	Prospective, preventive, randomized	90	None, IV milrinone for 21 days	Intravenous magnesium for 21 days	TCD flow velocity <120 cm/s, DCI	Magnesium better in terms of TCD and occurrence of DCI
Rouanet, 2021 [19]	Prospective, observational	21	None	Norepinephrine	TCD values and NIHSS at 45 and 90 minutes	TCD value lower in milrinone group, no clinical difference
Labeyrie, 2021 [13]	Retrospective two-site comparison	200	Balloon angioplasty	Induced hypertension	1-month mortality, 6-month mRS 0–2, brain infarction	No or minimal difference between strategies
Lakhal, 2021 [14]	Retrospective historical comparison	94	Induced hypertension	Hypertension alone	6-month mRS 2–6, brain infarction	mRS 2–6 and infarction 75% lower in treatment group

Note: *IV* intravenous, *NIHSS* National Institutes of Health Stroke Scale

subarachnoid hemorrhage [24]. The study included 90 patients with aneurysmal subarachnoid hemorrhage randomly classified into two groups. Magnesium sulfate was given as an infusion of 500 mg daily for 21 days, or milrinone was given as an infusion of 0.5 µg/kg/min for 21 days. Cerebral vasospasm was diagnosed via transcranial Doppler (TCD) (mean cerebral blood flow velocity in the involved cerebral artery ≥120 cm/s), neurological deterioration according to the Glasgow Coma Scale (GCS), or angiography (decrease in diameter of the involved cerebral artery >25%). The researchers found that mean TCD flow velocity decreased significantly in the magnesium group compared to the milrinone group through days 7, 14, and 21 ($p < 0.001$). The incidence of cerebral vasospasm was significantly lower with magnesium than with milrinone. GCS improved significantly in the magnesium group compared to the milrinone group through day 7, day 14, and day 21. The incidence of hypotension was higher with milrinone than with magnesium. In conclusion, the incidence of cerebral vasospasm after aneurysmal subarachnoid hemorrhage was significantly lower and GCS significantly better with magnesium when compared to milrinone. Milrinone was associated with a higher incidence of hypotension and needing dopamine and norepinephrine when compared to magnesium.

Rouanet and coauthors studied cerebral hemodynamics and clinical responses to induced hypertension with norepinephrine and inotropic therapy with milrinone as a rescue strategy for DCI [19]. Patients with SAH receiving rescue therapy with norepinephrine or milrinone for DCI treatment were retrospectively reviewed. TCD and the National Institutes of Health (NIH) Stroke Scale were evaluated before therapy initiation and 45 and 90 minutes after the onset of therapy. Ninety-eight patients with aneurysmal SAH were admitted during the study period. Twenty-one (21.4%) developed DCI, of whom six had DCI twice, leading to a total of 27 analyzed DCI events. Twelve events were treated with norepinephrine and 15 with milrinone. On average, patients treated with norepinephrine had their mean arterial pressure raised from 85 mm Hg at baseline to 112 mm Hg 90 minutes later, whereas those treated with milrinone had a significant decrease in mean arterial pressure over treatment, from 94 mm Hg to 88 mm Hg at 90 minutes. Among the patients treated with induced hypertension, there were no significant changes in TCD flow velocities (highest at baseline 163.2 cm/s, at 45 minutes 172.9 cm/s, and at 90 minutes 164 cm/s). Conversely, in those treated with milrinone, there was a significant decrease from baseline to 45 and 90 minutes (highest at baseline 197.1 cm/s, at 45 minutes 172.8 cm/s, and at 90 minutes 159 cm/s). In both groups, a significant improvement in mean NIH Stroke Scale scores was seen, from 17 at baseline to 15 at 90 minutes. In summary, flow velocities decreased after milrinone therapy only, not after norepinephrine, whereas clinical improvement was achieved with both treatment strategies.

Labeyrie et al. aimed to compare the overall efficacy of two center-driven strategies for the treatment of DCI, with or without vasospasm angioplasty [13]. Two hundred consecutive patients with aneurysmal SAH were enrolled in each of two northern European centers. In the interventional center, vasospasm balloon angioplasty was indicated as first line as a rescue treatment of DCI, combined with intravenous milrinone. In the noninterventional center, induced hypertension was the only rescue therapy for DCI. New cerebral infarcts, death at 1 month, and favorable outcome at 6 months (mRS ≤ 2) were retrospectively analyzed by independent observers and the two centers compared before and after propensity score matching for baseline characteristics. Baseline characteristics differed between centers only for age, the rate of smokers, and patients with chronic high blood pressure. In the interventional center, vasospasm angioplasty was performed in 38% of patients at a median time from bleeding of 8 days. There was no significant difference in the incidence of new infarcts (9% vs.14%, $p = 0.11$), death (8% vs. 9%, $p = 0.4$), and patients' outcomes were 74% favorable for interventional centers vs. 72% favorable for noninterventional centers ($p = 0.4$) before and after propensity matching.

Lakhal and coauthors compared intravenous milrinone, in combination with induced hypertension, as a rescue strategy for DCI, where also a historical control group received hypertension alone [14]. This was a controlled observational study conducted in an academic hospital with prospectively and retrospectively collected data. In the milrinone group, patients with cerebral vasospasm following SAH were treated with intravenous milrinone (0.5 µg/kg/min) and induced hypertension. The historical control group had been managed with induced hypertension alone. Endovascular balloon angioplasty was considered in both groups as an additional measure. The end points were 6-month functional disability (defined as an mRS score between 2 and 6) and vasospasm-related brain infarction, the rate of first-line or rescue endovascular angioplasty for vasospasm, and the immediate tolerance to milrinone. In total, 94 patients were analyzed (41 and 53 in the milrinone and the control group, respectively). Milrinone infusion was independently associated with a lower likelihood of 6-month functional disability (adjusted odds ratio (aOR) = 0.28, 95% confidence interval (CI) = 0.10–0.77) and vasospasm-related brain infarction (aOR = 0.19, 95% CI 0.04–0.94). Endovascular angioplasty was less frequent in the milrinone group (6 (15%) vs. 28 patients (53%), $p = 0.0001$, aOR = 0.12, 95% CI 0.04–0.38). The administration of milrinone (a median duration of infusion = 5 (2–8) days) was prematurely discontinued owing to poor tolerance in 12 patients, mostly ($n = 10$) for hypotension (mean arterial blood pressure <100 mm Hg despite 1.5 µg/kg/min-1 of norepinephrine). However, this event was similarly observed in milrinone and control patients ($n = 10$ (24%) vs. $n = 11$ (21%), respectively; $p = 0.68$). Milrinone was associated with a higher incidence of polyuria and hyponatremia or hypokalemia, whereas arrhythmia, myocardial ischemia, and thrombocytopenia were infrequent. In conclusion, despite milrinone's premature discontinuation in 29% of patients as a result of its poor tolerance, it was associated with a lower rate of endovascular angioplasty and a positive impact on long-term neurological and radiological outcomes.

Discussion

The prevention and management of symptomatic vasospasm has undoubtedly made great progress over the past decades, although the scientific evidence, particularly for preventive measures, remains relatively thin. Only oral nimodipine and intravenous fasudil could be convincingly shown to reduce the rate of symptomatic vasospasm and poor outcome in randomized trials [2, 23]. Later, in smaller prospective trials, cilostazol, like milrinone, a selective phosphodiesterase-3 inhibitor, also showed promising results [15, 22]. Regarding the management of symptomatic vasospasm, the most convincing argument for a specific strategy often comes not from randomized trials focusing on long-term outcome but rather from the immediately visible effect on the neurological deficits. Immediate improvement in symptoms and neurological deficits after the institution of a rescue therapy leaves little doubt regarding efficacy. At our institution, the often strikingly visible clinical improvement was also the reason for accepting intravenous milrinone as the standard rescue therapy following initial use as a measure of last resort. Clinical improvement was judged on the basis of focal neurological symptoms, the level of consciousness, and headache. The high degree of suspicion may well have led to the initiation of a rescue therapy in some cases who would also have recovered with less. On the other hand, the good tolerability of milrinone in light of the severe and irreversible consequences of occurring infarction justified a relatively generous indication in our view.

When summarizing the results of the few comparative clinical studies, we noticed that intravenous milrinone is obviously effective in improving cerebral perfusion but also that milrinone induces hypotension, which reduces the positive effect if left uncorrected. This, together with the fact that the control groups also were treated with active management, explains the marginal, unconvincing group differences in the cited studies (Table 3).

Around 40 years ago, triple-H (hypervolemia, hypertension, and hemodilution) therapy became the mainstay of treatment for vasospasm following subarachnoid hemorrhage [16, 20, 26]. Volume expansion using crystalloid and colloid solutions was subsequently discredited in a number of settings, and further analysis for the case of subarachnoid hemorrhage indicated that hemodilution and plasma expansion added little to the effect of induced hypertension or were even counterproductive [4, 18]. Milrinone became popular as an inotropic agent because of its associated vasodilation effects [12]. While improvement in angiographic cerebral vasospasm has be shown after intra-arterial application, the effect following intravenous application remains unclear [1, 3, 10]. A few case reports and the abovementioned comparative study by Rouanet et al. demonstrated decreasing flow velocities after intravenous milrinone therapy as measured with transcranial Doppler [11, 19, 21]. The effect on TCD values suggests a direct effect of milrinone on the cerebral vasculature. Clarifying the effect of intravenous milrinone on cerebral perfusion and macroscopic vasospasm was the main aim of our analysis in Aarau. We saw an immediate improvement in brain perfusion after the administration of intravenous milrinone. Because additional norepinephrine was used to maintain the desired level of arterial pressure, our analysis can obviously not differentiate between the effects of milrinone and those of norepinephrine.

In our series, although patients suffering DCI still had a somewhat less favorable outcome at 6 months compared to patients without secondary neurological decline, the difference was relatively modest (median mRS 1, IQR 1–3 compared to median mRS 1, IQR 0–2). We must assume that without a very effective rescue therapy, the difference would have been more pronounced. Lacking a control group, however, our data cannot prove or disprove this hypothesis.

The use of CT perfusion in our series clearly showed the immediate positive hemodynamic effect of the used hyperdynamic rescue therapy. Median T4 volumes of 40 cc at the time of decline could be reduced to 10 cc with hyperdynamic therapy, and the average focal TTP delay of 2.5 sec to 1.7 sec. Although, as mentioned above, several reports have described a direct effect on the vasospasm of larger arteries following an intra-arterial and intra-cisternal application of milrinone, reports on cerebral perfusion and vasospasm after intravenous (IV) application are scarce [3, 21]. The mentioned study by Rouanet showed decreasing TCD flow velocities after intravenous milrinone [19], and Zeiler and colleagues described a case of the angiographic resolution of vasospasm with intravenous milrinone [27]. In the Aarau series, we saw visible a reduction in macroscopic vasospasm on CTA more frequently but not exclusively in patients undergoing additional intra-arterial spasmolysis using nimodipine.

In summary, current evidence suggests that intravenous milrinone plays a beneficial part in the rescue therapy for DCI. Cntrolling arterial pressure with additional norepinephrine appears important. On the other hand, a whole number of strategies and medications seem to be available today for effective preventive and rescue therapy for DCI. Proving that a specific one is much better than others appears difficult, and randomized controlled trials in the field appear to be rarely brought to a successful end. Currently, four randomized controlled trials are mentioned on the platform https://clinicaltrials.gov, two of them terminated and the other two still recruiting.

Acknowledgments The authors express their gratitude to Dr. Rolf Ensner, MD, from the Surgical ICU, Kantonsspital Aarau, without whom our original study would not have been possible, as well as to our neuroradiological colleagues Jatta Berberat, MSc, PhD, and Luca Remonda, MD, PhD, from the Kantonsspital Aarau for their constant support and help with the initial analysis.

Author Contributions Conception and design: Steiger, Marbacher. Acquisition of data: Steiger, Marbacher, Andereggen. Analysis and interpretation of data: Steiger, Andereggen, Marbacher. Drafting of the chapter: Steiger. Critical revision of the chapter: Marbacher, Andereggen.

Funding Information No external funding was used for the current analysis.

Declarations

Conflicts of interests: The authors report no conflict of interest concerning the materials or methods used in this study or the findings specified in this chapter.

Compliance with ethical standards: The information shared is not based on human studies and/or animal studies. The analysis was conceived as a quality assessment based on existing data.

References

1. Abulhasan YB, Ortiz Jimenez J, Teitelbaum J, Simoneau G, Angle MR. Milrinone for refractory cerebral vasospasm with delayed cerebral ischemia. J Neurosurg. 2020;27:1–12. https://doi.org/10.3171/2020.1.JNS193107. Epub ahead of print. PMID: 32217799
2. Allen GS, Ahn HS, Preziosi TJ, Battye R, Boone SC, Boone SC, Chou SN, Kelly DL, Weir BK, Crabbe RA, Lavik PJ, Rosenbloom SB, Dorsey FC, Ingram CR, Mellits DE, Bertsch LA, Boisvert DP, Hundley MB, Johnson RK, Strom JA, Transou CR. Cerebral arterial spasm--a controlled trial of nimodipine in patients with subarachnoid hemorrhage. N Engl J Med. 1983;308(11):619–24. https://doi.org/10.1056/NEJM198303173081103. PMID: 6338383
3. Arakawa Y, Kikuta K, Hojo M, Goto Y, Ishii A, Yamagata S. Milrinone for the treatment of cerebral vasospasm after subarachnoid hemorrhage: report of seven cases. Neurosurgery. 2001;48(4):723–8; discussion 728–30. https://doi.org/10.1097/00006123-200104000-00004. PMID: 11322432
4. Bercker S, Winkelmann T, Busch T, Laudi S, Lindner D, Meixensberger J. Hydroxyethyl starch for volume expansion after subarachnoid haemorrhage and renal function: results of a retrospective analysis. PLoS One. 2018;13(2):e0192832. https://doi.org/10.1371/journal.pone.0192832. PMID: 29447255; PMCID: PMC5813956
5. Bernier TD, Schontz MJ, Izzy S, Chung DY, Nelson SE, Leslie-Mazwi TM, Henderson GV, Dasenbrock H, Patel N, Aziz-Sultan MA, Feske S, Du R, Abulhasan YB, Angle MR. Treatment of subarachnoid hemorrhage-associated delayed cerebral ischemia with milrinone: a review and proposal. J Neurosurg Anesthesiol. 2021;33(3):195–202. https://doi.org/10.1097/ANA.0000000000000755. PMID: 33480639; PMCID: PMC8192346
6. Castle-Kirszbaum M, Lai L, Maingard J, Asadi H, Danks RA, Goldschlager T, Chandra RV. Intravenous milrinone for treatment of delayed cerebral ischaemia following subarachnoid haemorrhage: a pooled systematic review. Neurosurg Rev. 2021;44(6):3107–24. https://doi.org/10.1007/s10143-021-01509-1. Epub 2021 Mar 8. PMID: 33682040
7. Crespy T, Heintzelmann M, Chiron C, Vinclair M, Tahon F, Francony G, Payen JF. Which protocol for milrinone to treat cerebral vasospasm associated with subarachnoid Hemorrhage? J Neurosurg Anesthesiol. 2019;31(3):323–9. https://doi.org/10.1097/ANA.0000000000000527. PMID: 30015694
8. Connolly ES Jr, Rabinstein AA, Carhuapoma JR, Derdeyn CP, Dion J, Higashida RT, Hoh BL, Kirkness CJ, Naidech AM, Ogilvy CS, Patel AB, Thompson BG, Vespa P, American Heart Association Stroke Council; Council on Cardiovascular Radiology and Intervention; Council on Cardiovascular Nursing; Council on Cardiovascular Surgery and Anesthesia; Council on Clinical Cardiology. Guidelines for the management of aneurysmal subarachnoid hemorrhage: a guideline for healthcare professionals from the American Heart Association/american Stroke

Association. Stroke. 2012;43(6):1711–37. https://doi.org/10.1161/STR.0b013e3182587839. Epub 2012 May 3. PMID: 22556195

9. Cooper DJ, Myburgh J, Heritier S, Finfer S, Bellomo R, Billot L, Murray L, Vallance S, SAFE-TBI Investigators; Australian and New Zealand Intensive Care Society Clinical Trials Group. Albumin resuscitation for traumatic brain injury: is intracranial hypertension the cause of increased mortality? J Neurotrauma. 2013;30(7):512–8. https://doi.org/10.1089/neu.2012.2573. Epub 2013 Mar 21. PMID: 23194432; PMCID: PMC3636581

10. Fraticelli AT, Cholley BP, Losser MR, Saint Maurice JP, Payen D. Milrinone for the treatment of cerebral vasospasm after aneurysmal subarachnoid hemorrhage. Stroke. 2008;39(3):893–8. https://doi.org/10.1161/STROKEAHA.107.492447. Epub 2008 Jan 31. PMID: 18239182

11. Katyal N, George P, Nattanamai P, Raber LN, Beary JM, Newey CR. Improvement in sonographic vasospasm following intravenous milrinone in a subarachnoid hemorrhage patient with normal cardiac function. Cureus. 2018;10(7):e2916. https://doi.org/10.7759/cureus.2916. PMID: 30186721; PMCID: PMC6122655

12. Khajavi K, Ayzman I, Shearer D, Jones SC, Levy JH, Prayson RA, Skibinski CI, Hahn JF, Chyatte D. Prevention of chronic cerebral vasospasm in dogs with milrinone. Neurosurgery. 1997;40(2):354–62; discussion 362–3. https://doi.org/10.1097/00006123-199702000-00025. PMID: 9007870

13. Labeyrie MA, Simonato D, Gargalas S, Morisson L, Cortese J, Ganau M, Fuschi M, Patel J, Froelich S, Gaugain S, Chousterman B, Houdart E. Intensive therapies of delayed cerebral ischemia after subarachnoid hemorrhage: a propensity-matched comparison of different center-driven strategies. Acta Neurochir (Wien). 2021;163(10):2723–31. https://doi.org/10.1007/s00701-021-04935-8. Epub 2021 Jul 24. PMID: 34302553

14. Lakhal K, Hivert A, Alexandre PL, Fresco M, Robert-Edan V, Rodie-Talbere PA, Ambrosi X, Bourcier R, Rozec B, Cadiet J. Intravenous milrinone for cerebral vasospasm in subarachnoid Hemorrhage: the MILRISPASM controlled before-after study. Neurocrit Care. 2021; https://doi.org/10.1007/s12028-021-01331-z. Epub ahead of print. PMID: 34478028

15. Matsuda N, Naraoka M, Ohkuma H, Shimamura N, Ito K, Asano K, Hasegawa S, Takemura A. Effect of cilostazol on cerebral vasospasm and outcome in patients with aneurysmal subarachnoid Hemorrhage: a randomized, double-blind, Placebo-Controlled Trial. Cerebrovasc Dis. 2016;42(1–2):97–105. https://doi.org/10.1159/000445509. Epub 2016 Apr 13. PMID: 27070952

16. McDougall CG, Spetzler RF, Zabramski JM, Partovi S, Hills NK, Nakaji P, Albuquerque FC. The Barrow ruptured aneurysm trial. J Neurosurg. 2012;116(1):135–44. https://doi.org/10.3171/2011.8.JNS101767. Epub 2011 Nov 4. PMID: 22054213

17. Padda IS, Tripp J. Phosphodiesterase inhibitors. Treasure Island: StatPearls Publishing [Internet]; 2023. Available from: https://www.ncbi.nlm.nih.gov/books/NBK559276/.

18. Raabe A, Beck J, Keller M, Vatter H, Zimmermann M, Seifert V. Relative importance of hypertension compared with hypervolemia for increasing cerebral oxygenation in patients with cerebral vasospasm after subarachnoid hemorrhage. J Neurosurg. 2005;103(6):974–81. https://doi.org/10.3171/jns.2005.103.6.0974. PMID: 16381183

19. Rouanet C, Chaddad F, Freitas F, Miranda M, Vasconcellos N, Valiente R, Muehlschlegel S, Silva GS. Kinetics of cerebral blood flow velocities during treatment for delayed cerebral ischemia in aneurysmal subarachnoid hemorrhage. Neurocrit Care. 2021; https://doi.org/10.1007/s12028-021-01288-z. Epub ahead of print. PMID: 34286467

20. Rosenwasser RH, Delgado TE, Buchheit WA, Freed MH. Control of hypertension and prophylaxis against vasospasm in cases of subarachnoid hemorrhage: a preliminary report. Neurosurgery. 1983;12:658–61.

21. Santos-Teles AG, Passos RH, Panerai RB, Ramalho C, Farias S, Rosa JG, Gobatto A, Benigno P, Caldas JR. Intravenous administration of milrinone, as an alternative approach to treat vasospasm in subarachnoid hemorrhage: a case report of transcranial Doppler monitoring. Clin Case Rep. 2019;7(4):648–52. https://doi.org/10.1002/ccr3.2034. PMID: 30997055; PMCID: PMC6452455

22. Senbokuya N, Kinouchi H, Kanemaru K, Ohashi Y, Fukamachi A, Yagi S, Shimizu T, Furuya K, Uchida M, Takeuchi N, Nakano S, Koizumi H, Kobayashi C, Fukasawa I, Takahashi T, Kuroda K, Nishiyama Y, Yoshioka H, Horikoshi T. Effects of cilostazol on cerebral vasospasm after aneurysmal subarachnoid hemorrhage: a multicenter prospective, randomized, open-label blinded end point trial. J Neurosurg. 2013;118(1):121–30. https://doi.org/10.3171/2012.9.JNS12492. Epub 2012 Oct 5. PMID: 23039152

23. Shibuya M, Suzuki Y, Sugita K, Saito I, Sasaki T, Takakura K, Nagata I, Kikuchi H, Takemae T, Hidaka H, et al. Effect of AT877 on cerebral vasospasm after aneurysmal subarachnoid hemorrhage. Results of a prospective placebo-controlled double-blind trial. J Neurosurg. 1992;76(4):571–7. https://doi.org/10.3171/jns.1992.76.4.0571. PMID: 1545249

24. Soliman R, Zohry G. Efeitos do sulfato de magnésio e da milrinona sobre o vasoespasmo cerebral após hemorragia subaracnoidea por aneurisma: estudo randômico [Effect of magnesium sulphate and milrinone on cerebral vasospasm after aneurysmal subarachnoid hemorrhage: a randomized study]. Braz J Anesthesiol. 2019;69(1):64–71. Portuguese. https://doi.org/10.1016/j.bjan.2018.09.005. Epub 2018 Nov 6. PMID: 30409409.

25. Steiger HJ, Ensner R, Andereggen L, Remonda L, Berberat J, Marbacher S. Hemodynamic response and clinical outcome following intravenous milrinone plus norepinephrine-based hyperdynamic hypertensive therapy in patients suffering secondary cerebral ischemia after aneurysmal subarachnoid hemorrhage. Acta Neurochir. 2022;164(3):811–21. https://doi.org/10.1007/s00701-022-05145-6.

26. Treggiari MM, Deem S. Which H is the most important in triple-H therapy for cerebral vasospasm? Curr Opin Crit Care. 2009;15(2):83–6. https://doi.org/10.1097/MCC.0b013e32832922d1. PMID: 19276798

27. Zeiler FA, Silvaggio J. Early angiographic resolution of cerebral vasospasm with high dose intravenous milrinone therapy. Case Rep Crit Care. 2015;2015:164597. https://doi.org/10.1155/2015/164597. Epub 2015 Sep 17. PMID: 26457209; PMCID: PMC4589610

Open Access This chapter is licensed under the terms of the Creative Commons Attribution 4.0 International License (http://creativecommons.org/licenses/by/4.0/), which permits use, sharing, adaptation, distribution and reproduction in any medium or format, as long as you give appropriate credit to the original author(s) and the source, provide a link to the Creative Commons license and indicate if changes were made.

The images or other third party material in this chapter are included in the chapter's Creative Commons license, unless indicated otherwise in a credit line to the material. If material is not included in the chapter's Creative Commons license and your intended use is not permitted by statutory regulation or exceeds the permitted use, you will need to obtain permission directly from the copyright holder.

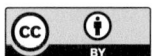

Tenascin-C as a Target for Intervention in Delayed Cerebral Ischemia After Subarachnoid Hemorrhage

Hidenori Suzuki, Fumihiro Kawakita, Hideki Nakajima, Hiroki Oinaka, Mai Nampei, and Yume Suzuki

Introduction

The outcomes of aneurysmal subarachnoid hemorrhage (SAH) are still extremely poor [27]. A patient with SAH who survives early brain injury (EBI) and has a ruptured intracranial aneurysm secured by clipping or coiling remains at risk for delayed cerebral ischemia (DCI), an important treatable factor leading to worse outcomes [53, 79]. The mechanisms of DCI are complicated and consist of at least three major causes: cerebral vasospasm (CVS), microcirculatory disturbance with or without CVS, and neuroelectric disturbance [62, 68]. As the loss of consciousness at onset, severe initial neurological status, heavy bleeding, and the presence of global cerebral edema are surrogate makers of EBI, as well as predictors of DCI and poor outcome [1, 6, 47, 58], EBI may directly cause DCI with or without CVS or be a precursor with increased tissue vulnerability to a secondary insult DCI. Another possibility is that common triggers may cause EBI as an early manifestation and DCI as a late manifestation. Candidates of the common triggers or mediators between EBI and DCI include blood breakdown products, neuroinflammatory molecules, matricellular proteins, and glutamates [22, 43, 54, 55, 69]. Among these candidates, a matricellular protein (MCP), tenascin-C (TNC), has been involved in all three major causes of DCI, specifically CVS, microcirculatory disturbances, and neuroelectric disturbances [20, 21, 44, 50], and is a target in this review article.

H. Suzuki (✉)
Department of Neurosurgery, Mie University Graduate School of Medicine, Tsu, Mie, Japan

Research Center for Matrix Biology, Mie University Graduate School of Medicine, Tsu, Mie, Japan
e-mail: suzuki02@med.mie-u.ac.jp

F. Kawakita · H. Nakajima · H. Oinaka · M. Nampei · Y. Suzuki
Department of Neurosurgery, Mie University Graduate School of Medicine, Tsu, Mie, Japan

What Is TNC?

TNCs are representative of MCPs, which belong to extracellular matrix glycoproteins but are different from classical ones: MCPs have nonstructural, inducible, and secretory properties as well as diverse biological functions depending on cell types and biological scenarios or situations surrounding their induction [28, 59, 75]. TNC biologically modulates or mediates many cellular functions and morphological changes [28, 67]. A variety of stimuli control expressions of TNCs, which transiently appear in almost any tissue and cell [30].

An intact monomer of TNCs is a huge approximately 220–400 kDa molecule, and consists of four domains, namely a N-terminal assembly domain with heptad repeats, 14.5 epidermal growth factor (EGF)-like repeats, eight fibronectin type III (FNIII) repeats, and a C-terminal fibrinogen-like globular domain, each of which binds to a specific partner to exert various functions [28, 46]. TNCs typically form hexamers within the N-terminal domains, from which six monomers emanate [46]. An alternative splicing of messenger ribonucleic acid results in the insertion of one or more extra FNIII domains (A1, A2, A3, A4, B, AD2, AD1, C, or D), producing a lot of different isoforms [14, 46]. Many isoforms of TNC with diverse functions and sizes were also produced by post-translational modifications and proteolytic processes or the destruction of TNC: the functions of hexameric, monomeric, and protease-cleaved TNCs differ by hindering or destructing existing binding sites or by generating smaller TNC fragments with a new binding site [8, 14, 30].

In patients with DCI after SAH, the pH in the cerebrospinal fluid (CSF) was reported to be higher [76]. This suggests that an active form of TNC—that is, a larger molecular mass of TNC isoform with more than one alternatively spliced FNIII repeats—may be produced more after SAH, especially in patients with DCI [14]. SAH upregulates and activates matrix metalloproteinases (MMPs) [52], which readily cleave larger TNC isoforms at alternatively spliced regions and other sites and which release smaller fragments of TNC [14, 28]. As a result, multiple TNC isoforms with different functions and diverse interactions with other molecules may be simultaneously produced to enhance the complexity of TNC's functions, leading to a variety of pathologies after SAH.

Post-SAH Upregulation of TNC

The rupture of an intracranial aneurysm rapidly spreads arterial blood into the subarachnoid space, sometimes associated with mechanical brain injuries by acute hydrocephalus and intracerebral hemorrhage, and increases intracranial pressure to cause transient global cerebral ischemia. All global cerebral ischemia cases, mechanical brain injuries, and blood breakdown products can trigger a variety of cascades, including inflammatory ones, leading to EBI and DCI with or without CVS [53]. Extravasated blood components, including thrombin, platelet, and leukocyte activate microglia, generate and release proinflammatory cytokines and MCPs, including TNCs [39]. A pattern-recognition receptor such as Toll-like receptor 4 (TLR4) is expressed on almost any cell in brain parenchyma, vascular walls, and peripheral blood [19, 42], and it is activated by many endogenous ligands with damage-associated molecular patterns, such as extravasated blood components (e.g., heme and fibrinogen), intracellular components released by tissue injuries, newly synthesized MCPs (e.g., TNC and galectin-3), and other inflammatory molecules, all of which increase following aneurysmal rupture (Fig. 1) [19, 39, 67]. The post-SAH activation of TLR4 may be an initial step of cascades to neuroinflammation, and the subsequent tissue injuries may further activate and upregulate TLR4 in brain and cerebral arteries, leading to EBI and DCI with or without CVS [32, 42, 57].

TLR4 is considered as able to mediate maximal inflammatory reactions by activating two major transcriptional factors, nuclear factor-kappa B (NF-κB), and activator protein-1, and the latter functions mainly via mitogen-activated protein kinase (MAPK) [42]. NF-κB and MAPK are reported to induce proinflammatory molecules and MCPs [41, 42]. As an MCP, TNC is one of the agonists for TLR4 in that it provides positive feedback mechanisms on the upregulation of TNC itself and TLR4 via both NF-κB and MAPK, leading to the further activation of TNC-TLR4 signaling and consequently the development or aggravation of EBI or DCI with or without CVS [13, 51, 57]. Products of TNC-TLR4 pathways such as proinflammatory cytokines and mediators, including reactive oxygen species, can also induce TNCs through NF-κB- and MAPK-independent pathways [30]. In addition, although TNC and TLR4 were upregulated by experimental SAH, upregulated TNC activated EGF receptors, through which TLR4 and TNC were induced in cerebral arteries in SAH mice [32]. As TNC is known to activate NF-κB-, MAPK-, and RhoA-mediated pathways, all of which not only upregulate TNC at the transcriptional level but also cause EBI and/or CVS [4, 9, 42], TNC signaling may positively feedback on the upregulation of TNC itself to further activate the signaling transduction, inducing EBI and DCI with or without CVS (Fig. 2). Our experimental studies showed that a specific TLR4 antagonist not only inhibited EBI development by inactivating MAPKs to downregulate TNCs [40, 41] but also suppressed CVS [19].

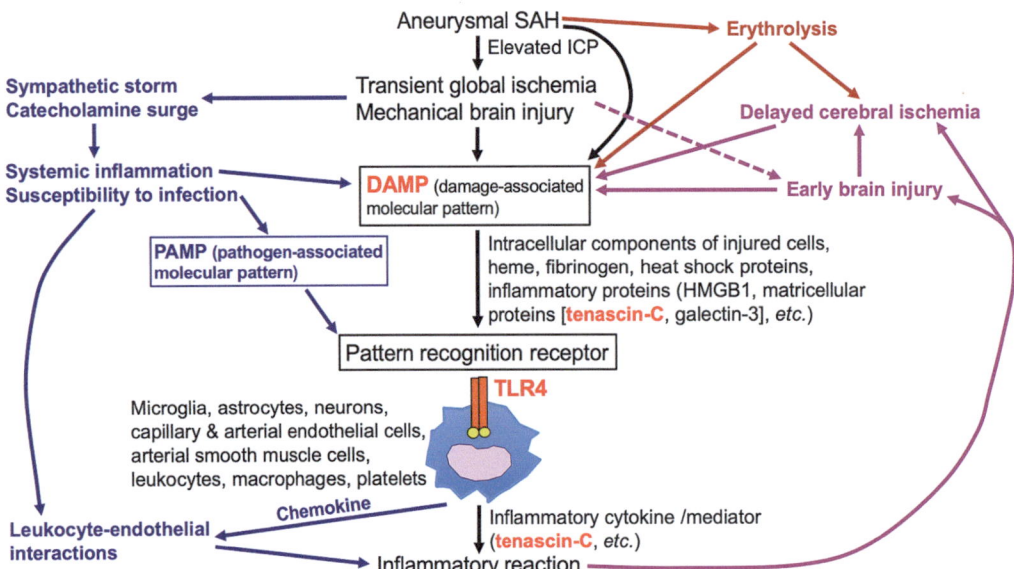

Fig. 1 Developmental mechanisms of inflammation after subarachnoid hemorrhage (SAH): HMGB1 high mobility group box 1, ICP intracranial pressure, TLR4 Toll-like receptor 4

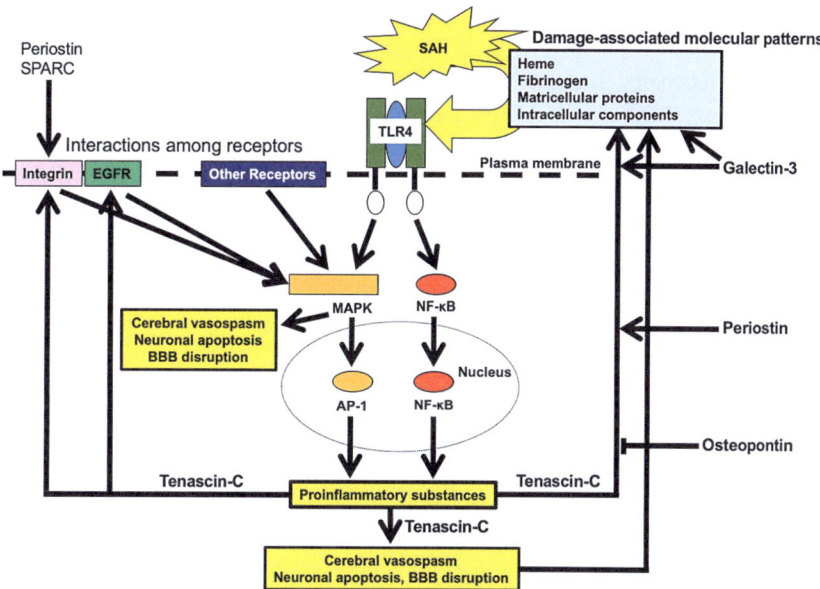

Fig. 2 Toll-like receptor 4 (TLR4) and tenascin-C signaling in early brain injury and delayed cerebral ischemia after subarachnoid hemorrhage (SAH): AP-1 activator protein-1, BBB blood-brain barrier, EGFR epidermal growth factor receptor, MAPK mitogen-activated protein kinase, NF-κB nuclear factor-kappa B, SPARC secreted protein acidic, and rich in cysteine

TNC as a Biomarker for DCI

In a clinical setting, patients with aneurysmal SAH had an increased TNC level in both CSF and peripheral blood [65, 74]. In CSF, levels of large-splice variants of TNC containing C domain in the FNIII repeats peaked within the first 3 days of SAH and decreased over time [70]. Worse admission neurological status, a higher amount of SAH, and the association of acute hydrocephalus caused higher CSF levels of TNC, followed by the occurrence of angiographic CVS, DCI, chronic shunt-dependent hydrocephalus, and resultantly worse outcome [63, 64]. The findings support the concept that TNC may mediate between more-severe SAH or EBI and DCI with or without CVS [67].

The plasma levels of a large-splice variant of TNC containing C domain in the FNIII repeats also transiently increased in SAH patients with the subsequent development of angiographic CVS [65]. The post-SAH plasma level of TNC peaked at days 4–6 [66], which were an average of 2.4 days before the occurrence of CVS on transcranial Doppler (TCD) and an average of 3.6 days before the onset of DCI [65].

How Does TNC Develop DCI?

TNCs were upregulated in brain parenchyma (astrocytes, neurons, and brain capillary endothelial cells), cerebral arterial walls (endothelial, smooth muscle, and adventitial cells), and inflammatory cells in the subarachnoid space after SAH in rats and mice [12, 49, 65]. SAH itself and SAH-induced TNC upregulate or activate MMPs and serine proteases, which in turn cleave TNCs [42]. In cleaved TNCs, a cryptic site is released and binds to several receptors, such as TLR4, EGF receptors, and various integrins, depending on the domains, through which different signaling pathways may be activated, followed by the development of EBI and DCI with or without CVS [10, 30, 31, 42]. In addition to positive feedback loops between the TNC-induced upregulation of MMPs and MMP-induced cleavage of TNCs [30], the crosstalk among TNC's receptors—that is, TLR4, EGF receptors, and integrins—was reported to augment each receptor-mediating signaling [7, 32].

After experimental SAH, TNCs disrupted Blood-brain barrier (BBB) by activating MAPK and then MMP-9 in brain capillary endothelial cells in mice [11, 45]. Although SAH causes both caspase-dependent and -independent neuronal apoptosis [33], TNCs induced apoptosis in neurons at least through caspase-dependent pathways with the activation of NF-κB and MAPKs as well as the upregulation of TLR4 in mice [25, 49]. In addition, the TNC-induced activation of MAPK in the arterial smooth muscle cells caused CVS in rats [10, 67]. TNCs can regulate arterial wall remodeling associated with CVS, which consists of changes in cell phenotypes, proliferations of smooth muscle cells, depositions of extracellular matrix such as collagen, matrix contractions [5, 78], and periarterial infiltrations of inflammatory cells [12]. Post-SAH inflammation may also be promoted by TNCs through the modulation of the activation, adhesion, rolling, and infiltration of an inflammatory cell via diverse signaling pathways [30].

TNCs can upregulate some receptors, such as vascular endothelial growth factor receptors-2 in brain with EBI and platelet-derived growth factor receptors in cerebral arteries with CVS after experimental SAH [24, 67]. TNCs also modulate pathways related to calcium/calmodulin kinase, protein kinase C, phospholipase C, and RhoA in addition to activating NF-κB- and MAPK-mediated pathways, and they induce endothelin receptors type A as well as proinflammatory cytokines and growth factors [30]. All the receptors and molecules have been reported to induce EBI and DCI with or without CVS [9, 42]. In addition, TNC can adhere to platelets or directly interact with von Willebrand factors to activate platelets [48], and they can mediate the deposition or accumulation of fibrins via their negative transcriptional control of a tissue plasminogen activator in injured arteries [29]: These reactions form microthrombi within the blood vessels and microvessels, potentially contributing to the development of DCI [29, 48].

TNC also interacts with other MCPs, such as periostin, galectin-3, and osteopontin [3, 15, 18, 23]. TNC and periostin, the latter of which was induced in brain capillary endothelial cells, regulated each other's expressions and downstream NF-κB- and MAPK-mediated signaling pathways, forming a positive feedback mechanism to develop and worsen EBI in SAH mice [17, 26, 38]. Increased plasma periostin levels were related to the development of DCI with and without CVS in a clinical setting of aneurysmal SAH [16, 77]. TNC can bind to and activate galectin-3, which has caused neuroinflammation and the acute disruption of BBB in SAH mice [36, 39]. In a clinical setting of SAH, delayed cerebral infarction without CVS was associated with increased plasma galectin-3 levels [37]. Experimental and clinical SAH induced osteopontin in a delayed fashion [2, 35, 61], which inactivated NF-κB [56] and activated an endogenous MAPK inhibitor in SAH rats [60], antagonizing TNC's functions and exerting neuroprotective effects [3]. Given that TNC and osteopontin are known to share some receptors, osteopontin may also inhibit TNC's binding to the receptor competitively [30].

Drugs Antagonizing TNC's Functions

The expression of TNC can be inhibited by a lot of medications, including steroids, nonsteroidal anti-inflammatory drugs, aldosterone receptor antagonists, drugs that block angiotensin II (e.g., angiotensin II type 1 receptor antagonists and angiotensin converting enzyme inhibitors), antioxidants, Rho-kinase inhibitors, platelet-derived growth factor receptor inhibitors, and cilostazol [58]. Some new therapeutic drugs that target TNC are also being developed and are expected to be applied clinically [58]. However, drugs that have been clinically proven to suppress TNC expression are very limited in aneurysmal SAH. As far as we know, only the combined administration of a Rho-kinase inhibitor fasudil hydrochloride and a selective inhibitor of phosphodiesterase type III cilostazol has reduced plasma levels of large-splice variants of TNC containing B and C domains in the FNIII repeats, and it has been associated with decreased incidences of chronic hydrocephalus requiring shunting surgery [34] and delayed cerebral infarction leading to a poor outcome [73], respectively. Although whether the combination effects of fasudil hydrochloride and cilostazol on TNC's expressions and post-SAH pathologies are additive, synergistic, or interactive remains unknown, our study showed that cilostazol, a pleiotropic antiplatelet, dose-dependently reduced the development of delayed cerebral infarction without decreasing the incidence of CVS after SAH in a clinical setting [73].

Recently, an experimental study reported that a selective antagonist of α-amino-3-hydroxy-5-methyl-4-isoxazole propionate receptor perampanel inhibited the post-SAH upregulation of TNC expression in brain capillary endothelial cells and prevented acute BBB disruption after SAH in mice [20]. As perampanel is a clinically approved antiepileptic drug, it is readily available for clinical application. A recent clinical study showed promising results, where perampanel inhibited the post-SAH development of delayed cerebral microinfarction, although perampanel did not suppress the incidence of CVS [71].

Perspective

TNC has been involved in several levels of pathophysiological processes of SAH, and the vicious cycle through positive feedback mechanisms to furthermore induce TNC may lead to DCI with and without CVS. Therefore, TNC would be promising as a target for intervention in DCI after aneurysmal SAH. Until technological progress develops new TNC-targeting drugs or strategies that can translate our knowledge regarding TNC into the management of DCI, trying existing drugs or repurposing old drugs to prevent and/or to treat DCI after SAH is worthwhile. Although further meticulous translational studies are needed [72], cilostazol and perampanel are at the moment considered to be useful for post-SAH DCI management.

Author Contributions Hidenori Suzuki conceived the idea for the article and drafted the work. All authors contributed to the literature search, data analysis, and critical revision of the work. All authors read and approved the final manuscript.

Funding Information This work was funded by the Japan Society for the Promotion of Science KAKENHI (grant number JP20K17963). The Sanikai Foundation (Grant Number N/A) funded Dr. Kawakita and the Taiju Life Social Welfare Foundation (Grant Number N/A) funded Dr. H. Suzuki.

Declarations

Competing Interests: Dr. H. Suzuki reports personal fees from Eisai and Kowa and a research fund from Japan Blood Products Organization outside the submitted work. The other authors declare that they have no conflict of interest.

References

1. Ahn SH, Savarraj JP, Pervez M, Jones W, Park J, Jeon SB, Kwon SU, Chang TR, Lee K, Kim DH, Day AL, Choi HA. The subarachnoid hemorrhage early brain edema score predicts delayed cerebral ischemia and clinical outcomes. Neurosurgery. 2018;83:137–45.
2. Asada R, Nakatsuka Y, Kanamaru H, Kawakita F, Fujimoto M, Miura Y, Shiba M, Yasuda R, Toma N, Suzuki H, pSEED Group. Higher plasma osteopontin concentrations associated with subsequent development of chronic shunt-dependent hydrocephalus after aneurysmal subarachnoid hemorrhage. Transl Stroke Res. 2021;12:808–16.
3. Asada R, Suzuki H. Osteopontin in post-subarachnoid hemorrhage pathologies. J Integr Neurosci. 2022;21:62. https://doi.org/10.31083/j.jin2102062.
4. Chiquet M, Gelman L, Lutz R, Maier S. From mechanotransduction to extracellular matrix gene expression in fibroblasts. Biochim Biophys Acta. 2009;1793:911–20.
5. Chiquet-Ehrismann R, Chiquet M. Tenascins: regulation and putative functions during pathological stress. J Pathol. 2003;200:488–99.
6. Claassen J, Carhuapoma JR, Kreiter KT, Du EY, Connolly ES, Mayer SA. Global cerebral edema after subarachnoid hemorrhage: frequency, predictors, and impact on outcome. Stroke. 2002;33:1225–32.
7. Eberwein P, Laird D, Schulz S, Reinhard T, Steinberg T, Tomakidi P. Modulation of focal adhesion constituents and their downstream events by EGF: on the cross-talk of integrins and growth factor receptors. Biochim Biophys Acta. 2015;1853:2183–98.
8. Faissner A, Roll L, Theocharidis U. Tenascin-C in the matrisome of neural stem and progenitor cells. Mol Cell Neurosci. 2017;81:22–31.
9. Fan R, Enkhjargal B, Camara R, Yan F, Gong L, ShengtaoYao TJ, Chen Y, Zhang JH. Critical role of EphA4 in early brain injury after subarachnoid hemorrhage in rat. Exp Neurol. 2017;296:41–8.
10. Fujimoto M, Shiba M, Kawakita F, Liu L, Nakasaki A, Shimojo N, Imanaka-Yoshida K, Yoshida T, Suzuki H. Epidermal growth factor-like repeats of tenascin-C-induced constriction of cerebral arteries via activation of epidermal growth factor receptors in rats. Brain Res. 2016;1642:436–44.
11. Fujimoto M, Shiba M, Kawakita F, Liu L, Shimojo N, Imanaka-Yoshida K, Yoshida T, Suzuki H. Deficiency of tenascin-C and attenuation of blood-brain barrier disruption following experimental subarachnoid hemorrhage in mice. J Neurosurg. 2016;124:1693–702.
12. Fujimoto M, Shiba M, Kawakita F, Liu L, Shimojo N, Imanaka-Yoshida K, Yoshida T, Suzuki H. Effects of tenascin-C knockout on cerebral vasospasm after experimental subarachnoid hemorrhage in mice. Mol Neurobiol. 2018;55:1951–8.
13. Fujimoto M, Suzuki H, Shiba M, Shimojo N, Imanaka-Yoshida K, Yoshida T, Kanamaru K, Matsushima S, Taki W. Tenascin-C induces prolonged constriction of cerebral arteries in rats. Neurobiol Dis. 2013;55:104–9.
14. Giblin SP, Midwood KS. Tenascin-C: form versus function. Cell Adhes Migr. 2015;9:48–82.
15. Kanamaru H, Kawakita F, Asada R, Suzuki H. The role of periostin in brain injury caused by subarachnoid hemorrhage. OBM Neurobiol. 2019;3:15. https://doi.org/10.21926/obm.neurobiol.1903035.
16. Kanamaru H, Kawakita F, Nakano F, Miura Y, Shiba M, Yasuda R, Toma N, Suzuki H, pSEED Group. Plasma periostin and delayed cerebral ischemia after aneurysmal subarachnoid hemorrhage. Neurotherapeutics. 2019;16:480–90.
17. Kanamaru H, Kawakita F, Nishikawa H, Nakano F, Asada R, Suzuki H. Clarithromycin ameliorates early brain injury after subarachnoid hemorrhage via suppressing periostin-related pathways in mice. Neurotherapeutics. 2021;18:1880–90.
18. Kanamaru H, Suzuki H. Potential therapeutic molecular targets for blood-brain barrier disruption after subarachnoid hemorrhage. Neural Regen Res. 2019;14:1138–43.
19. Kawakita F, Fujimoto M, Liu L, Nakano F, Nakatsuka Y, Suzuki H. Effects of toll-like receptor 4 antagonists against cerebral vasospasm after experimental subarachnoid hemorrhage in mice. Mol Neurobiol. 2017;54:6624–33.
20. Kawakita F, Kanamaru H, Asada R, Imanaka-Yoshida K, Yoshida T, Suzuki H. Inhibition of AMPA (α-amino-3-hydroxy-5-methyl-4-isoxazole propionate) receptor reduces acute blood-brain barrier disruption after subarachnoid hemorrhage in mice. Transl Stroke Res. 2022;13:326–37.
21. Kawakita F, Kanamaru H, Asada R, Suzuki H. Potential roles of matricellular proteins in stroke. Exp Neurol. 2019;322:113057. https://doi.org/10.1016/j.expneurol.2019.113057.
22. Kawakita F, Kanamaru H, Asada R, Suzuki Y, Nampei M, Nakajima H, Oinaka H, Suzuki H. Roles of glutamate in brain injuries after subarachnoid hemorrhage. Histol Histopathol. 2022;37:1041–51.
23. Kawakita F, Suzuki H. Periostin in cerebrovascular disease. Neural Regen Res. 2020;15:63–4.
24. Liu L, Fujimoto M, Kawakita F, Nakano F, Imanaka-Yoshida K, Yoshida T, Suzuki H. Anti-vascular endothelial growth factor treatment suppresses early brain injury after subarachnoid hemorrhage in mice. Mol Neurobiol. 2016;53:4529–38.
25. Liu L, Fujimoto M, Nakano F, Nishikawa H, Okada T, Kawakita F, Imanaka-Yoshida K, Yoshida T, Suzuki H. Deficiency of tenascin-C alleviates neuronal apoptosis and neuroinflammation after experimental subarachnoid hemorrhage in mice. Mol Neurobiol. 2018;55:8346–54.
26. Liu L, Kawakita F, Fujimoto M, Nakano F, Imanaka-Yoshida K, Yoshida T, Suzuki H. Role of periostin in early brain injury after subarachnoid hemorrhage in mice. Stroke. 2017;48:1108–11.
27. Macdonald RL, Schweizer TA. Spontaneous subarachnoid haemorrhage. Lancet. 2017;389:655–66.
28. Midwood KS, Chiquet M, Tucker RP, Orend G. Tenascin-C at a glance. J Cell Sci. 2016;129:4321–7.
29. Midwood KS, Hussenet T, Langlois B, Orend G. Advances in tenascin-C biology. Cell Mol Life Sci. 2011;68:3175–99.
30. Midwood KS, Orend G. The role of tenascin-C in tissue injury and tumorigenesis. J Cell Commun Signal. 2009;3:287–310.
31. Nakano F, Kawakita F, Liu L, Nakatsuka Y, Nishikawa H, Okada T, Kanamaru H, Pak S, Shiba M, Suzuki H. Anti-vasospastic effects of epidermal growth factor receptor inhibitors after subarachnoid hemorrhage in mice. Mol Neurobiol. 2019;56:4730–40.
32. Nakano F, Kawakita F, Liu L, Nakatsuka Y, Nishikawa H, Okada T, Shiba M, Suzuki H. Link between receptors that engage in developing vasospasm after subarachnoid hemorrhage in mice. Acta Neurochir Suppl. 2020;127:55–8.

33. Nakano F, Liu L, Kawakita F, Nakatsuka Y, Nishikawa H, Okada T, Shiba M, Suzuki H. Possible involvement of caspase-independent pathway in neuronal death after subarachnoid hemorrhage in mice. Acta Neurochir Suppl. 2020;127:43–6.
34. Nakatsuka Y, Kawakita F, Yasuda R, Umeda Y, Toma N, Sakaida H, Suzuki H, pSEED Group. Preventive effects of cilostazol against the development of shunt-dependent hydrocephalus after subarachnoid hemorrhage. J Neurosurg. 2017;127:319–26.
35. Nakatsuka Y, Shiba M, Nishikawa H, Terashima M, Kawakita F, Fujimoto M, Suzuki H, pSEED Group. Acute-phase plasma osteopontin as an independent predictor for poor outcome after aneurysmal subarachnoid hemorrhage. Mol Neurobiol. 2018;55:6841–9.
36. Nishikawa H, Liu L, Nakano F, Kawakita F, Kanamaru H, Nakatsuka Y, Okada T, Suzuki H. Modified citrus pectin prevents blood-brain barrier disruption in mouse subarachnoid hemorrhage by inhibiting galectin-3. Stroke. 2018;49:2743–51.
37. Nishikawa H, Nakatsuka Y, Shiba M, Kawakita F, Fujimoto M, Suzuki H, pSEED Group. Increased plasma galectin-3 preceding the development of delayed cerebral infarction and eventual poor outcome in non-severe aneurysmal subarachnoid hemorrhage. Transl Stroke Res. 2018;9:110–9.
38. Nishikawa H, Suzuki H. Implications of periostin in the development of subarachnoid hemorrhage-induced brain injuries. Neural Regen Res. 2017;12:1982–4.
39. Nishikawa H, Suzuki H. Possible role of inflammation and galectin-3 in brain injury after subarachnoid hemorrhage. Brain Sci. 2018;8:30. https://doi.org/10.3390/brainsci8020030.
40. Okada T, Liu L, Nishikawa H, Nakano F, Nakatsuka Y, Suzuki H. TAK-242, toll-like receptor 4 antagonist, attenuates brain edema in subarachnoid hemorrhage mice. Acta Neurochir Suppl. 2020;127:77–81.
41. Okada T, Kawakita F, Nishikawa H, Nakano F, Liu L, Suzuki H. Selective toll-like receptor 4 antagonists prevent acute blood-brain barrier disruption after subarachnoid hemorrhage in mice. Mol Neurobiol. 2019;56:976–85.
42. Okada T, Suzuki H. Toll-like receptor 4 as a possible therapeutic target for delayed brain injuries after aneurysmal subarachnoid hemorrhage. Neural Regen Res. 2017;12:193–6.
43. Okada T, Suzuki H. Mechanisms of neuroinflammation and inflammatory mediators involved in brain injury following subarachnoid hemorrhage. Histol Histopathol. 2020;35:623–36.
44. Okada T, Suzuki H. The role of tenascin-C in tissue injury and repair after stroke. Front Immunol. 2021;11:607587. https://doi.org/10.3389/fimmu.2020.607587.
45. Okada T, Suzuki H, Travis ZD, Zhang JH. The stroke-induced blood-brain barrier disruption: current progress of inspection technique, mechanism, and therapeutic target. Curr Neuropharmacol. 2020;18:1187–212.
46. Reinhard J, Roll L, Faissner A. Tenascins in retinal and optic nerve neurodegeneration. Front Integr Neurosci. 2017;11:30. https://doi.org/10.3389/fnint.2017.00030.
47. Savarraj J, Parsha K, Hergenroeder G, Ahn S, Chang TR, Kim DH, Choi HA. Early brain injury associated with systemic inflammation after subarachnoid hemorrhage. Neurocrit Care. 2018;28:203–11.
48. Schaff M, Receveur N, Bourdon C, Wurtz V, Denis CV, Orend G, Gachet C, Lanza F, Mangin PH. Novel function of tenascin-C, a matrix protein relevant to atherosclerosis, in platelet recruitment and activation under flow. Arterioscler Thromb Vasc Biol. 2011;31:117–24.
49. Shiba M, Fujimoto M, Imanaka-Yoshida K, Yoshida T, Taki W, Suzuki H. Tenascin-C causes neuronal apoptosis after subarachnoid hemorrhage in rats. Transl Stroke Res. 2014;5:238–47.
50. Shiba M, Suzuki H. Lessons from tenascin-C knockout mice and potential clinical application to subarachnoid hemorrhage. Neural Regen Res. 2019;14:262–4.
51. Shiba M, Suzuki H, Fujimoto M, Shimojo N, Imanaka-Yoshida K, Yoshida T, Kanamaru K, Matsushima S, Taki W. Imatinib mesylate prevents cerebral vasospasm after subarachnoid hemorrhage via inhibiting tenascin-C expression in rats. Neurobiol Dis. 2012;46:172–9.
52. Söderholm M, Nordin FG, Nilsson J, Engström G. High serum level of matrix metalloproteinase-7 is associated with increased risk of spontaneous subarachnoid hemorrhage. Stroke. 2018;49:1626–31.
53. Suzuki H. What is early brain injury? Transl Stroke Res. 2015;6:1–3.
54. Suzuki H. Inflammation: a good research target to improve outcomes of poor-grade subarachnoid hemorrhage. Transl Stroke Res. 2019;10:597–600.
55. Suzuki H. How to promote hemoglobin scavenging or clearance and detoxification in hemorrhagic stroke. Transl Stroke Res. 2023; https://doi.org/10.1007/s12975-022-01075-8.
56. Suzuki H, Ayer R, Sugawara T, Chen W, Sozen T, Hasegawa Y, Kanamaru K, Zhang JH. Protective effects of recombinant osteopontin on early brain injury after subarachnoid hemorrhage in rats. Crit Care Med. 2010;38:612–8.
57. Suzuki H, Fujimoto M, Kawakita F, Liu L, Nakano F, Nishikawa H, Okada T, Imanaka-Yoshida K, Yoshida T, Shiba M. Toll-like receptor 4 and tenascin-C signaling in cerebral vasospasm and brain injuries after subarachnoid hemorrhage. Acta Neurochir Suppl. 2020;127:91–6.
58. Suzuki H, Fujimoto M, Kawakita F, Liu L, Nakatsuka Y, Nakano F, Nishikawa H, Okada T, Kanamaru H, Imanaka-Yoshida K, Yoshida T, Shiba M. Tenascin-C in brain injuries and edema after subarachnoid hemorrhage: findings from basic and clinical studies. J Neurosci Res. 2020;98:42–56.
59. Suzuki H, Fujimoto M, Shiba M, Kawakita F, Liu L, Ichikawa N, Kanamaru K, Imanaka-Yoshida K, Yoshida T. The role of matricellular proteins in brain edema after subarachnoid hemorrhage. Acta Neurochir Suppl. 2016;121:151–6.
60. Suzuki H, Hasegawa Y, Chen W, Kanamaru K, Zhang JH. Recombinant osteopontin in cerebral vasospasm after subarachnoid hemorrhage. Ann Neurol. 2010;68:650–60.
61. Suzuki H, Hasegawa Y, Kanamaru K, Zhang JH. Mechanisms of osteopontin-induced stabilization of blood-brain barrier disruption after subarachnoid hemorrhage in rats. Stroke. 2010;41:1783–90.
62. Suzuki H, Kanamaru H, Kawakita F, Asada R, Fujimoto M, Shiba M. Cerebrovascular pathophysiology of delayed cerebral ischemia after aneurysmal subarachnoid hemorrhage. Histol Histopathol. 2021;36:143–58.
63. Suzuki H, Kanamaru K, Shiba M, Fujimoto M, Imanaka-Yoshida K, Yoshida T, Taki W. Cerebrospinal fluid tenascin-C in cerebral vasospasm after aneurysmal subarachnoid hemorrhage. J Neurosurg Anesthesiol. 2011;23:310–7.
64. Suzuki H, Kanamaru K, Shiba M, Fujimoto M, Kawakita F, Imanaka-Yoshida K, Yoshida T, Taki W. Tenascin-C is a possible mediator between initial brain injury and vasospasm-related and -unrelated delayed cerebral ischemia after aneurysmal subarachnoid hemorrhage. Acta Neurochir Suppl. 2015;120:117–21.
65. Suzuki H, Kanamaru K, Suzuki Y, Aimi Y, Matsubara N, Araki T, Takayasu M, Kinoshita N, Imanaka-Yoshida K, Yoshida T, Taki W. Tenascin-C is induced in cerebral vasospasm after subarachnoid hemorrhage in rats and humans: a pilot study. Neurol Res. 2010;32:179–84.
66. Suzuki H, Kanamaru K, Suzuki Y, Aimi Y, Matsubara N, Araki T, Takayasu M, Takeuchi T, Okada K, Kinoshita N, Imanaka-Yoshida K, Yoshida T, Taki W. Possible role of tenascin-C in cerebral vasospasm after aneurysmal subarachnoid haemorrhage. In: Kırış T, Zhang JH, editors. Cerebral vasospasm. (Acta Neurochirurgica Supplement, vol 104). Vienna: Springer; 2008. https://doi.org/10.1007/978-3-211-75718-5_35.

67. Suzuki H, Kawakita F. Tenascin-C in aneurysmal subarachnoid hemorrhage: deleterious or protective? Neural Regen Res. 2016;11:230–1.
68. Suzuki H, Kawakita F, Asada R. Neuroelectric mechanisms of delayed cerebral ischemia after aneurysmal subarachnoid hemorrhage. Int J Mol Sci. 2022;23:3102. https://doi.org/10.3390/ijms23063102.
69. Suzuki H, Kawakita F, Asada R, Nakano F, Nishikawa H, Fujimoto M. Old but still hot target, glutamate-mediated neurotoxicity in stroke. Transl Stroke Res. 2022;13:216–7.
70. Suzuki H, Kinoshita N, Imanaka-Yoshida K, Yoshida T, Taki W. Cerebrospinal fluid tenascin-C increases preceding the development of chronic shunt-dependent hydrocephalus after subarachnoid hemorrhage. Stroke. 2008;39:1610–2.
71. Suzuki H, Miura Y, Yasuda R, Yago T, Mizutani H, Ichikawa T, Miyazaki T, Kitano Y, Nishikawa H, Kawakita F, Fujimoto M, Toma N. Effects of new-generation antiepileptic drug prophylaxis on delayed neurovascular events after aneurysmal subarachnoid hemorrhage. Transl Stroke Res. 2023; https://doi.org/10.1007/s12975-022-01101-9.
72. Suzuki H, Nakano F. To improve translational research in subarachnoid hemorrhage. Transl Stroke Res. 2018;9:1–3.
73. Suzuki H, Nakatsuka Y, Yasuda R, Shiba M, Miura Y, Terashima M, Suzuki Y, Hakozaki K, Goto F, Toma N. Dose-dependent inhibitory effects of cilostazol on delayed cerebral infarction after aneurysmal subarachnoid hemorrhage. Transl Stroke Res. 2019;10:381–8.
74. Suzuki H, Nishikawa H, Kawakita F. Matricellular proteins as possible biomarkers for early brain injury after aneurysmal subarachnoid hemorrhage. Neural Regen Res. 2018;13:1175–8.
75. Suzuki H, Shiba M, Fujimoto M, Kawamura K, Nanpei M, Tekeuchi E, Matsushima S, Kanamaru K, Imanaka-Yoshida K, Yoshida T, Taki W. Matricellular protein: a new player in cerebral vasospasm following subarachnoid hemorrhage. Acta Neurochir Suppl. 2013;115:213–8.
76. Suzuki H, Shiba M, Nakatsuka Y, Nakano F, Nishikawa H. Higher cerebrospinal fluid pH may contribute to the development of delayed cerebral ischemia after aneurysmal subarachnoid hemorrhage. Transl Stroke Res. 2017;8:165 73.
77. Tanioka S, Ishida F, Nakano F, Kawakita F, Kanamaru H, Nakatsuka Y, Nishikawa H, Suzuki H, pSEED Group. Machine learning analysis of matricellular proteins and clinical variables for early prediction of delayed cerebral ischemia after aneurysmal subarachnoid hemorrhage. Mol Neurobiol. 2019;56:7128–35.
78. Toma N, Imanaka-Yoshida K, Takeuchi T, Matsushima S, Iwata H, Yoshida T, Taki W. Tenascin-C coated on platinum coils accelerates organization of cavities and reduces lumen size in a rat aneurysm model. J Neurosurg. 2005;103:681–6.
79. Vergouwen MD, Vermeulen M, van Gijn J, Rinkel GJ, Wijdicks EF, Muizelaar JP, Mendelow AD, Juvela S, Yonas H, Terbrugge KG, Macdonald RL, Diringer MN, Broderick JP, Dreier JP, Roos YB. Definition of delayed cerebral ischemia after aneurysmal subarachnoid hemorrhage as an outcome event in clinical trials and observational studies: proposal of a multidisciplinary research group. Stroke. 2010;41:2391–5.

Open Access This chapter is licensed under the terms of the Creative Commons Attribution 4.0 International License (http://creativecommons.org/licenses/by/4.0/), which permits use, sharing, adaptation, distribution and reproduction in any medium or format, as long as you give appropriate credit to the original author(s) and the source, provide a link to the Creative Commons license and indicate if changes were made.

The images or other third party material in this chapter are included in the chapter's Creative Commons license, unless indicated otherwise in a credit line to the material. If material is not included in the chapter's Creative Commons license and your intended use is not permitted by statutory regulation or exceeds the permitted use, you will need to obtain permission directly from the copyright holder.

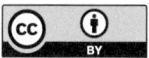

Introducing Bayesian Analysis for Clinicians: Sex-Associated Risk Assessment of Intracranial Aneurysms

Philippe Bijlenga, Georg Ralph Spinner, Marco Scutari, Matteo Delucchi, and Sven Hirsch

Introduction

Intracranial aneurysms (IAs), prevalent cerebrovascular disorders, pose significant challenges in diagnosis and treatment. Characterized by irregular, dilated blood vessels within the cranial cavity, IAs are critical to understanding due to their impact on the brain's blood supply [12]. The formation of these aneurysms can arise from several factors, including imbalances in vascular remodeling, the stress exerted by blood flow, and impaired repair mechanisms of the vessel wall [17]. Typically developing at major intracranial arterial bifurcations near the circle of Willis, these aneurysms vary in location, dimensions, and morphology [25]. Despite their potential severity, IAs are often asymptomatic, discovered incidentally during imaging for unrelated medical conditions [14].

In some cases, IAs may undergo morphological changes, growing in size and thus significantly increasing the risk of rupture. Rupture can have severe consequences, such as aneurysmal subarachnoid hemorrhage (aSAH), intracerebral hemorrhage, or intraventricular hemorrhage, potentially causing stroke or death [11, 32]. Interestingly, reductions in IA size, though rare, have been observed. These reductions often follow diminished arterial blood flow, resulting from the occlusion of arteriovenous shunts in vascular malformations or the application of flow-diverting stents [6, 8, 22, 24, 26].

Risk factors for the development of IAs include genetic predispositions [2], a family history of aneurysms [7, 29, 30], tobacco consumption [5, 33, 40], hypertension [41], specific medical conditions like polycystic kidney disease [15], and certain connective tissue disorders [9]. Notably, women are twice as likely as men to develop IAs and suffer from an aSAH [11, 25].

The management of IAs involves a range of treatment options, from surgical interventions (clipping) to endovascular procedures (coiling, stenting, and flow diversion). In some instances, consistent monitoring through imaging tests is preferable to detect any changes in the aneurysm or signs of cranial nerve or brain damage. The decision-making process for screening and treatment is complex, balancing economic, ethical, and clinical considerations [28]. Given the lack of reliable models and precise risk quantifications, we can take only a multidisciplinary approach, combining insights from the literature, expert guidelines, and local evidence [1, 13].

The high stakes involved in decision-making for IAs, ranging from full recovery to severe disability or death, make the process susceptible to cognitive biases. Biases, such as loss aversion, framing effects, and varying perspectives, can lead to suboptimal outcomes. The complexity of decision-making in the context of IAs is further compounded by the multistage nature of the process, influenced by factors such as cumulative value and event partitioning. The application of prospect theory, initially proposed by Daniel Kahneman and Amos Tversky, provides a framework for understanding these decision-making processes under uncertainty. Kahneman's work, particularly in his book *Thinking, Fast and Slow*, delves into the influence of heuristics and mental shortcuts on decision-making, highlighting systematic deviations from rational judgment [18, 19, 34].

The evaluation of event probabilities is significantly influenced by heuristic availability, a cognitive process that assesses the ease of recalling certain events or categories from memory. This heuristic can lead to biases such as representativeness, where the frequency or likelihood of events is overestimated on the basis of how memorable they are. Such biases have profound impacts on judgment and decision-making processes, emphasizing the need for awareness and mitigation strategies [35].

In the medical field, assessing associations between symptoms and diseases is a common practice that involves measuring their strength, direction, specificity, consistency, and plausibility. However, the estimates of symptom and disease frequencies are often skewed by the availability heuristic. In many cases, little is known about the occurrence of a symptom in isolation or the incidence of a disease without the presence of a specific symptom. This lack of comprehensive data, along with the rarity of truly pathognomonic signs or symptoms, poses a challenge in accurately diagnosing and treating medical conditions.

Furthermore, medical decision-making is frequently hindered by gaps in understanding underlying disease mechanisms and treatment effects. The necessity of providing answers, often with incomplete information, further exacerbates the reliance on heuristic availability and leads to a biased perception of symptom–disease relationships, compounded by insufficient data on symptom and disease prevalence in broader populations.

These challenges highlight the need for a conscientious approach in medical decision-making that acknowledges cognitive biases and knowledge gaps. Developing strategies to enhance awareness and mitigate these biases is crucial for improving diagnostic accuracy and patient outcomes. This approach is exemplified by revisiting Kahneman's classic experiment, which demonstrates how new evidence should update but not completely determine beliefs. In this experiment, the likelihood of Steve's being a librarian or his being a farmer is assessed on the basis of his characteristics and the proportion of librarians and farmers in the population. The conclusion underscores the importance of considering all relevant information in the decision-making process [31, 36].

Bayes's theorem, a cornerstone of probabilistic inference, offers a methodological approach to quantify the likelihood of events on the basis of new information. This theorem, formulated by eighteenth-century statistician Reverend Thomas Bayes, calculates the probability of an event occurring given the occurrence of another event. The theorem is defined as $P(A|B) = (P(A) * P(B|A))/P(B)$, where $P(A|B)$ represents the posterior probability, $P(B|A)$ the likelihood, $P(A)$ the prior probability, and $P(B)$ the overall probability of event B [3, 4, 21]. By applying Bayes's theorem, decision-making processes can be modeled in the context of IAs, particularly when considering the cumulative prospect theory and its implications for sequential event interactions.

In this work, we use Bayes's theorem to estimate the prevalence of IAs and the incidence of IA rupture in different demographics, utilizing data from the literature and resources like the International Stroke Genetics Consortium (ISGC) intracranial aneurysm databank (AneuX databank). This approach allows for the development of methodologies that not only estimate the risk of IA rupture but also enhance decision-making strategies through Bayesian networks. These networks provide a visual map of the interdependencies between various risk factors, offering a more comprehensive understanding of IA dynamics [10].

In summary, this manuscript provides a comprehensive overview of intracranial aneurysms, from their formation and risk factors to the complexities of treatment decision-making. It highlights the importance of understanding cognitive biases in medical judgments and the role of Bayesian analysis in refining these processes.

Estimating Recruitment Population and At-Risk Demographics in Intracranial Aneurysm (IA)

Rupture Cases

Our study applies Bayes's theorem to assess the impact of aneurysmal subarachnoid hemorrhage (aSAH) incidence on IA diagnosis probability, with a focus on sex-based risk variations. This approach helps estimate the IA rupture risk in diagnosed patients on the basis of sex while considering prior probability, likelihood, and trait probability.

We highlight a framing bias due to the unnoticed nature of asymptomatic IAs versus the more detectable ruptured IAs. Although most IA ruptures are diagnosed when receiving medical attention, about 10% are missed due to sudden death, symptom misinterpretation, or healthcare access barriers [16, 20].

Using aSAH data as a less biased source, we based our model on data gathered over a decade from renowned institutions. The data indicate an aSAH incidence of 6.1 per 100,000 person-years [11]. The ISGC-IA cohort comprises 7992 patients, with 5434 diagnosed post-rupture (3653 women and 1781 men) and 2558 diagnosed incidentally (1823 women and 735 men) (Fig. 1). We estimate the recruitment population to be around 8.9 million, not accounting for the 10% of cases featuring undiagnosed aSAH.

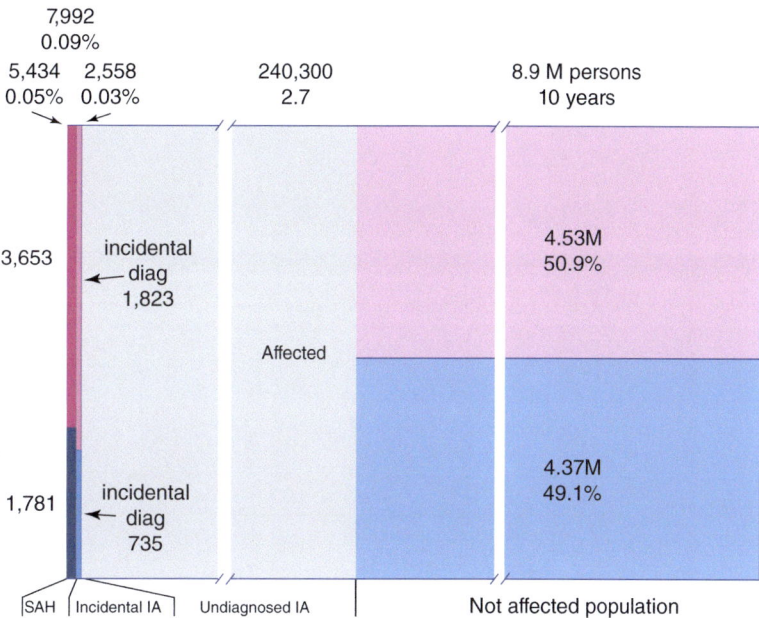

Fig. 1 Graphic representation of the size of the ISGC cohort, estimated recruitment population, and population affected by an IA but undiagnosed (in gray). Note the breaks. At scale, the gray area should be twice as wide and the whole rectangle 253 times wider

According to United Nations 2010 statistics, the sex ratio in the study countries is approximately 50.9% women and 49.1% men [42]. The Rotterdam study suggests a 1.8% IA prevalence, while other sources propose about a 3% one [27, 37, 38]. Our study adopts a 2.7% IA prevalence, as agreed by the @neurIST community in 2010.

Out of 8.9 million, we estimate 240,300 individuals might have an IA, with only 7,992 diagnosed. The diagnosed cohort reveals 5,434 post-aSAH diagnoses and 2,558 incidental diagnoses.

Risk Estimations for Intracranial Aneurysm

Our analysis of ISGC-IA data shows the likelihood of being diagnosed as an IA patient and being a woman can be estimated between 67.2% and 71.3% and overall at 68.5%. Setting the a priori IA risk hypothesis at 2.7% and employing the country-wide sex ratio as the probability of being a woman, we estimate the posterior probability to be diagnosed with an IA for a woman at 3.6% and male diagnosis probability at 1.7%.

Formally:

$$P(H = \text{"IA diagnosis"} | E = \text{"female"}) = P(H = \text{"IA diagnosis"}) *$$
$$P(E = \text{"female"} | H = \text{"IA diagnosis"}) / P(E = \text{"female"}) = 0.027 * 0.68 / 0.509 = 3.6\%.$$

and

$$P(H = \text{"IA diagnosis"} | E = \text{"male"}) = 0.027 * 0.31 / 0.491 = 1.7\%.$$

The estimated population affected by the disease thus involves 163,650 women and 75,650 men (Fig. 2).

The actual number of incidentally IA-diagnosed women in the cohort was 1823, representing about 1% of the potentially affected population (163650). Similarly, the actual number of incidentally IA-diagnosed men was 735, representing 1% of the potentially affected population (75650).

Sex-Associated Risks in IA Diagnosis and Rupture

The probability of a female being diagnosed with ruptured IA (aSAH) is 67.22%, while for men, it's 32.77%. Using Bayes's theorem, we find the relative risk of women being diagnosed with ruptured IA to be about 1.97 times higher than men.

Formally:

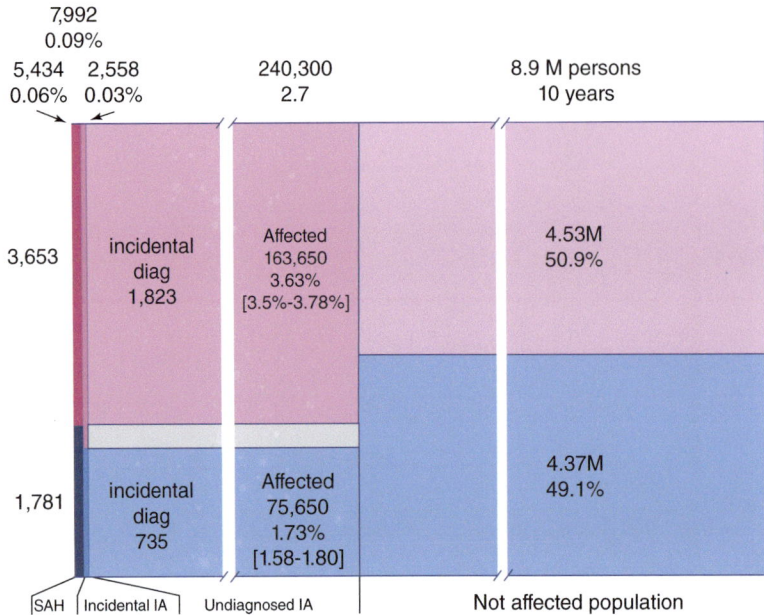

Fig. 2 Graphical representation of the female and male number and proportions in the population of recruitment, population of affected patients, and cohort diagnosed with unruptured IA and after IA rupture. The difference in likelihood of women in the SAH and incidental diagnosed population is illustrated in gray Note the breaks

$$P\left(H = \text{"IA diagnosis"} | E = \text{"female"}\right) = 6.1/100{,}000 * 67.2\%$$
$$/ 50.9\% = 8.03/100{,}000.$$

$$P\left(H = \text{"IA diagnosis"} | E = \text{"male"}\right) = 6.1/100{,}000 * 32.8\%$$
$$/49.1\% = 4.07/100{,}000.$$

$$\frac{P\left(H = \text{"IA diagnosis"} | E = \text{"female"}\right)}{P\left(H = \text{"IA diagnosis"} | E = \text{"male"}\right)} = 1.97$$

Considering the ISGC cohort composition (67.99% aSAH), the probability being diagnosed with an incidental IA being a women (67.2%) and diagnosis likelihood post-rupture (67.2% women), the posterior probability of a aSAH diagnosis given the patient is a female affected by an IA is 6.4%. For men, this probability is 77.6%, indicating a slightly higher risk of rupture diagnosis in men compared to women, with a relative risk of approximately 0.82 for women as compared to men.

Formally:

$$P\left(H = \text{"IA diagnosis"} | E = \text{"female"}\right) = 68\% * 67.2\% / 68.5\%$$
$$= 66.7\%.$$

$$P\left(H = \text{"IA diagnosis"} | E = \text{"male"}\right) = 68\% * 32.8\% / 31.5\%$$
$$= 70.8\%.$$

$$\frac{P\left(H = \text{"IA diagnosis"} | E = \text{"female"}\right)}{P\left(H = \text{"IA diagnosis"} | E = \text{"male"}\right)} = 0.95$$

Our study offers insights into the sex-based differences in IA diagnosis and rupture risk through Bayesian analysis and demographic data utilization. The findings underline the importance of considering sex-specific factors in IA risk assessment and healthcare planning (Fig. 3).

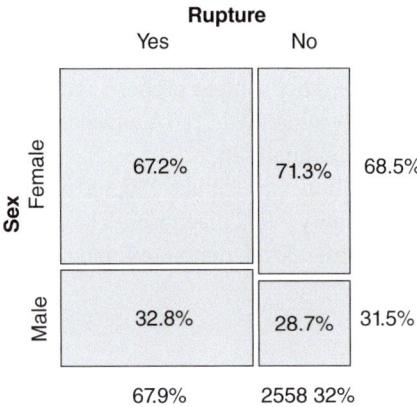

Fig. 3 The likelihood to be diagnosed with at least one aneurysm is more than twice as high in women as in men, but the likelihood for both men and women to be diagnosed either with an unruptured IA or after IA rupture are not statistically different. Therefore, the risk of the rupture of IA is most likely very similar in men and women

Discussion

This study demonstrates the application of Bayes's theorem in constructing a model that integrates diverse data sources and perspectives, thus minimizing framing effects. It clarifies our model's assumptions, highlighting its limitations, and reveals the higher prevalence of intracranial aneurysm (IA) in women and their increased risk of suffering from aneurysmal subarachnoid hemorrhage (aSAH). However, once diagnosed with an IA, women and men share similar rupture risks.

Our findings indicate that sex plays a role in IA diagnosis incidence, but assessing rupture risk requires caution due to potential cofactors influencing IA initiation, progression, and rupture. We note that only 1% of those affected by IA in the Western world from 2000 to 2010 were diagnosed, pointing to a significant undiagnosed population. Most diagnosed aneurysms undergo interventions, which might not always be necessary, leading to a potentially biased understanding of the affected population. The rise in diagnostic imaging is likely increasing the detection of incidental IAs, thus changing the epidemiological landscape.

There is a noticeable disparity in IA prevalence and aSAH incidence, with rates twice as high in women as in men. This calls for further investigation into the sex-based risk of rupture versus aneurysm initiation. The strongest known predictor of aneurysm rupture is its location [12, 14, 25]. A recent study suggests differing aneurysm locations and other factors between sexes [39].

Deciphering IA Complexity with Bayesian Networks

Bayesian methods, applied to individual or multiple interacting factors, can simplify complex systems. This approach involves modeling dependencies in a Bayesian network (BN), a directed acyclic graph (DAG) representing factors as nodes and relationships as edges (Fig. 4). Conditional probabilities quantify node dependencies, with the joint probability distribution informed by data and prior knowledge.

An exploratory BN from Geneva University Hospital data [10] shows that the influence of sex on IA rupture is indirect, affected by factors like IA location, blood pressure awareness, and smoking behavior. Interactive BNs help explore factor effects and their interactions, comparing multiple BNs representing distinct patient groups (Fig. 4).

Using a BN addresses interdependencies among factors, and a limitation in standard multivariate regression or principal component analysis is that they assume factor independence. These advanced tools must undergo robust validation and be user-friendly and efficient to encourage clinical adoptions.

Conclusions

This chapter introduced Bayes's theorem, Bayesian analysis, and modeling tailored to clinicians. It highlighted their practicality in assessing the risk of IA and the nuanced role of sex in these outcomes. We know that the prevalence of IA and incidence of aSAH are twice as high in women as in men. However, we often misinterpret this information when estimating the risk of IA rupture in diagnosed patients.

Our application of Bayesian analysis reveals that the risk of IA rupture is similar between men and women once diagnosed. Despite this, the disparities in prevalence and incidence underscore the importance of considering sex as a significant risk factor in IA management decisions.

Furthermore, we advocate for data sharing and for the adoption of Bayesian modeling in clinical practice. This methodology synthesizes data from various studies, acknowledging the interconnected nature of influencing factors, and presents them within an integrated network. Such an approach not only facilitates comprehensive risk assessments but also champions personalized patient care strategies.

However, the utility of Bayesian models in everyday clinical scenarios hinges on their accessibility and ease of use. Therefore, a concerted effort is required to develop interfaces that clinicians can navigate intuitively and confidently. Equally paramount is the rigorous validation of these tools, ensuring their reliability and efficacy in real-world medical settings.

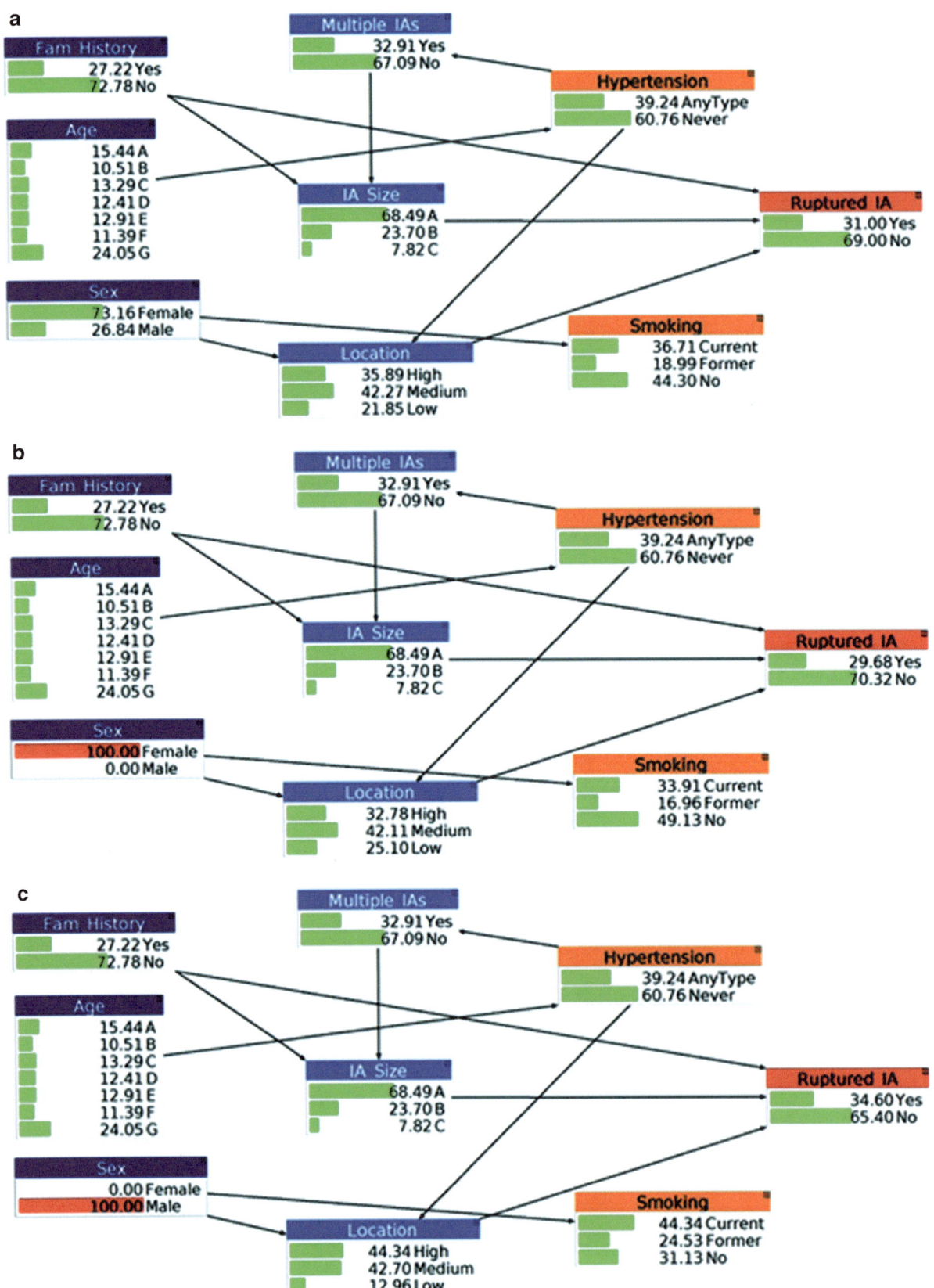

Fig. 4 An interactive Bayesian network (BN) based on the discrete BN model of Delucchi et al. [10], illustrated with HUGIN lite [23] Panel (**a**) illustraes the distribution of cases among categories of each variable and arrows the interactions between variables. Panels (**b**) and (**c**) illustrate how conditioning the "Sex" node as "Female" or "Male," respectively, alters the conditional probability distributions of associated nodes such as "Smoking," "Location," and "Ruptured IA." Comparing panel (**b**) and (**c**) shows that the probability of being diagnosed with a ruptured IA is ~5% higher in men than in women

Acknowledgments We thank Jason Parry for carefully revising the manuscript and English language editing.

Funding Information This work has been made possible by previous studies funded by the following: the FP6 Framework Program of the European Commission Information Society Technologies IST (IST-2004-027703) and the AneuX project, funded by the Swiss Initiative for Systems Biology SystemsX.ch and evaluated by the Swiss National Research Fund; the contribution of the ISGC community, funded by the European Research Council under the European Union's Horizon 2020 research and innovation program (PRYSM, grant agreement No. 852173); the Netherlands Cardiovascular Research Initiative (an initiative with the support of the Dutch Heart Foundation, CVON2015-08 ERASE); NIH funding; the French Regional Council of Pays-de-la-Loire (VaCaRMe program) and the Agence Nationale de la Recherche (ANR-15-CE17-0008-01 to G.L); the French Ministry of Health (Clinical trial CT02848495 to HD); the Genavie Foundation, the Société Française de Radiologie, and the Société Française de Neuroradiologie; Spain's Ministry of Health (Instituto de Salud Carlos III Fondo de Investigaciones sanitarias P19/00011 and by "RICORS-ICTUS RD21/0006/0021); the Canadian Institutes of Health Research; the Helsinki University Central Hospital EVO grant TYH2018316; and the Stroke Association. Funders were not involved in the study design, in the analysis of the data, or in the interpretation of the results.

Declarations

Conflict of interest: The authors declare that they have no conflict of interest.

References

1. Algra AM, Lindgren A, Vergouwen MDI, Greving JP, van der Schaaf IC, van Doormaal TPC, Rinkel GJE. Procedural clinical complications, case-fatality risks, and risk factors in endovascular and neurosurgical treatment of unruptured intracranial aneurysms: a systematic review and meta-analysis. JAMA Neurol. 2018; https://doi.org/10.1001/jamaneurol.2018.4165.
2. Bakker MK, van der Spek RAA, van Rheenen W, et al. Genome-wide association study of intracranial aneurysms identifies 17 risk loci and genetic overlap with clinical risk factors. Nat Genet. 2020; https://doi.org/10.1038/s41588-020-00725-7.
3. Bayes T. An essay towards solving a problem in the doctrine of chances. London: Philosophical Transactions of the Royal Society of London; 1763.
4. Bellhouse D. The Reverend Thomas Bayes: a guide to his works. Int Stat Rev. 2011;79(2):208–25.
5. Bennett P, Aguiar GB, RCD S. the relationship between smoking and brain aneurysms: from formation to rupture. Rev Assoc Med Bras (1992). 2021;67(6):895–9.
6. Berge J, Biondi A, Machi P, Brunel H, Pierot L, Gabrillargues J, Kadziolka K, Barreau X, Dousset V, Bonafe A. Flow-diverter silk stent for the treatment of intracranial aneurysms: 1-year follow-up in a multicenter study. AJNR Am J Neuroradiol. 2012;33(6):1150–5.
7. Broderick JP, Sauerbeck LR, Foroud T, Huston J, Pankratz N, Meissner I, Brown RD. The familial intracranial aneurysm (FIA) study protocol. BMC Med Genet. 2005;6:17.
8. Byrne JV, Beltechi R, Yarnold JA, Birks J, Kamran M. Early experience in the treatment of intra-cranial aneurysms by endovascular flow diversion: a multicentre prospective study. PLoS One. 2010; https://doi.org/10.1371/journal.pone.0012492.
9. Clarke M. Systematic review of reviews of risk factors for intracranial aneurysms. Neuroradiology. 2008;50(8):653–64.
10. Delucchi M, Spinner GR, Scutari M, Bijlenga P, Morel S, Friedrich CM, Furrer R, Hirsch S. Bayesian network analysis reveals the interplay of intracranial aneurysm rupture risk factors. Comput Biol Med. 2022;147:105740.
11. Etminan N, Chang HS, Hackenberg K, de Rooij NK, Vergouwen MDI, Rinkel GJE, Algra A. Worldwide incidence of aneurysmal subarachnoid Hemorrhage according to region, time period, blood pressure, and smoking prevalence in the population: a systematic review and meta-analysis. JAMA Neurol. 2019;76(5):588–97.
12. Etminan N, Rinkel GJ. Unruptured intracranial aneurysms: development, rupture and preventive management. Nat Rev Neurol. 2016;12(12):699–713.
13. Etminan N, de Sousa DA, Tiseo C, et al. European Stroke Organisation (ESO) guidelines on management of unruptured intracranial aneurysms. Eur Stroke J. 2022;7(3):V.
14. Gondar R, Gautschi OP, Cuony J, et al. Unruptured intracranial aneurysm follow-up and treatment after morphological change is safe: observational study and systematic review. J Neurol Neurosurg Psychiatry. 2016;87(12):1277–82.
15. Haemmerli J, Morel S, Georges M, et al. Characteristics and distribution of intracranial aneurysms in autosomal dominant polycystic kidney disease patients compared to the general population: a meta-analysis. Kidney360. 2023; https://doi.org/10.34067/KID.0000000000000092.
16. Huang J, van Gelder JM. The probability of sudden death from rupture of intracranial aneurysms: a meta-analysis. Neurosurgery. 2002;51(5):1101–7.
17. Humphrey JD. Coupling hemodynamics with vascular wall mechanics and mechanobiology to understand intracranial aneurysms. Int J Comut Fluid Dyn. 2009;23(8):569–81.
18. Kahneman D. Thinking, fast and slow. New York: Farrar, Straus and Giroux; 2011.
19. Kahneman D, Tversky A. Prospect theory: an analysis of decision under risk. Econometrica. 1979;47(2):263–91.
20. Koffijberg H, Buskens E, Granath F, Adami J, Ekbom A, Rinkel GJE, Blomqvist P. Subarachnoid haemorrhage in Sweden 1987-2002: regional incidence and case fatality rates. J Neurol Neurosurg Psychiatry. 2008;79(3):294–9.
21. Laplace PS. Théorie analytique des probabilités. Paris: Courcier; 1812.
22. Lylyk P, Miranda C, Ceratto R, Ferrario A, Scrivano E, Luna HR, Berez AL, Tran Q, Nelson PK, Fiorella D. Curative endovascular reconstruction of cerebral aneurysms with the pipeline embolization device: the Buenos Aires experience. Neurosurgery. 2009;64(4):632–42; discussion 642-3; quiz N6
23. Madsen AL, Lang M, Kjærulff UB, Jensen F. The Hugin tool for learning Bayesian networks. In: Nielsen TD, Zhang NL, editors. Symbolic and quantitative approaches to reasoning with uncertainty. Berlin, Heidelberg: Springer; 2003. p. 594–605.
24. Meisel HJ, Mansmann U, Alvarez H, Rodesch G, Brock M, Lasjaunias P. Cerebral arteriovenous malformations and associated aneurysms: analysis of 305 cases from a series of 662 patients. Neurosurgery. 2000;46(4):793–800; discussion 800-2
25. Morel S, Hostettler IC, Spinner GR, et al. Intracranial aneurysm classifier using phenotypic factors: an international pooled analysis. J Pers Med. 2022; https://doi.org/10.3390/jpm12091410.
26. Nelson PK, Lylyk P, Szikora I, Wetzel SG, Wanke I, Fiorella D. The pipeline embolization device for the intracranial treatment of aneurysms trial. AJNR Am J Neuroradiol. 2011;32(1):34–40.
27. Rinkel GJ, Djibuti M, Algra A, van Gijn J. Prevalence and risk of rupture of intracranial aneurysms: a systematic review. Stroke. 1998;29(1):251–6.

28. Rinkel GJ, Ruigrok YM. Preventive screening for intracranial aneurysms. Int J Stroke Off J Int Stroke Soc. 2022;17(1):30–6.
29. Ronkainen A, Hernesniemi J, Puranen M, Niemitukia L, Vanninen R, Ryynanen M, Kuivaniemi H, Tromp G. Familial intracranial aneurysms. Lancet. 1997;349(9049):380–4.
30. Ruigrok YM, Rinkel GJ, Algra A, Raaymakers TW, Van Gijn J. Characteristics of intracranial aneurysms in patients with familial subarachnoid hemorrhage. Neurology. 2004;62(6):891–4.
31. Sanderson G. Bayes theorem, the geometry of changing beliefs, 2019.
32. Schatlo B, Fung C, Stienen MN, et al. Incidence and outcome of aneurysmal subarachnoid hemorrhage: the Swiss Study on Subarachnoid Hemorrhage (Swiss SOS). Stroke. 2021;52(1):344–7.
33. Schatlo B, Gautschi OP, Friedrich CM, Ebeling C, Jagersberg M, Kulscar Z, Pereira VM, Schaller K, Bijlenga P. Association of single and multiple aneurysms with tobacco abuse: an @neurIST risk analysis. Neurosurg Focus. 2019;47(1):E9.
34. Sheshinski E, Viscusi WK. Cumulative prospect theory. J Risk Uncertain. 1992;5(4):307–32.
35. Tversky A, Kahneman D. Availability: a heuristic for judging frequency and probability. Cogn Psychol. 1973;5(2):207–32.
36. Tversky A, Kahneman D. Judgment under uncertainty: heuristics and biases: biases in judgments reveal some heuristics of thinking under uncertainty. Science. 1974;185(4157):1124–31.
37. Vernooij MW, Ikram MA, Tanghe HL, Vincent AJPE, Hofman A, Krestin GP, Niessen WJ, Breteler MMB, van der Lugt A. Incidental findings on brain MRI in the general population. N Engl J Med. 2007;357(18):1821–8.
38. Vlak MH, Algra A, Brandenburg R, Rinkel GJ. Prevalence of unruptured intracranial aneurysms, with emphasis on sex, age, comorbidity, country, and time period: a systematic review and meta-analysis. Lancet Neurol. 2011;10(7):626–36.
39. Wälchli T, Ndengera M, Constanthin PE, et al. Sex-dependent manifestations of intracranial aneurysms. Stroke Vasc Interv. 2023; https://doi.org/10.1101/2023.03.29.23287441.
40. Woo D, Khoury J, Haverbusch MM, Sekar P, Flaherty ML, Kleindorfer DO, Kissela BM, Moomaw CJ, Deka R, Broderick JP. Smoking and family history and risk of aneurysmal subarachnoid hemorrhage. Neurology. 2009;72(1):69–72.
41. Zhong P, Lu Z, Li T, Lan Q, Liu J, Wang Z, Chen S, Huang Q. Association between regular blood pressure monitoring and the risk of intracranial aneurysm rupture: a Multicenter retrospective study with propensity score matching. Transl Stroke Res. 2022; https://doi.org/10.1007/s12975-022-01006-7.
42. UNdata export on global popualtion by country, 2018.

Open Access This chapter is licensed under the terms of the Creative Commons Attribution 4.0 International License (http://creativecommons.org/licenses/by/4.0/), which permits use, sharing, adaptation, distribution and reproduction in any medium or format, as long as you give appropriate credit to the original author(s) and the source, provide a link to the Creative Commons license and indicate if changes were made.

The images or other third party material in this chapter are included in the chapter's Creative Commons license, unless indicated otherwise in a credit line to the material. If material is not included in the chapter's Creative Commons license and your intended use is not permitted by statutory regulation or exceeds the permitted use, you will need to obtain permission directly from the copyright holder.

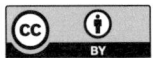

Challenges of the Endovascular Approach for Difficult Cerebral Aneurysms

Shigeru Miyachi

Introduction

Initially, endovascular embolization was only considered as an alternative treatment option to clipping for cerebral aneurysms. However, with an increase in the safety and reliability of coiling, patients began to prefer less-invasive approaches and request an endovascular treatment, resulting in a gradual increase in the rate of coiling. Nowadays, half of aneurysm patients are treated with coiling in Japan and more than 70–80% in Western countries [1]. Such remarkable progress has been brought about by the rapid and evolutional improvement in imaging technology, devices, treatment skills, and perioperative management. Recent novel devices that do not use coils, such as the flow diverter and the flow disruptor, may open the door to changing the basic concept of endovascular treatment.

Here, the transition of endovascular treatment methods is introduced and discussed on the basis of my experiences with and challenges when facing difficult aneurysms.

Transition in the Endovascular Treatment Methods Over 20 Years

Over the past 20 years, dramatic changes in technological development have seemed to occur every 5 years, bringing about new devices and novel techniques. The 20-year period from 2001 to 2020 can be divided into fours periods, and my strategies for unruptured aneurysms include key factors and clinical results that fall into these periods. We treated a total of 1461 unruptured aneurysms in this period.

In the first period (2001–2005: $n = 236$) 2D or 3D types of shape-memory coils as well as the various sizes and softness levels were lined up. The balloon-assist technique was introduced in this period, but balloon catheters were applied only to specific cases because of their stiffness and large diameter. Because of this, two-thirds of aneurysms were treated with simple methods using a single microcatheter.

Antiplatelet management in perioperative terms was established in the second period (2006–2010: $n = 339$). The surgical consensus during this time was to take the preloading of dual antiplatelet agents from at least 1 week before the operation and to continue them for several months postoperatively. Such antiplatelet agents contributed to the decrease in perioperative ischemic complications. In this period, a bi-plane angiography machine with three-dimensional digital subtraction angiography (3D-DSA) and roadmap technology were developed and improved our understanding of the angioarchitecture. The balloon neck-plasty technique was generalized, and half of the aneurysms were embolized with balloon-assisted coiling.

In the third period (2010–2014: $n = 433$), the double catheter technique was developed first in Japan, and it was adopted for use in difficult aneurysms with branch involvement. Neck bridge stents increased the indication of very broad-necked aneurysms, and half of the cases with the indication of balloon-assisted embolization were switched to stent-assisted coiling.

In the fourth and most recent period (2015–2020: $n = 453$), a breakthrough occurred with the introduction of flow diverter stents. Flow diverters were applied to large aneurysms in the carotid artery and yielded good clinical and angiographic effects. The numbers of internal trapping and simple coiling remarkably decreased. The various historical changes to our techniques and methods for aneurysms are shown in Fig. 1.

As for the location of treated aneurysms, posterior circulation aneurysms accounted for 39% in the first period. However, its rate gradually decreased over time, to 16% in the fourth period. This change resulted from the expanded

S. Miyachi (✉)
Department of Neurological Surgery, Aichi Medical University, Nagakute, Aichi, Japan
e-mail: miyachi.shigeru.752@mail.aichi-med-u.ac.jp

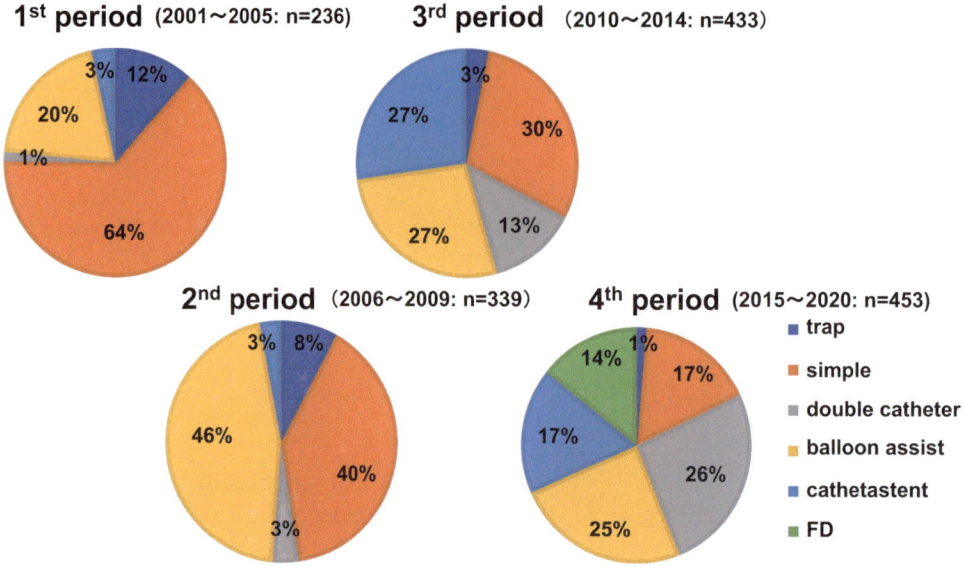

Fig. 1 Embolization methods in each period

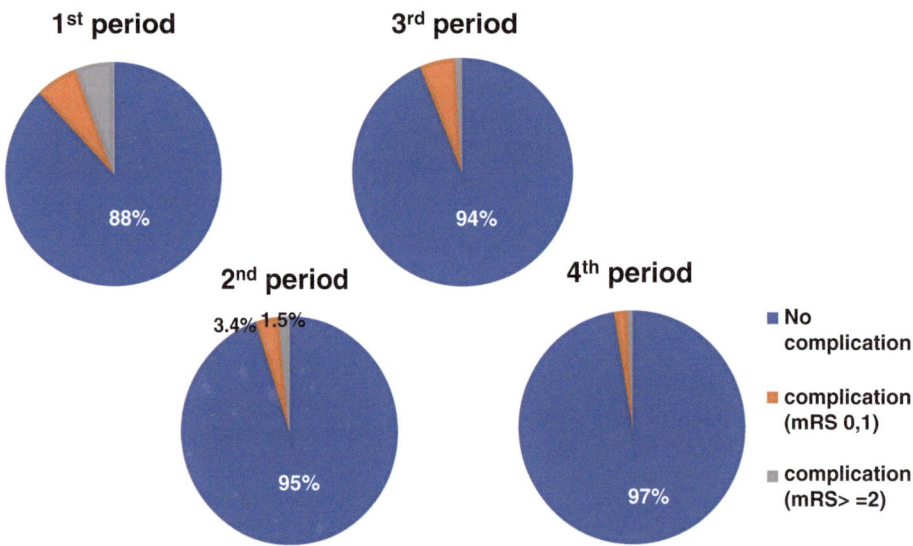

Fig. 2 Complications in each period

indication for the embolization of anterior circulation aneurysms in later periods. The complication rate also decreased over these periods (Fig. 2). The total complication rate was 12% in the first period but 2.7% in the fourth period. Particularly, the rate of serious complications was substantially decreased: from 5.7% in the first period to 0.7% in the fourth period. This good outcome was yielded mainly thanks to improvements in technology and devices. The evolution of imaging technology, such as high-resolution fluoroscopy, clear roadmaps in biplane systems, 3D-reconstruction images, and cone-beam computed tomography (CT) improved our understanding of the fine angioarchitecture and made the maneuver as safe and precise as possible. Improvements in devices, including access catheters, microcatheters, balloon catheters, stents, coils, and flow diverters, and a new strategy using such new devices have contributed to enabling the embolization of difficult aneurysms [1].

Challenges for Large Aneurysms

Flow diverters (FDs) were introduced as alternative options for treating large cerebral aneurysms. FDs can promote aneurysm occlusion by diverting blood flow away from the aneurysm sac, after which the orifice can be closed with dense woven mesh, conserving the diseased parent artery. This promotes natural aneurysmal thrombosis and shrinkage and allows the remodeling of the parent artery through a process of endoluminal reconstruction [2]. The re-establishment of homeostasis may contribute to a favorable angiographic and physical state and to the amelioration of symptoms (Fig. 3).

The use of a flow diverter was more beneficial in terms of safety, efficacy, and cost compared to conventional parent artery occlusion and saccular coil-packing techniques [3, 4]. Particularly for large carotid cavernous aneurysms (CCAs), conventional coil embolization has limited utility due to its inability to prevent recurrences and reduce mass effect. The trapping of the parent artery may risk introducing ischemic complications due to intracranial perfusion disorders. Flow diverters for large CCAs have shown promising clinical and radiological efficacy in the literature, including our reports [4, 5]. However, the side effects due to the high metal coverage rate of FDs pose some problems, such as thrombotic complications inducing in-stent thrombosis, causing the occlusion of the parent artery or jailed branches. Perioperative strong antiplatelet management is essential to prevent this complication. Another delayed complication is aneurysmal rupture. It occurs due to shifted wall shear stress or the partial strong jet of inflow caused by partial aneurysmal thrombosis. Particularly, large symptomatic paraclinoid aneurysms with a narrow neck come with a high risk of delayed rupture [6, 7]. Although absolute effective prophylactic measures have not been established, preceded saccular coil placement and overlapping stents are now tried as treatment measures, which have not reached consensus level.

Challenge for Blood Blister–Like Aneurysms

A ruptured blood blister–like aneurysm (BBA) is one of the most difficult aneurysms for any radical treatment. Traditionally, wrapping and clipping or trapping with/without an external–internal arterial bypass by taking direct approach have been recommended for anterior wall (so-called dorsal) BBAs at the internal carotid artery. However, the wall of a BBA is usually very thin and fragile, and its shape is too shallow to clip because this aneurysm is thought to be formed after focal arterial dissection. That is why it easily brings about catastrophic ruptures during the surgical approach. Further, in the case of slow backflow to the distal carotid artery after successful trapping, the retrograde thrombosis of the anterior choroidal artery occasionally occurs, resulting in ischemic complications.

Endovascular treatments with balloon- or stent-assisted coiling have often failed because of intraoperative coil penetration or rupture and fewer effects for the regrowth of the aneurysm [8]. The ideal treatment strategy was thought to be neck coverage without touching the aneurysm itself. According to this concept, tight mesh stents such as flow

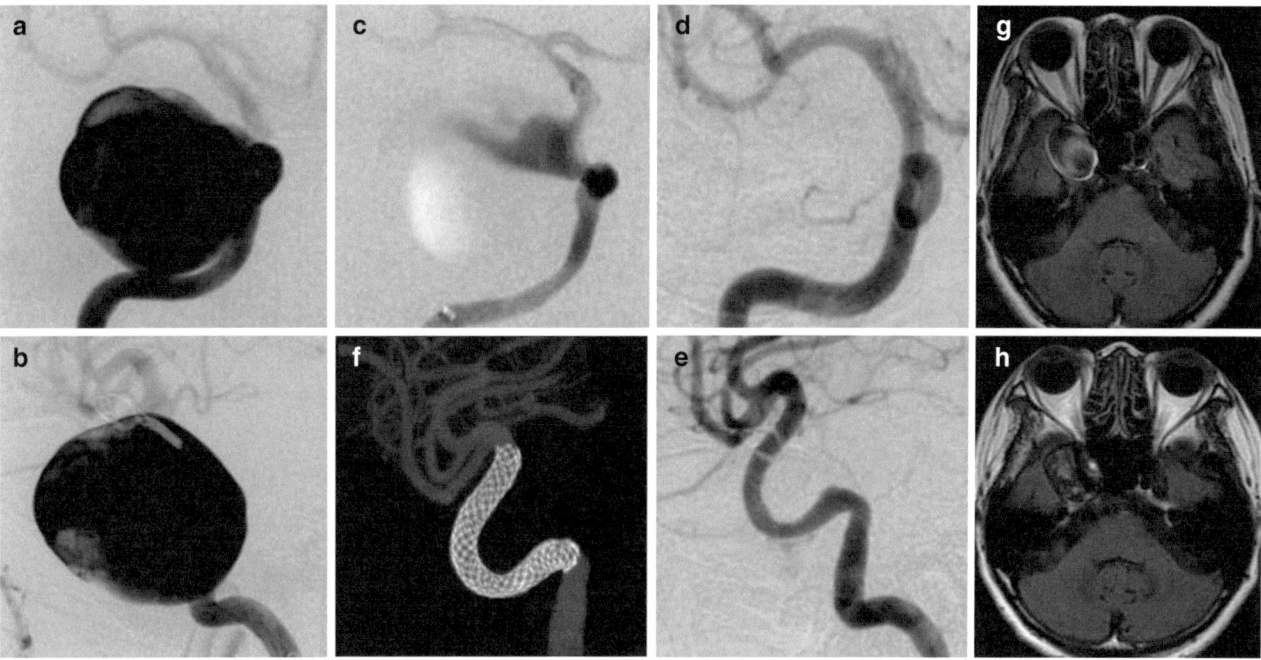

Fig. 3 A case of a flow diverter for a large carotid aneurysm. The patient was a 68-year-old woman with right abducens palsy. Carotid angiogram shows a large carotid cavernous aneurysm ((**a**) A-P view, (**b**) lateral view). After Pipeline (Medtronic) was deployed, remarkable reduction in inflow to the aneurysm was noted (**c**). Follow-up angiogram after 6 months shows complete occlusion of the aneurysm and the patency of the parent artery ((**d**) A-P view, (**e**) lateral view, (**f**) cone beam CT). MRI shows the thrombosis inside the aneurysm and a decrease in size ((**g**) preoperation and (**h**) postoperation). The patient symptom is completely resolved

diverters have been introduced (Fig. 4). Particularly, the overlapped flow diverter yielded better results than stent-assisted coiling and a direct surgical approach [9–11]. Shah et al. reported that endovascular therapy may have a better safety profile and provide better functional outcomes than surgery [10]. Rouchaud also described surgical deconstructive techniques as having higher rates of initial complete occlusion than endovascular techniques (77.3% versus 33.0%) but a higher risk for perioperative stroke (29.1% versus 5.0%) [9]. An FD is significantly superior to surgical treatment in decreasing the incidence of perioperative rebleeding, hydrocephalus, postoperative infarction, and postoperative vasospasm [10]. However, this novel arterioplastic option for BBAs has the following two risks: the first is perioperative thrombogenesis because of no preload of antiplatelet agents and the second is uncertain hemostatic effects because the inflow to the aneurysm continues through the mesh just after the procedure. For safer and proper treatment, further improvements in devices and techniques are essential.

Challenge with Robotics

Robotics is one of the most celebrated technological innovations. Some endovascular treatment robots are capable of simple 2D movements, such as pushing, pulling, and twisting devices like catheters, whereas others are capable of complicated 3D conventional surgeries. The range of

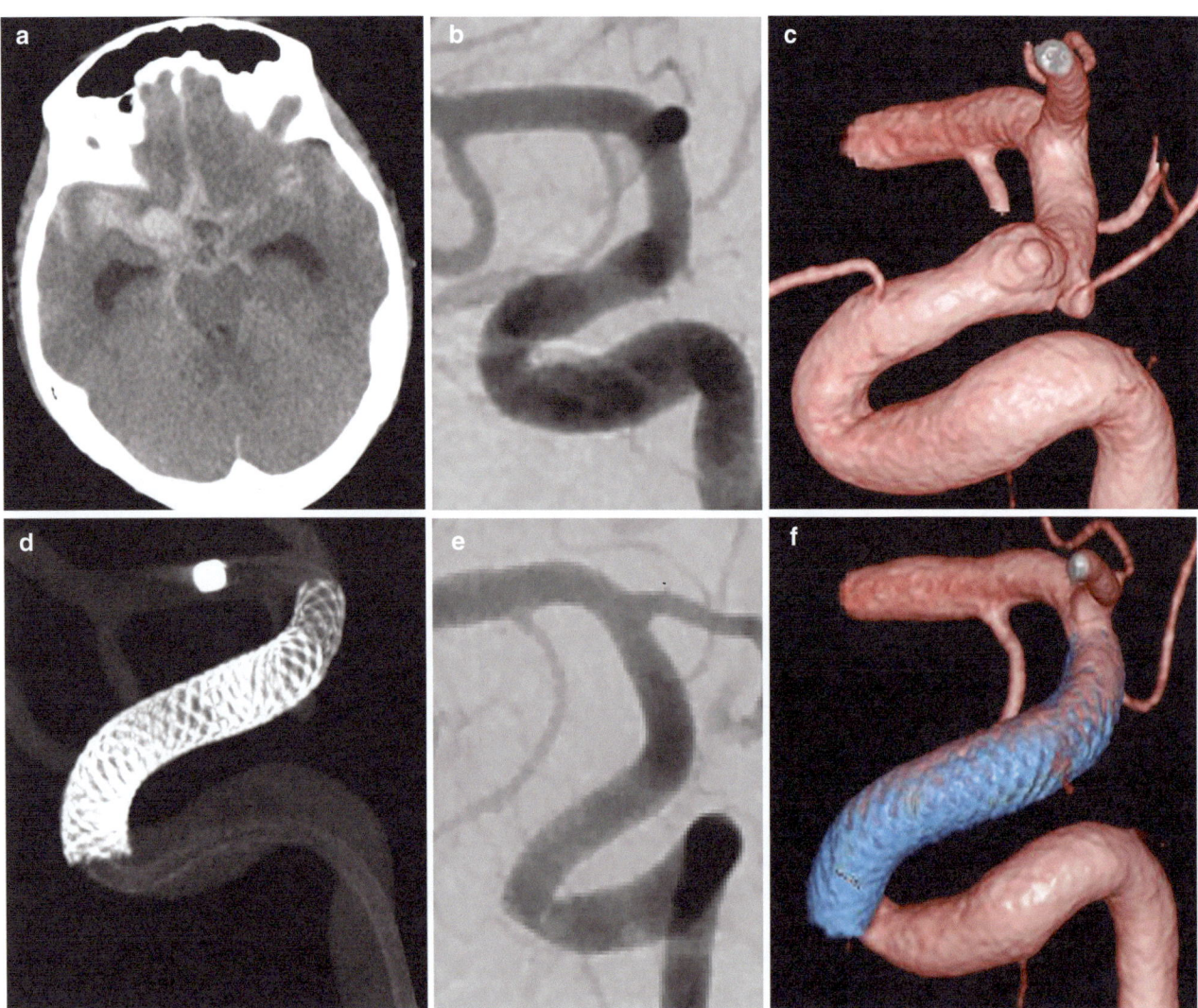

Fig. 4 A case of a flow diverter for blood blister–like aneurysm (BBA). The patient was a 54-year-old woman with a high-grade SAH and in comatose state. CT shows a massive SAH (**a**) and right carotid angiogram shows a shallow BBA beside the origin of posterior communicating artery ((**b**) lateral view, (**c**) 3D-CTA). Two Pipelines are overlapped, covering the neck ((**d**) cone beam CT). The angiogram taken 2 months later shows the patency of the internal carotid artery and the complete disappearance of the aneurysm ((**e**) lateral view, (**f**) 3D-DSA). The patient was discharged without neurological deficits

movement allowed is extremely small while maintaining stability. Thus, the implementation of robotics in the routine clinical practice of endovascular procedure could be possible in the near future. Although the CorPath GRX vascular robotic system (Siemens Healthineers, Erlangen, Germany) has already been introduced and clinically used in advance in the cardiovascular field [12, 13], its application in neuroendovascular intervention is challenging because the access routes are usually tortuous and small and because a very gentle maneuver is required to ensure that no injury occurs to the extremely fragile cerebral arteries.

Meanwhile, in cerebral embolisms, recanalization should be performed promptly because treatment delay causes serious cerebral infarction. However, if physicians performing the mechanical thrombectomy are unavailable, the patient will be transported to another stroke center via the drip and ship method or stroke specialists will be called. In such cases, a remote emergency surgery by a specialist using the remote surgery system can be beneficial to reduce the time lost due to waiting or transportation.

Because fluoroscopy is used, there can be a problem with the surgeon's and the staff's cumulative exposure; therefore, the ability to operate in a separate room without exposure can also contribute to the medical staff's safety and health.

Further, this system seems extremely promising for preventing virus infection and radiation exposure to the medical staff.

Therefore, we developed a new robot system with the function of the sensory feedback system and simultaneous control of the catheter and guidewire [8].

Structure

Our robotic support system is designed with the structure of a master and a slave within a closed-loop system [14, 15]. The surgeon's console is the master side, and the catheter manipulator is the slave side of the system. Our system has two independent slaves manipulating the microcatheter and micro-guidewire connected with the remote master driver with two joysticks. This design can be used in performing the usual catheterization in neuroendovascular intervention with both hands. The slave manipulator has sufficient output power, more than 1 newton, to reproduce the exact master intervention without slippage or delay. Successful microcatheterization and insertion into the aneurysm model can be performed in the wet vascular model corresponding to the 3D handling without excessive stress to the vascular or aneurysmal wall. This machine has a unique function that indicates the reactive force of resistance on a wire that is stuck using the sensor system [16, 17]. It enables sensing feedback by using an originally developed insertion-force measuring device, which detects the pressure stress on the vessel wall and alerts the operator by using an audible scale. This system is useful in preventing the overaction of the machine (Fig. 5).

Remote Telesurgery

Telesurgery between remote areas is simulated [18]. The slave robot in the angiography room was an original machine, and the master side was set in a separate room. They were connected via hypertext transfer protocol (HTTP) communication using a local area network system. The surgeon operated by looking at a personal computer monitor that shared an angiography monitor. The slave robot catheterized and inserted a coil for the aneurysm into the silicon blood-vessel model in the angiography room (Fig. 6). Our robot promptly responded to the surgeon's operations and quite accurately responded to the joystick's swift movements. The surgeon could control the operation, such as stopping the operation and reinserting the device by listening to the pitch indicating the insertion force picked up by the microphone in the angiography room PC in real time.

However, the following improvements and countermeasures are necessary for practical clinical use. The network needs to be strengthened as a countermeasure against delays in a higher-performance transmission control system. Although the operator's motion could be well reproduced in the simple model, its exact correspondence with the rapid action and within the acutely curved vessel was difficult to determine. The ethical issues regarding responsibility in the event of complications during the procedure due to hardware difficulties and transmission errors need to be clarified [19]. Importantly, independent specified maneuver training is required to operate the robot, and training time should be

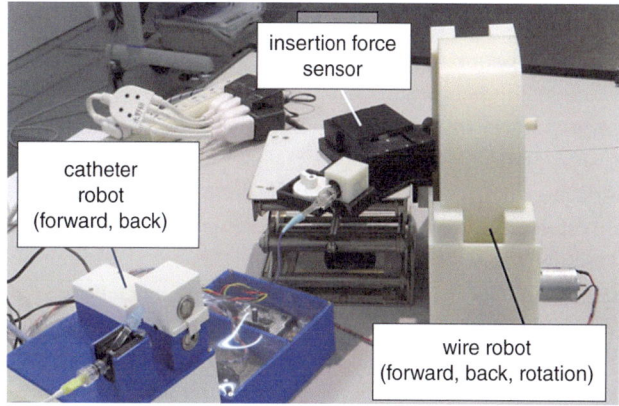

Fig. 5 Slave robot system with a catheter, a wire robot, and an insertion force sensor. The catheter and the guidewire are separately and simultaneously operated. They are combined with an insertion force-measuring device

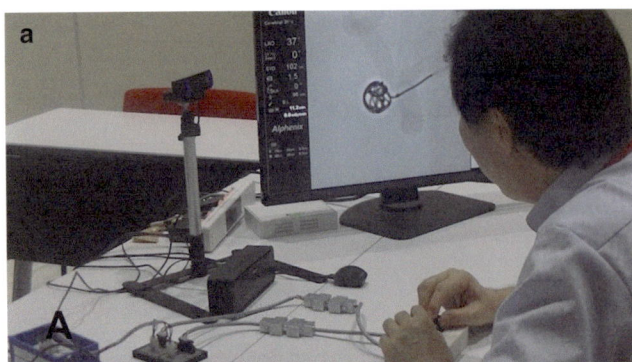 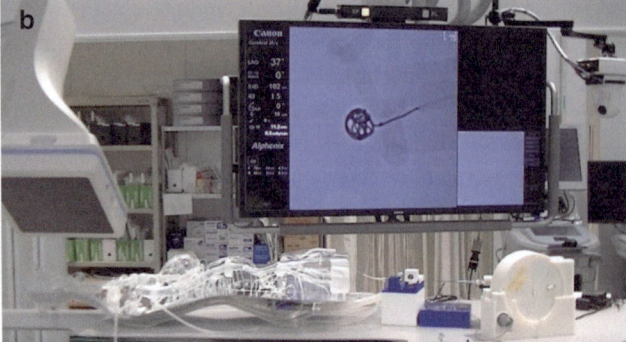

Fig. 6 Remote experimental telesurgery of aneurysm embolization. The operation of coiling in the master side (**a**), at 50 m distance from the angiography room, corresponded exactly with the slave side (**b**)

shared to deploy novel robotic technologies in clinical practice. Diminished relationships between patients and their treating physicians due to the remote contact may cause communication problems.

This new style of remote intervention will help professionals perform neuroendovascular interventions without the presence of neuroendovascular specialists. Although the motion of the slave side is completely controlled like a puppet by the master surgeon for now, automatic control of the slave action will be equipped with and thus controlled by artificial intelligence with deep learning in the future. Robotic intelligence may help in performing not only actual surgeries but also automatic surgeries under the vigilant observation of real surgeons. This system seems extremely promising for preventing viral infections and radiation exposure to the medical staff. It will also enable medical professionals to operate in remote areas and create a ubiquitous medical environment.

Conclusions

Indications pointing to using the endovascular approach as a certain treatment option for aneurysms is increasing. Complete radical results have not been completely achieved for extremely difficult aneurysms, such as thrombotic aneurysms, BBAs, and dolichoectasia, among others [20]. Additionally, when using noncoiled methods, namely flow diverters or flow disruptors, the higher device costs of endovascular tools should be taken into consideration. Further improvements to these devices and technologies are essential, but conventional effective treatments, such as trapping with bypass, should be re-evaluated in cases without such indications or cases where endovascular treatments have been clinically shown to be less effective.

Disclosures The authors declare no potential conflicts of interest.

References

1. The Japan Neurosurgeucal Society. Japan neurosurgical database, 2022. https://jnd.mincs-res.jp/jnd.web/ (in Japanese).
2. Kim BM, Shin YS, Baik MW, Lee DH, Jeon P, Baik SK, Lee TH, Kang DH, Suh SI, Byun JS, Jung JY, Kwon K, Kim DJ, Park KY, Kim BS, Park JC, Kim SR, Kim YW, Kim H, Jo K, Yoon CH, Kim YS. Pipeline embolization device for large/Giant or fusiform aneurysms: an initial multi-Center experience in Korea. Neurointervention. 2016;11:10–7.
3. Zanaty M, Chalouhi N, Starke RM, Barros G, Saigh MP, Schwartz EW, Ajiboye N, Tjoumakaris SI, Hasan D, Rosenwasser RH, Jabbour P. Flow diversion versus conventional treatment for carotid cavernous aneurysms. Stroke. 2014;45:2656–61.
4. Miyachi S, Ohnishi H, Hiramatsu R, Izumi T, Matsubara N, Kuroiwa T. Innovations in endovascular treatment strategies for large carotid cavernous aneurysms-the safety and efficacy of a flow diverter. J Stroke Cerebrovasc Dis. 2017;26:1071–80.
5. Miyachi S, Hiramatsu R, Ohnishi H, Yagi R, Kuroiwa T. Usefulness of the pipeline embolic device for large and giant carotid cavernous aneurysms. Neurointervention. 2018;12:83–90.
6. Rouchaud A, Brinjikji W, Lanzino G, Cloft HJ, Kadirvel R, Kallmes. Delayed hemorrhagic complications after flow diversion for intracranial aneurysms: a literature overview. Neuroradiology. 2016;58:171–7.
7. Brinjikji W, Lanzino G, Cloft HJ, Siddiqui AH, Kallmes DF. Risk factors for hemorrhagic complications following pipeline embolization device treatment of intracranial aneurysms: results from the international retrospective study of the pipeline embolization device. AJNR Am J Neuroradiol. 2015;36:2308–13.
8. Matsubara N, Miyachi S, Tsukamoto N, Izumi T, Naito T, Haraguchi K, Wakabayashi T. Endovascular coil embolization for saccular-shaped blood blister-like aneurysms of the internal carotid artery. Acta Neurochir. 2011;153:287–94.
9. Rouchaud A, Brinjikji W, Cloft HJ, Kallmes DF. Endovascular treatment of ruptured blister-like aneurysms: a systematic review and meta-analysis with focus on deconstructive versus reconstructive and flow-diverter treatments. AJNR Am J Neuroradiol. 2015;36:2331–9.
10. Shah SS, Gersey ZC, Nuh M, Ghonim HT, Elhammady MS, Peterson EC. Microsurgical versus endovascular interventions for blood-blister aneurysms of the internal carotid artery: systematic review of literature and meta-analysis on safety and efficacy. J Neurosurg. 2017;127:1361–73.
11. Sanchez VE, Haider AS, Rowe SE, Wahood W, Sagoo NS, Ozair A, El Ahmadieh TY, Kan P, Johnson JN. Comparison of blister

aneurysm treatment techniques: a systematic review and meta-analysis. World Neurosurg. 2021;154:e82–e101.
12. Weisz G, Metzger DC, Caputo RP, Delgado JA, Marshall JJ, Vetrovec GW, Reisman M, Waksman R, Granada JF, Novack V, Moses JW, Carrozza JP. Safety and feasibility of robotic percutaneous coronary intervention: precise (percutaneous robotically-enhanced coronary intervention) study. J Am Coll Cardiol. 2013;61:1596–600.
13. Harrison J, Ang L, Naghi J, Behnamfar O, Pourdjabbar A, Patel MP, Reeves RR, Mahmud E. Robotically-assisted percutaneous coronary intervention: reasons for partial manual assistance or manual conversion. Cardiovasc Revasc Med. 2018;9:526–31.
14. Haraguchi K, Miyachi S, Matsubara N, Nagano Y, Yamada H, Marui N, Sano A, Fujimoto H, Izumi T, Yamanouchi T, Asai T, Wakabayashi T. A mechanical coil insertion system for endovascular coil embolization of intracranial aneurysms. Interv Neuroradiol. 2013;19:159–66.
15. Miyachi S, Nagano Y, Hironaka T, Kawaguchi R, Ohshima T, Matsuo N, Maejima R, Takayasu M. Novel operation support robot with sensory-motor feedback system for neuroendovascular intervention. World Neurosurg. 2019;127:e617–23.
16. Matsubara N, Miyachi S, Nagano Y, Ohshima T, Hososhima O, Izumi T, Tsurumi A, Wakabayashi T, Sakaguchi M, Sano A, Fujimoto H. A novel pressure sensor with an optical system for coil embolization of intracranial aneurysms. Laboratory investigation. J Neurosurg. 2009;111:41–7.
17. Matsubara N, Miyachi S, Izumi T, Yamada H, Marui N, Ota K, Tajima H, Shintai K, Ito M, Imai T, Nishihori M, Wakabayashi T. Clinical application of insertion force sensor system for coil embolization of intracranial aneurysms. World Neurosurg. 2017;105:857–63.
18. Miyachi S, Nagano Y, Kawaguchi R, Ohshima T, Tadauchi H. Remote surgery using a neuroendovascular intervention support robot equipped with a sensing function: experimental verification. Asian J of Neurosurg AJNS. 2021;16:363–6.
19. Nogueira RG, Sachdeva R, Al-Bayati AR, Mohammaden MH, Frankel MR, Haussen DC. Robotic assisted carotid artery stenting for the treatment of symptomatic carotid disease: technical feasibility and preliminary results. J Neurointerv Surg. 2020;12(3):41–344.
20. Miyachi S. Tactics, techniques & spirits of neuroendovascular therapy – Miyachi's style. 2nd ed. Osaka: Medicus Shuppan, Publishers Co., Ltd; 2022.

Open Access This chapter is licensed under the terms of the Creative Commons Attribution 4.0 International License (http://creativecommons.org/licenses/by/4.0/), which permits use, sharing, adaptation, distribution and reproduction in any medium or format, as long as you give appropriate credit to the original author(s) and the source, provide a link to the Creative Commons license and indicate if changes were made.

The images or other third party material in this chapter are included in the chapter's Creative Commons license, unless indicated otherwise in a credit line to the material. If material is not included in the chapter's Creative Commons license and your intended use is not permitted by statutory regulation or exceeds the permitted use, you will need to obtain permission directly from the copyright holder.

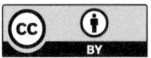

Part II
AVM and dAVF

An Evaluation of Motor Function in Surgery for Cerebral Arteriovenous Malformations via 3-Tesla Magnetic Resonance Tractography

Ayumi Akazawa, Yoshifumi Higashino, Makoto Isozaki, Takahiro Yamauchi, Satoshi Kawajiri, Munetaka Yomo, Ken Matsuda, Hidetaka Arishima, Shintaro Yamada, Miduki Oiwa, Tsutomu Okada, Yasutaka Fushimi, Nobuyuki Miki, Yoshiki Arakawa, and Kenichiro Kikuta

Abbreviations

MRT	magnetic resonance tractography
AVM	arteriovenous malformation
SMG	Spetzler–Martin grade
MDACST	minimal distance between AVM and corticospinal tract
MRI	magnetic resonance imaging
DTT	diffusion tensor tractography
OR	optic radiation
FA	fractional anisotropic
CST	corticospinal tract
3 T	3 tesla

Introduction

The achievement of complete resection is ideal in surgery for brain AVMs. Thus, the risk evaluation of the occurrence of postoperative deficits following the achievement of complete resection is essential in the surgery of brain AVMs [1]. Recent advances in magnetic resonance imaging (MRI) technology have allowed major neural tracts in white matter to be visualized via diffusion tensor tractography (DTT) [2, 3]. We previously showed that a 3-tesla (3 T) magnetic resonance (MR) unit can describe most neural tracts more clearly than a 1.5 T unit can [4]. The location of the corticospinal tract (CST) identified using the intraoperative navigation system integrated via 3 T MR tractography (MRT) was almost colocalized to the responded site via intraoperative electrophysiological white matter stimulation mapping [5]. We also demonstrated the 3 T MRT findings regarding the optic radiation (OR) was related to pre- and postoperative visual symptoms in patients with arteriovenous malformations (AVMs) in and around the visual pathway [6]. The asymmetry index (AI) of the mean fractional anisotropic (FA) values of the affected side to the contralateral side helped to evaluate the status of OR [7]. In this study, we investigate the effectiveness of the 3 T DTT of the corticospinal tract (CST) for the estimation of motor function in surgery for cerebral AVMs.

Materials and Methods

Characteristics of Patients

Out of 112 patients with brain AVM operated on by the senior author (K.K.) between 2000 and 2022 in the Department of Neurosurgery, Kyoto Graduate School of Medicine and University of Fukui, in consecutive 30 patients a pre- and postoperative evaluation of neural tracts via 3 T MRT was performed before and after surgery. Two patients with cerebellar or brainstem AVM and six patients with occipital AVMs adjacent to the optic pathway were excluded. Further, 22 patients adjacent to the CST were included in this study. The patients included 12 men and 10 women ranging in age from 4 to 45 years (mean age 29.0 ± 13.6 years). Here, 14 patients presented with hemorrhage, five patients with epileptic seizure, and three with ischemic symptoms. The locations of the AVMs were in the frontal lobe in seven patients, the temporal lobe in eight, the parietal lobe in eight, the sylvian fissure in two, and the insular in two. SMG values were I in six patients, II in nine, III in six, and IV in one. Preoperative feeder embolization was performed in five cases. There was no embolization-related complication. The microsurgical resection of the AVMs achieved total removal in all 22 patients. Complete obliteration was confirmed via postoperative angiography, and no one received additional surgery or stereotactic radiosurgery. The characteristics of the patients are shown in Table 1. This study was approved by the ethical committees of the University of Fukui (20190157).

Imaging Protocol

MR imaging was performed before surgery and at 1 month after surgery with a 3 T MR scanner (Trio; Siemens, Erlargen, Germany). Data acquisition, the data processing of diffusion tensor imaging, and fiber tractography reconstruction proceeded as follows. By using the integrated parallel acquisition technique (iPAT) and a receiver-only-8-channer phased array head coil, a single-shot spin-echo planner sequence was applied with the following parameters: repetition time (TR), 7000 ms; echo time (TE), 79 ms; motion-probing gradient (MPG) in 40 noncolinear directions and four non-diffusion-weighted scans; b value, 700 s/mm^2; matrix, 128 × 104; voxel size, 2 mm × 2 mm × 2 mm; no interslice gap; single averaging; quadruple averaging with the GRAPPA algorithm with a reduction factor of 2 and 24 additional autocalibrating phase-encoding lines in the center of k-space. In total, 60 transverse slices covering the whole brain were acquired within 5 min 30 s. In the same session, an MR study with axial T1-weighted three-dimensional magnetization-prepared rapid acquisition gradient-echo sequences (MPRAGE) (TR/TE/TI = 2000/4.4/990 ms; flip angle, 8 degrees; matrix, 256 × 240; field of view, 24 cm; and 208 slices with slice thickness of 1 mm, no interslice gap, and single averaging), axial T2-weighted turbo spin-echo sequences (TR/TE = 8400/108 ms; flip angle, 150 degrees; matrix, 512 × 448; field of view, 22 cm; and 40 slices with a slice thickness of 2.3 mm, a interslice gap of 0.7 mm, and double averaging), three-dimensional time-of-flight MR angiography (3D TOF MRA) (TR, 22 ms; flip angle, 20

Table 1 Character of the patients

Case	Sex	Age	Location	SMG	Size (mm)	Onset symptom	Findings of postoperative angiography	mRS at 3 months after surgery
1	M	45	Frontal	2	30	Epilepsy	Total removal	0
2	M	45	Frontal	2	27	Ischemia	Total removal	2
3	M	31	Frontal	1	20	Hemorrhage	Total removal	0
4	F	23	Frontal	2	30	Hemorrhage	Total removal	0
5	M	40	Frontal	1	29	Asymptomatic	Total removal	0
6	M	38	Frontal	2	30	Epilepsy	Total removal	0
7	M	28	Frontal	2	35	Epilepsy	Total removal	1
8	F	27	Temporal	3	30	Hemorrhage	Total removal	0
9	F	29	Temporal	1	5	Hemorrhage	Total removal	0
10	F	22	Temporal	2	30	Epilepsy	Total removal	0
11	M	25	Parietal	3	40	Headache	Total removal	1
12	F	22	Parietal	1	20	Hemorrhage	Total removal	1
13	F	27	Parietal	1	20	Hemorrhage	Total removal	1
14	M	48	Parietal	3	40	Hemorrhage	Total removal	1
15	M	45	Parietal	2	35	Hemorrhage	Total removal	3
16	M	38	Parietal	1	25	Asymptomatic	Total removal	0
17	F	4	Parietal	1	20	Epilepsy	Total removal	0
18	F	2	Parietal	4	50	Hemorrhage	Total removal	2
19	M	49	Sylvian	2	25	Hemorrhage	Total removal	0
20	M	21	Sylvian	3	45	Hemorrhage	Total removal	0
21	F	6	Insular	3	28	Hemorrhage	Total removal	2
22	F	23	Insular	3	15	Hemorrhage	Total removal	2

Note: *SMG* Spetzler-Martin grade = X and *mRS* modified Rankin Scale = X

degrees; single-slice acquisition; slice thickness, 0.8 mm; matrix, 512 × 208; and acquisition time, 4 min 8 s) was performed. After a fractional anisotropy (FA) map and a directional color-coded map were synthesized from the diffusion-tensor data by using DTI Studio 2.03 software (h Jiang. Mori; Department of Radiology, Johns Hopkins University), eigenvectors were translated into neuronal trajectories with the fiber assignment via the continuous tracking (FACT) method. As described previously, multiple regions of interest (ROIs) were used for tract reconstruction with three types of operation: AND; OR; and NOT. The ROIs were segmented by one author (T.O.) on $b = 0$ images. To reconstruct CST tractography, the first ROI was segmented at the cerebral peduncle of the medulla, followed by an "OR" operation. The second ROI was placed at the ipsilateral precentral gyrus, followed by an "AND" operation. Tracking was terminated when it reached a pixel with a low FA (< 0.20).

Measurement of the Size of the Nidus and the Minimal Distance Between the Nidus and the CST

The largest diameter of the nidus was measured on T2-weighted images (Fig. 1a). The minimal distance between the margin of the nidus and the margins of the CST (MDACST) was measured on transverse non-diffusion-weighted images (Fig. 1b). In cases with hematoma or with small AVMs, CST was identified on MRT imaging (Fig. 1c) and the exact location of the nidus was identified via MRA (Fig. 1d).

Evaluation of Tract Injury on MRT

For a qualitative assessment of tract injury, we prepared the criteria for the estimation of the tracts through visual inspection as follows: C (continuous): tracts were visualized continuously between the two ROIs (Fig. 2a: axial image, b: coronal image); I (involved): tracts were visualized continuously between the two ROIs but were contiguous to or involved in the lesion, such as AVMs, edema, and hematomas (Fig. 2c: axial image, d: coronal image); D (disrupted): tracts were not described continuously between the two ROIs (Fig. 2e: axial image, f: coronal image). "I" and "D" were defined as "tract injury." Tract injury was determined through majority decision by three independent neuroradiologists in a blind fashion. For a quantitative assessment of tract injury, mean FA values along with the tractography and asymmetry index (AI) of FA between the tract in the affected side and the unaffected side (AI = (affected - unaffected) / (affected + unaffected) ÷ 2) were also calculated.

Evaluation of Motor Disfunctions

Motor weakness in the upper or lower extremities was evaluated before surgery, at 1 month after surgery, and at 3 months after surgery via manual muscle tests (MMTs). Symptoms that resolved within 1 month after surgery were defined as "transient symptoms" and symptoms that persisted 3 months after surgery were defined as "permanent symptoms." The worsening of motor function was defined as the postoperative worsening of the motor function compared to the preoperative one.

Statistical Analysis

For univariate analysis, Pearson's chi-squared test or Fisher's exact test was used for categorical variables and the Mann–Whitney U test for numeric variables. Forward and backward stepwise logistic regression analyses with the Akaike information criterion (AIC) were carried out to determine the associations of potential confounders with age, sex, MDACST, the presence of hematoma before surgery, tract injury on preoperative MRT or postoperative MRT, the size of the AVM, and the presence of preoperative motor dysfunction. Cutoff value at receiver operating characteristic (ROC) analysis using area under the curve (AUC) was calculated via Benis's method. All statistical analysis including ROC analysis was performed by using JMP 15.2.0 (SAS Institute, Cary, NC, United States of America) and R (R Foundation for Statistical Computing, Vienna, Austria), with an error probability of < 0.05.

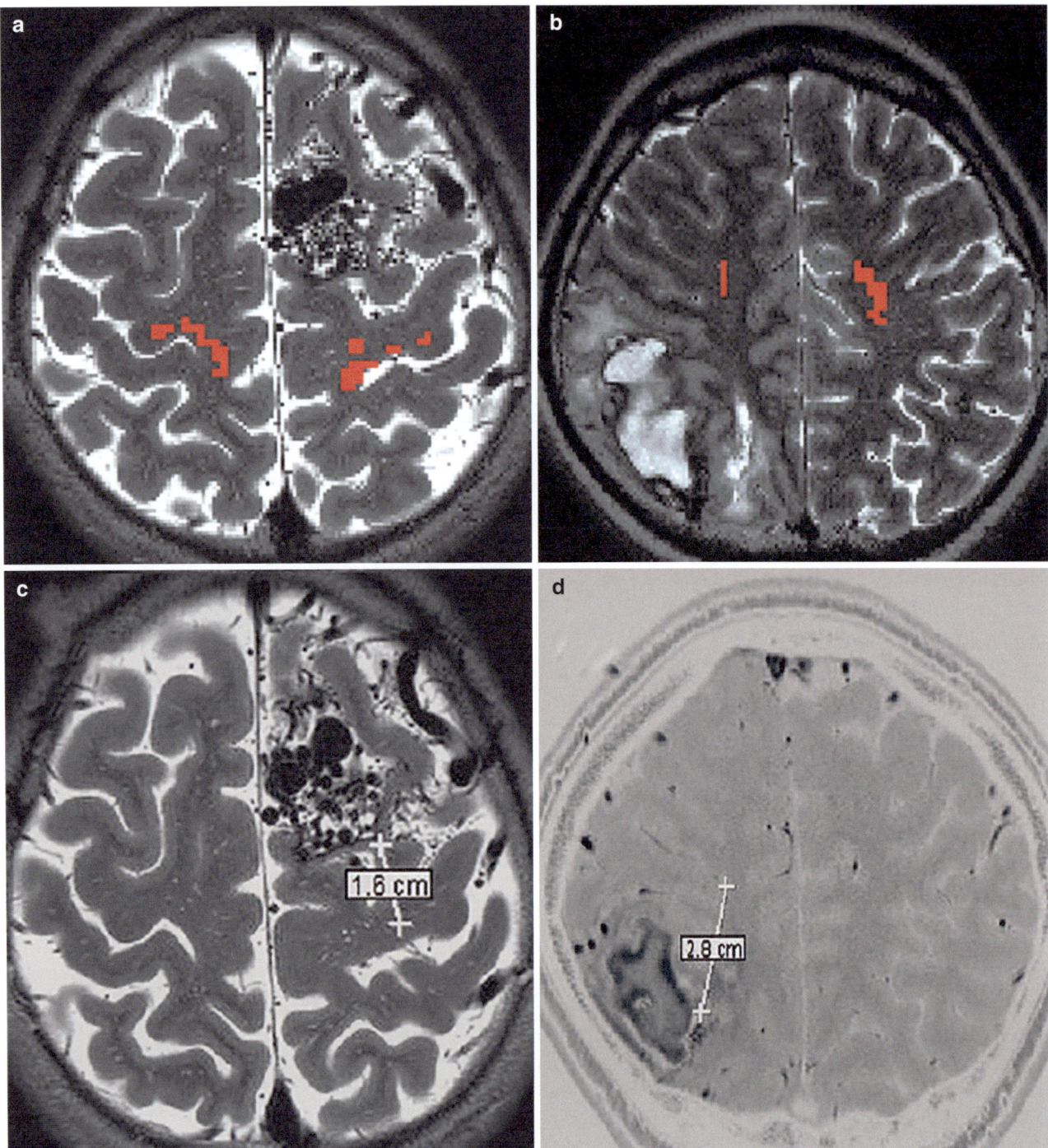

Fig. 1 The largest diameter of the nidus was measured on T2-weighted images (**a**), and the minimal distance between the AVM and the corticospinal tract (CST) was measured on transverse non-diffusion-weighted images (**b**). In cases with hematoma or with small AVMs, the exact location of the nidus was identified via MRT imaging (**c**) and MRA (**d**)

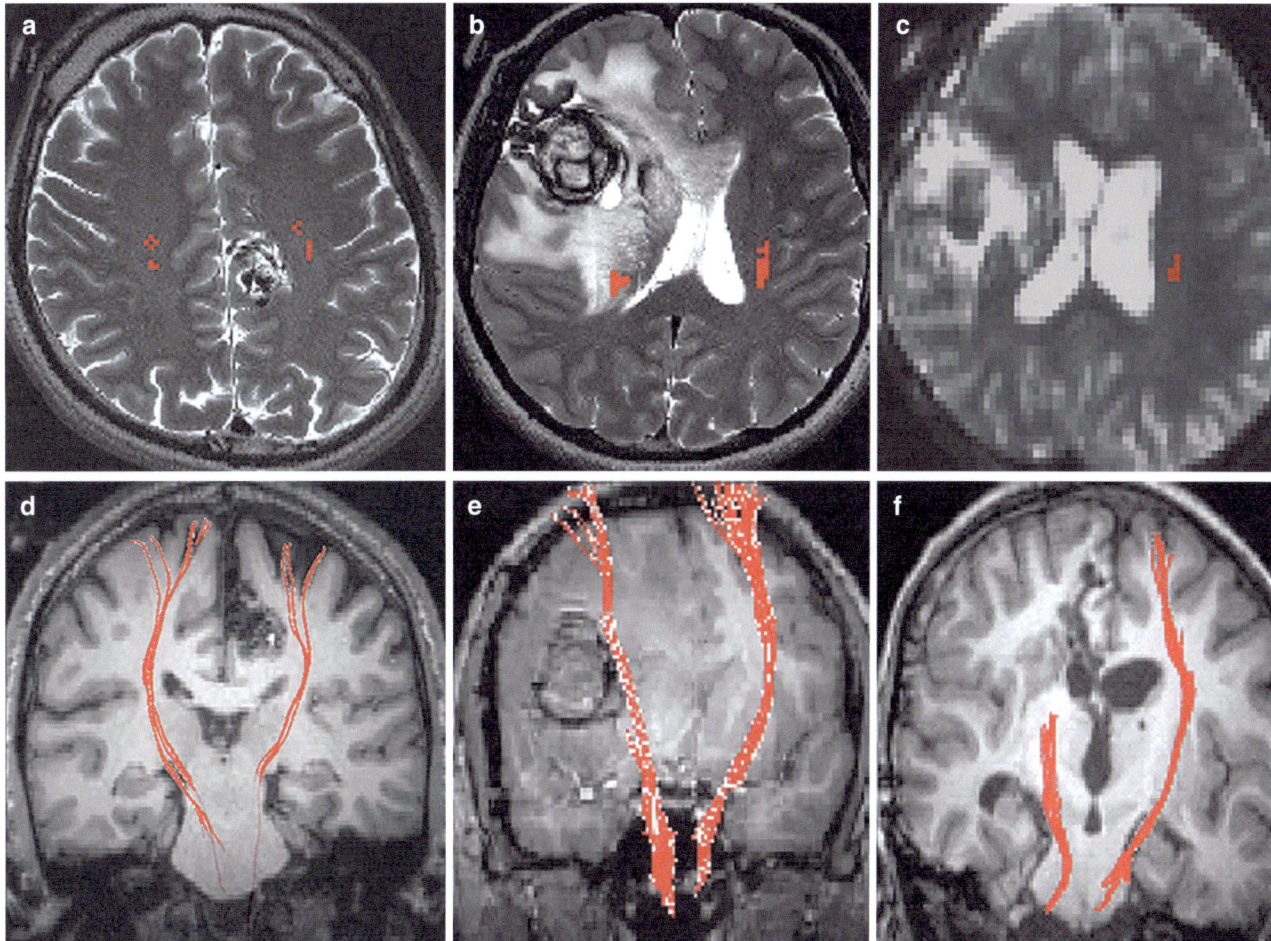

Fig. 2 A qualitative assessment of tract injury was determined by using three categorizations. C (continuous): tracts were visualized continuously between the two ROIs ((**a**) axial, (**b**) coronal); I (involved): tracts were visualized continuously between the two ROIs but were contiguous to or involved in the lesion, such as AVMs, edema, and hematomas ((**c**) axial, (**d**) coronal); D (disrupted): tracts were not described continuously between the two ROIs ((**e**) axial, (**f**) coronal image). "I" and "D" were defined as "tract injury"

Results

Criteria for Estimation of the CST via Visual Inspection

In this study, 44 CSTs were estimated on MRT via visual inspection by three observers according to our proposed criteria. A majority decision on tract injury was obtained in all tracts (100%), and a unanimous decision was achieved in 52 tracts (76%) (kappa value).

Preoperative Motor Dysfunction and Findings on MRT

Six of the 22 patients presented with motor weakness before surgery. Among radiological factors, univariate analysis revealed that the presence of hematoma ($p = 0.0316$) and tract injury via visual inspection ($p = 0.0050$) were significantly related to preoperative motor dysfunction. The MDACST was significantly smaller in patients with preoperative motor dysfunction than in patients without preoperative motor dysfunction ($p = 0.005$) (Table 2).

Transient Motor Dysfunction and Findings on MRT

Motor dysfunction within 1 month after surgery was observed in 10 patients. Univariable analysis revealed that the presence of preoperative motor dysfunction was significantly related to the occurrence of transient motor dysfunction ($p = 0.0289$). The MDACST was significantly smaller in patients with transient motor dysfunction than in patients without transient dysfunction ($p = 0.0133$) (Table 3).

Table 2 Factors affecting preoperative motor dysfunction

		Preoperative motor dysfunction		
		Presence (n = 6)	Absence (n = 16)	p
SMG	I	1	6	0.0991
	II	1	7	
	III, IV	4	3	
Size of AVM (mm)		31.3 +/− 13.0	27.6 +/− 9.1	0.6286
Minimal distance between AVM and CST (mm)		8.50 +/− 8.34	24.6 +/− 13.9	*0.0050**
Mean FA value		0.545 +/− 0.0394	0.581 +/− 0.0449	0.1197
Asymmetry index (AI) of FA		−0.0356 +/− 0.0420	−0.0246 +/− 0.0465	0.6851
Presence of hematoma		4	3	*0.0316**
Tract injury on MRT		5	3	*0.0050**

Note: *SMG* Spetzler-Martin grade, *AVM* arteriovenous malformation, *CST* corticospinal tract, *FA* fractional anisotropic, *AI* asymmetry index, *MRT* magnetic resonance tractography
* Significant at p < 0.05

Table 3 Factors affecting postoperative transient motor dysfunction

		Transient motor disfunction		
		Presence (n = 10)	Absence (n = 12)	p
Preoperative findings				
SMC	I	1	6	0.0947
	II	4	4	
	III, IV	5	2	
Size of AVM (mm)		32.0 +/− 10.26	25.8 +/− 9.46	0.1724
Minimal distance between AVM and CST (mm)		13.9 +/− 14.7	25.4 +/− 12.4	*0.0133**
Mean FA value		0.561 +/− 0.0372	0.579 +/− 0.0516	0.6909
Asymmetry index of FA (A.I.)		−0.0321 +/− 0.0371	−0.0238 +/− 0.0513	0.6681
Presence of preop. Motor dysfunction		5	1	*0.0289**
Tract injury on preop. MRT		5	3	0.2248
Presence of preop. Hematoma		3	3	0.7932
Postoperative findings at 1 mo.				
Presence of postop. Hematoma		4	3	0.4520
Tract injury on postop. MRT		6	3	0.0964

Note: *SMG* Spetzler-Martin grade, *AVM* arteriovenous malformation, *CST* corticospinal tract, *FA* fractional anisotropic, *AI* asymmetry index, *MRT* magnetic resonance tractography
* Significant at p < 0.05

Table 4 Factors affecting postoperative permanent motor dysfunction

		Permanent motor dysfunction		
		Presence (n = 8)	Absence (n = 14)	p-value
Preoperative findings				
SMG	I	0	7	0.0511
	II	4	4	
	III, IV	4	3	
Size of AVM (mm)		32.5 +/− 10.3	26.4 +/− 9.67	0.1905
Minimal distance between AVM and CST (mm)		9.37 +/− 7.54	26.4 +/− 13.9	*0.0024**
Mean FA value		0.554 +/− 0.0370	0.580 +/− 0.0483	0.3544
Asymmetry index (AI) of FA		−0.0341 +/− 0.0357	−0.0239 +/− 0.0500	0.6821
Preop. motor dysfunction		5	1	*0.0050**
Tract injury on MRT		4	4	0.3149
Presence of hematoma		3	3	0.4155
Postoperative findings at 1 mo.				
Presence of hematoma		4	3	0.1663
Tract injury on MRT		6	3	*0.0140**
Motor dysfunction		8	2	*0.0001**

Note: *SMG* Spetzler-Martin grade, *AVM* arteriovenous malformation, *CST* corticospinal tract, *FA* fractional anisotropic, *AI* asymmetry index, *MRT* magnetic resonance tractography
* Significant at p < 0.05

Permanent Motor Dysfunction and Findings on MRT

Motor dysfunction for 3 months after surgery was observed in eight patients. In the univariable analysis, the presence of preoperative motor dysfunction ($p = 0.0050$), tract injury on postoperative MRT ($p = 0.0140$), and the presence of transient motor dysfunction ($p = 0.001$) were significantly related to the occurrence of permanent motor dysfunction. The MDACST was significantly smaller in patients with permanent motor dysfunction than in patients without permanent dysfunction ($p = 0.0024$) (Table 4).

Multivariate Analysis Regarding Factors Predicting the Occurrence of Transient Motor Deterioration and Permanent Motor Dysfunction

Forward and backward stepwise logistic regression analyses with AIC to determine the associations of potential confounders with age, sex, MDACST, the presence of hematoma before surgery, tract injury on preoperative MRT or postoperative MRT, the size of the AVM, and the presence of preoperative motor dysfunction revealed that the occurrence of transient motor deterioration was most significantly predicted by the combination of age, MDACST, and tract injury on preoperative MRT with an AIC value of 19.55 (Table 5) and that the occurrence of permanent motor dysfunction was most significantly predicted by the combination of MDACST, tract injury on postoperative MRT, and tract injury on preoperative MRT with an AIC value of 8.0 (Table 6).

Table 5 Multivariate analysis indicating that the occurrence of transient motor deterioration was most significantly predicted by the combination of age, minimal distance between AVM and CST, and tract injury on preoperative MRT with an AIC value of 19.55

Variable	Estimate	p-value	OR	95% CI	
Age	−0.1128	0.1566	0.8933	0.72	1.01
Minimal distance between AVM and CST	−0.4735	0.0512	0.6228	0.30	0.86
Tract injury on preoperative MRT	−3.7049	0.1361	0.0246	0.00	1.28

Note: *AVM* arteriovenous malformation, *MRT* magnetic resonance tractography

Table 6 Multivariate analysis indicating that the occurrence of permanent motor dysfunction was most significantly predicted by the combination of minimal distance between AVM and CST, tract injury on postoperative MRT, and track injury on preoperative MRT with an AIC value of 8.0

Variable	Estimate	p-value	OR	95% CI	Infinity of the upper limit
Minimal distance between AVM and CST	−14.2400	0.999	6.52E−07	0	inf
Tract injury on postoperative MRT	117.3700	0.999	9.37E+50	0.00	inf
Tract injury on preoperative MRT	−145.9100	0.999	4.29E−64	0.00	inf

Note: *AVM* arteriovenous malformation, *MRT* magnetic resonance tractography

Receiver Operating Character (ROC) Analysis of the MDACST in Predicting the Occurrence of Transient Motor Deterioration and Permanent Motor Dysfunction

An ROC analysis revealed that the occurrence of transient motor deterioration was significantly related to MDACST ($p = 0.0003$, AUC = 0.90179, cutoff value 16 mm, sensitivity 100%, and specificity 79%) (Fig. 3a). The occurrence of permanent motor dysfunction was also significantly related to MDACST ($p < 0.001$, AUC = 0.96190, cutoff value 8 mm, sensitivity 85%, and specificity 100%) (Fig. 3b).

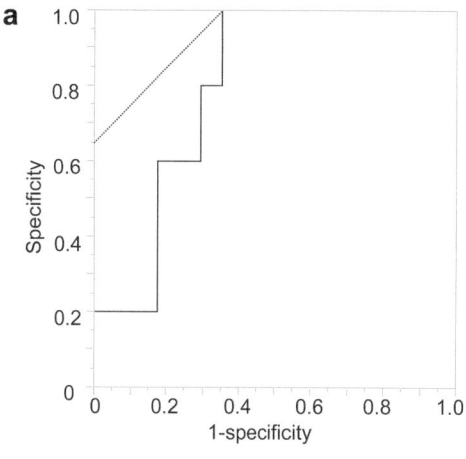

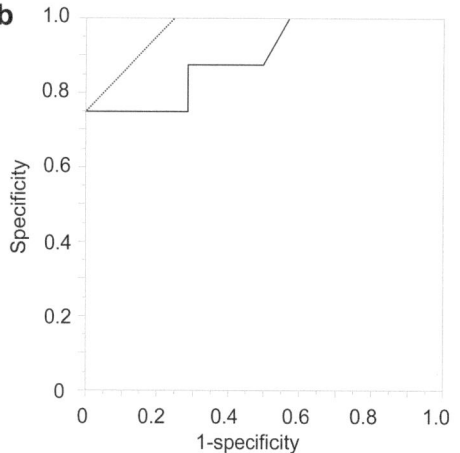

Fig. 3 An ROC analysis revealed that the occurrence of permanent motor dysfunction was significantly related to the minimal distance between the AVM and the corticospinal tract (CST) ($p = 0.0003$, AUC = 0.90179, cutoff value 16 mm, sensitivity 100%, and specificity 79%) (**a**). The occurrence of permanent motor function was significantly related to the minimal distance between the AVM and the CST ($p < 0.001$, AUC = 0.96190, cutoff value 8 mm, sensitivity 85%, and specificity 100%) (**b**)

Discussion

In general, the evaluation of the surgical risk of cerebral AVM has been performed by using Spetzler–Martin grading (SMG) reported in 1986 [8]. The occurrence rate of the postoperative morbidity and mortality of SMG I, II, III, IV, and V were 0%, 5%, 16–21.9%, 21.9–27%, and 16.7–31%, respectively. There was a statistically significant difference among grading [9]. Japan Stroke Society Guideline 2021 for the Treatment of Stroke recommended that SMG I and II AVMs be treated via surgery, SMG III AVMs be treated via surgery with endovascular embolization, and SMG IV and V AVMs be treated via conservative treatment [10]. The surgical outcome for SMG I, II, and III AVMs is favorable. Stein et al. reported that complete resection could be achieved in 97% of surgeries for 67 brain AVMs with a diameter less than 3 cm, and the complication rate was 1.5% [11]. Schaller et al. also reported that the complete resection rate was 98.4% in surgeries for 62 AVMs with a diameter less than 3 cm, and the complication rate was 3.2% [12]. The complication rate in surgeries for SMG I and II AVMs is quite low (less than 5%). The surgical risk of SMG I or II AVMs located in a noneloquent area was 0.6% and was only 5% when located even in an eloquent area [13]. However, the surgical risk of SMG III AVMs varied widely, ranging from 16% to 21.9% [8]. Lawton categorized SMG III AVMs into several types according to size (S), the presence of a deep drainer (V), and eloquence (E). The complication rates for surgery of S1V1E1 (small) AVMs, S2V1E0 (medium deep) AVMs, and S2V0E1 (medium eloquent) AVMs were 2.9%, 7.1%, and 14.8%, respectively. He pointed out that the surgical risk in surgery for SMG III AVMs was not the same. The size of AVM was the most important, and eloquence was the second-most important [14].

Surgical risk factors other than SMG have been reported. Du et al. showed that diffuse nidus configuration (odds ratio 3.6–5.74) and the presence of a deep perforation feeder (odds ratio 3.6–5.74) were independent predictive factors for postoperative deterioration [15]. The postoperative deterioration rate in surgery for unruptured AVM was 2.33 times higher than that for ruptured AVMs [16]. Those data suggest that not only SMG but also other risk factors should be taken into consideration in evaluating the surgical risk for SMG III AVMs.

Although recent MRI technology could describe the major neural tract around AVMs such as CST, the sensory pathway, and OR, there were a few reports applying the technology to evaluate patients with AVMs. We previously examined the status of CST and OR close to the nidus and found that they were less visualized in the affected hemisphere than were those distant from the nidus and that tracts were less visualized in patients with neurologic symptoms than in asymptomatic patients [17].

In this study, the presence of hematoma, tract injury on preoperative MRT, and the minimal distance between AVM and CST (MDACST) were significantly related to the presence of preoperative motor dysfunction. The presence of preoperative motor dysfunction and the MDACST were significantly related to the occurrence of transient motor dysfunction. The presence of preoperative motor dysfunction ($p = 0.0050$), tract injury on postoperative MRT ($p = 0.0140$), the presence of transient motor dysfunction ($p = 0.001$), and the MDACST were significantly related to the occurrence of permanent motor dysfunction. Multivariate analysis suggested that the MDACST was one of the most important factors predicting the occurrence of transient motor deterioration and the occurrence of permanent motor dysfunction as well. In addition, ROC analysis indicated that AVM surgery with an MDACST of less than 16 mm would yield transient motor deterioration and that less than 8 mm would yield permanent motor dysfunction. Those data might help to determine the surgical indication of AVM near CST. Li et al. recently analyzed the surgery of 90 patients with AVMs with a minimal distance between the AVM and the CST of less than 10 mm [18]. Postoperative permanent motor dysfunction was observed in 23.3%. They also revealed that the minimal distance between the AVM and the CST was the independent risk factor for postoperative permanent motor dysfunction. In addition, they indicated that not only closeness but also the closest CCT level, patient age, and AVM diffuseness were independent predictors for poor motor outcome. They established the CLAD (closeness, level, age, and diffuseness) grading score to predict poor motor outcome. They reported that AVM surgery with an MDACST of less than 10 mm was hazardous, with a permanent motor dysfunction rate of 23.3%. Our data suggest a significant risk of transient motor deterioration even in surgery of AVM with an MDACST of less than 16 mm.

The present study has some limitations, including the small number of patients enrolled in this study. Our results need to be confirmed by further prospective studies with a larger number of patients.

Conclusions

We conclude that surgery of AVM with a minimal distance between the AVM and the CST of less than 16 mm would yield postoperative transient motor dysfunction and that the same but with a minimal distance of less than 8 mm would yield permanent motor dysfunction.

Acknowledgments This study was supported by the Life Science Innovation Center, University of Fukui.

Funding Information This work was supported by a Grant-in-Aid for Scientific Research by the Japan Society for the Promotion of Science (JSPS) (No. 20K09344).

Declarations

Conflict of interest: The authors have no conflicting interests to declare that are relevant to the content of this chapter.

Ethical approval: This study was approved by the ethical committees of the University of Fukui (No. 20190157).

References

1. Hashimoto N. Microsurgery for cerebral arteriovenous malformations: a dissection technique and its theoretical implications. Neurosurgery. 2001;48:1278–60.
2. Kamada K, Todo T. Combined use of tractography-integrated functional neuronavigation and direct fiber stimulation. J Neurosurgy. 2005;102:664–72.
3. Yamada K, Kizu O. Tractography for arteriovenous malformations near the sensorimotor cortices. AJNR Am J Neuroradiol. 2005;26:598–602.
4. Okada T, Miki Y. Diffusion-tensor fiber tractography: intraindividual comparison of 3.0-T and 1.5-T MR imaging. Radiology. 2006;238:668–78.
5. Okada T, Mikuni N. Integration of diffusion tensor tractography of the corticospinal tract using 3T with intraoperative white matter stimulation mapping: preliminary results to validate corticospinal tract localization. Radiology. 2006;240:859–7.
6. Kikuta K, Takagi Y. Early experience with 3-T magnetic resonance tractography in the surgery of cerebral arteriovenous malformations in and around the visual pathway. Neurosurgery. 2006;58:331–7.
7. Bantis LE, Nakas CT, Reiser B. Construction of confidence regions in the ROC space after the estimation of the optimal Youden Index-based cut-off point. Biometrics. 2014;2014:212–23.
8. Spetzler RF, Martin NA. A proposed grading system for arteriovenous malformations. J Neurosurg. 1986;65:476–83.
9. Hamilton MG, Spetzler RF. The prospective application of a grading system for arteriovenous malformations. Neurosurgery. 1994;34:2–6.
10. Miyamoto S, Ogasawara K. Japan stroke society guideline 2021 for the treatment of stroke. Int J Stroke. 2022;17:1039–49.
11. Stein BM, Sisti MB. Microsurgery and radiosurgery in small AVMs. J Neurosurg. 1993;79:795–7.
12. Schaller C, Schramm J. Microsurgical results for small arteriovenous malformations accessible for radiosurgical or embolization treatment. Neurosurgery. 1997;40:664–72.
13. Morgan MK, Rochford AM. Surgical risks associated with the management of grade I and II brain arteriovenous malformations. Neurosurgery. 2007;61:417–22.
14. Lawton MT. Spetzler-Martin grade III arteriovenous malformations:surgical results and a modification of the grading scale. Neurosurgery. 2003;52:740–8.
15. Du R, Keyoung HM. The effects of diffuseness and deep perforating artery supply on outcomes after microsurgical resection of brain arteriovenous malformations. Neurosurgery. 2007;60:638–46.
16. Lawton MT, Du R. Effect of presenting hemorrhage on outcome after microsurgical resection of brain arteriovenous malformations. Neurosurgery. 2005;56:485–93.
17. Okada T, Miki Y. Diffusion tensor fiber tractography for arteriovenous malformations: quantitative analyses to evaluate the corticospinal tract and optic radiation. AJNR Am J Neuroradiol. 2007;28:1107–13.
18. Li M, Jiang P. A tractography-based grading scale of brain arteriovenous malformations close to the corticospinal tract to predict motor outcome after surgery. Front Neurol. 2019;10:1–9.

Open Access This chapter is licensed under the terms of the Creative Commons Attribution 4.0 International License (http://creativecommons.org/licenses/by/4.0/), which permits use, sharing, adaptation, distribution and reproduction in any medium or format, as long as you give appropriate credit to the original author(s) and the source, provide a link to the Creative Commons license and indicate if changes were made.

The images or other third party material in this chapter are included in the chapter's Creative Commons license, unless indicated otherwise in a credit line to the material. If material is not included in the chapter's Creative Commons license and your intended use is not permitted by statutory regulation or exceeds the permitted use, you will need to obtain permission directly from the copyright holder.

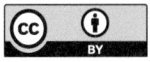

The Forefront of Gamma Knife Radiosurgery for Brain Arteriovenous Malformations: Our History of Treatment Optimisation Over 30 Years and the Modern Outcomes

Yuki Shinya, Hirotaka Hasegawa, Motoyuki Umekawa, Masahiro Shin, Mariko Kawashima, Satoshi Koizumi, Atsuto Katano, Yuichi Suzuki, Taichi Kin, and Nobuhito Saito

Introduction

Brain arteriovenous malformation (AVM) is a rare congenital intracranial vascular malformation, harbouring a lifelong risk of cerebral haemorrhage with a resultant mortality rate of 10.0–17.6% [4, 23]. Expert care at specialised facilities is reportedly important when managing AVMs because the risk of treatment-associated morbidity and mortality is non-negligible [14]. There are three primary treatment modalities to effectively manage this complex disease: surgical resection, endovascular treatment, and stereotactic radiosurgery (SRS), utilised either as standalone therapies or in combination [2, 11, 33]. Throughout the long history of AVM management, substantial progress has been achieved in both surgery and endovascular treatment [17, 19, 30, 34]. Concurrently, findings from the Randomized Trial of Unruptured Brain Arteriovenous Malformations (ARUBA) study advocated for the judicious application of therapeutic interventions when addressing unruptured AVMs [22].

Regarding SRS, numerous reports on the clinical outcomes have been provided from many experts in gamma knife radiosurgery (GKRS) [12, 24]. In general, 60–80% of AVMs are completely obliterated following a latency period of 3–5 years [8, 28, 29]. However, the risk of haemorrhagic stroke during the latency period is not negligible, with an annual rate of 0.9–1.4%, although the haemorrhage risk is almost completely eliminated after obliteration [3, 24]. Symptomatic radiation adverse events, such as post-SRS brain oedema, are possible but occur uncommonly – that is, in under 10% of the patients – with only 3% of them developing permanent deficits. The risk of a late adverse event is reported to be 2.8–7.7% at 10 years and 7.2–12.5% at 15 years [10].

Since the first introduction of GKRS in Japan in 1990, we have performed more than 1100 sessions of GKRS for AVM. Through the accumulation of treatment experiences and associated research over 30 years, we have endeavoured to sophisticate our treatment by understanding the long-term efficacies and limitations of GKRS, exploring factors associated with AVM obliteration, analysing what is important to prevent postradiosurgical haemorrhages, and incorporating new imaging technologies, enabling better visualisations of not only vascular anatomies but also functional neurofibres [8, 9, 11, 13, 15, 16, 18, 20, 21, 25–29]. This article aimed to provide brief introductions to our history of treatment optimisation and the latest treatment outcomes of GKRS for AVMs using our modern radiosurgical techniques.

Methods and Materials

Study Population

A retrospective analysis was conducted by using data obtained from 1032 patients with AVM who underwent GKRS at our institution from 1990 to 2022 to provide a comprehensive overview of our treatment advancement. Initially, we outlined our basic radiosurgical techniques and the advancement of GKRS at our institution. We subsequently analysed our modern radiosurgical outcomes from 2015 to 2020, excluding patients with less than 2 years of radiological follow-up, those who underwent volume-staged GKRS for large AVM, and those who had received previous radiotherapy for treated AVMs. Consequently, 90 patients treated with our modern radiosurgical techniques were identified. This study was approved by the institutional review board of our institution (approval number 2231), and all patients

---

Y. Shinya (✉) · H. Hasegawa · M. Umekawa · M. Shin
M. Kawashima · S. Koizumi · T. Kin · N. Saito
Department of Neurosurgery, The University of Tokyo Hospital, Tokyo, Japan

A. Katano · Y. Suzuki
Department of Radiology, The University of Tokyo Hospital, Tokyo, Japan

provided written informed consent for study participation in accordance with the principles of the Declaration of Helsinki.

Our Basic Radiosurgical Techniques

Our institution utilises the Leksell gamma knife (Elekta Instruments Inc., Stockholm, Sweden) for SRS. The procedure entails head fixation using a Leksell frame (Elekta Instruments Inc.) under local anaesthesia, followed by stereotactic imaging to obtain precise information on the shape, diameter, volume, and three-dimensional (3D) coordinates of the AVMs. Between June 1990 and February 1991, GKRS treatments at our institution relied primarily on two-dimensional (2D) digital subtraction angiography (DSA) images for defining and targeting the AVM nidus. From March 1991, the utilisation of computed tomography (CT) with DSA enabled axial-based treatment planning, thereby enhancing targeting accuracy. Subsequently, magnetic resonance imaging (MRI) was incorporated from August 1996 onwards. Radiosurgical planning was collaboratively conducted by dedicated neurosurgeons and radiation oncologists, utilising commercially available software. Until 1998, the KULA planning system (Elekta Instruments Inc.) was employed, while the Leksell GammaPlan (Elekta Instruments Inc.) has been implemented since 1999. The Leksell GammaPlan facilitated the visualisation of multiple radiographic images on a computer display, concurrently covering isodose lines and further enhancing targeting accuracy. These updates were carried out not only in our institution but also in facilities worldwide.

In principle, the optimal dose administered to the margin of each AVM nidus was 20 Gy. To mitigate potential complications when the nidus volume was either larger or in proximity to critical neuroanatomical structures, the marginal dose was cautiously reduced to 18 Gy. After treatment, patients were monitored at our institution or affiliate hospitals. MRI was conducted every 6 months until complete obliteration was confirmed, after which it was conducted annually. DSA was performed when these images strongly suggested AVM obliteration.

Our Radiosurgical Advancement

From 2004 onwards, our institution introduced new imaging techniques and novel treatment strategies to optimise GKRS treatment for AVMs.

Integration of Tractography

The potential risk of radiation-induced neurological deficits is notable for patients with AVMs located in critical or eloquent regions of the brain [15]. Therefore, we implemented the visualisation of critical brain white matter fibres by using tractography and integrating it into GKRS treatment [15, 16, 20]. Diffusion tensor imaging (DTI)–based tractography was integrated into the radiosurgical planning, beginning with the pyramidal tract in 2004 [20]. This integration was deemed essential due to the pyramidal tract's significance in reducing radiosurgical morbidity. As the methodology evolved, the DTI tractography of the optic radiation was incorporated in 2006, and further advancements led to the integration of DTI tractography for the arcuate fasciculus in 2007. Ultimately, Q-ball-based tractography emerged as a superior method for visualising each fibre compared to DTI-based tractography from 2015 onwards. DTI or Q-ball-based tractography was acquired on the day before treatment. The tractography-integrated images were subsequently imported into the treatment planning software on the day of the treatment, where the registration process was automated within GammaPlan. The integration was performed when the target lesion was located under 10 mm away from these fibres given the potential radiosurgical risks associated with such proximity. Until now, we have used these technologies in our GKRS for over 250 patients with AVMs in critical or eloquent areas. By integrating each neural fibre into the treatment plan, we could create an optimal treatment while constantly checking radiation doses to each critical neural fibre without uselessly reducing the dose to the nidus and suppressing excessive radiation exposure to the nerve fibres [15, 16].

Integration of Rotational Angiography (RA)

GKRS treatment relies entirely on imaging; therefore, enhancing image resolution and visualisation may theoretically contribute to improved treatment outcomes. RA is performed by using a cone-shaped X-ray beam and advanced flat-panel detectors on a contemporary C-arm system, and it delivers a superior spatial resolution of the angioarchitecture of vascular lesions. Consequently, RA integration substantially reduces suboptimal nidus coverage and excessive irradiation outside the nidus, potentially improving conformity and increasing the chance of obliteration [9, 29]. Beginning in 2015, we implemented RA-integrated GKRS (RA-GKRS) for all cerebrovascular malformations to provide high-resolution images and precise targeting of the nidus, further enhancing our radiosurgical outcomes [26, 29]. Prior to or on the day of treatment, RA is obtained by utilising the programmed acquisition protocol (3DRA and HiRes-XperCT modes) with conventional DSA. The 3DRA mode is generally employed for hemispheric AVMs and those presenting with potential metal artefacts (e.g. cases with previous embolisation), whereas HiRes-XperCT is applied for AVMs located deeply near the skull base (e.g. brainstem) and for faint, diffuse AVMs. The acquired volume dataset is automatically transferred to a preinstalled workstation (XtraVision; Philips Healthcare) for further reconstruction utilising a 256^3- or 512^3-resolution voxel matrix.

Subsequently, the DICOM "tag" is transformed from XA into CT in our software, allowing the GammaPlan to accurately identify the RA as a CT-like image. Once the RA has been incorporated into the GammaPlan, image coregistration with stereotactic CT and MR imaging (primarily time-of-flight MR angiography and gadolinium-enhanced T1 images, supplemented by T2) is automated by using the preinstalled coregistration function. To date, we have employed RA-GKRS for over 240 patients with AVMs. The integration of RA into the treatment plan enables more-optimal treatment planning while continuously monitoring prescribed radiation doses to even tiny nidus components and minimising excessive irradiation to surrounding brain tissues. We have previously reported the benefits of RA-GKRS in planning and clinical outcomes for cerebrovascular malformations [9, 26, 29].

Role of Endovascular Treatment

A combination of endovascular embolisation and GKRS is optional, particularly for large AVMs. [34] This combined approach was initially assumed to be ideal as embolisation could reduce nidus volume to a level suitable for GKRS application. However, subsequent studies have indicated that this strategy might be associated with a decrease in obliteration rates [10, 34]. Although entirely dismissing this combined approach would be premature, the obliteration rate for postembolised AVMs could be lower than that for nonembolised AVMs with similar volumes [13, 34]. In our institution, the trend of endovascular treatment for AVM has shifted towards less embolisation given the risk of postembolisation complications. Increased embolic material injection has been related to more haemorrhagic complications; in contrast, minimal targeting embolisation (MTE), limited to high-risk components such as an AVM-related aneurysm or a fistulous component, has proven effective in preventing AVM haemorrhage. In 2011, we introduced GKRS with MTE to target identified high-risk haemorrhage locations, especially for associated aneurysms, aiming to reduce the risk of post-GKRS haemorrhage during the latency period [17]. This treatment strategy is anticipated to contribute to acceptable therapeutic risk and effective haemorrhage prevention in contemporary complex AVM management. Moreover, the incorporation of flow analysis with phase contrast MRI, enabling the identification of high-risk bleeding sites, could be promising [10, 17, 31, 32].

Illustrative cases treated with our modern radiosurgical technique are shown in Figs. 1, 2, and 3.

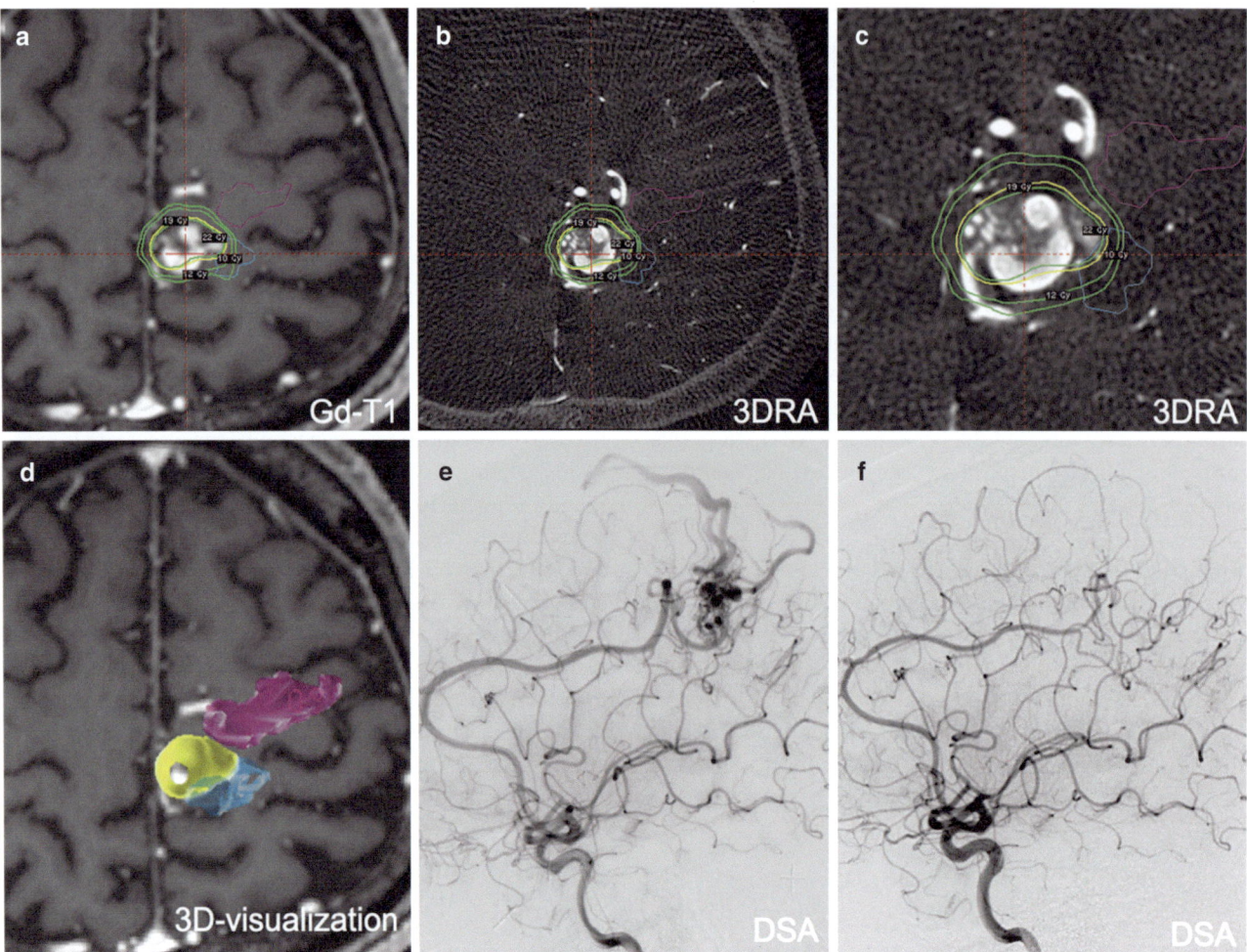

Fig. 1 Gamma knife radiosurgery after the integration of Q-ball tractography and rotational angiography (RA) for a 58-year-old man with an unruptured left parietal arteriovenous malformation (AVM). The nidus is 15 × 13 × 21 mm and close to the left corticospinal tract (CST) and spinothalamic tract (STT). The integration of Q-ball tractography enables the distinct delineation of the CST and STT, while the integration of RA can clearly visualise the detailed nidus components. The upper row (**a–c**) shows a radiosurgical dose planning after the integration of Q-ball tractography and RA, and the lower row (**d–f**) shows AVM before and after radiosurgery. Yellow line indicates the 50% isodose line for the prescribed treatment dose of 19 Gy, and green lines indicate marginal dose lines of 10, 12, and 22 Gy, in order from the outside, respectively. The purple shape indicates the left CST, and the cyan shape indicates the left STT. D shows the three-dimensional visualisation of target area, CST, and STT. Yellow shape indicates the targeted nidus, the purple shape indicates the left CST, and the cyan shape indicates the left STT. (**e**) shows the lateral aspect of the digital subtraction angiography before radiosurgery, and (**f**) shows the same after obliteration. (**a**) Gd-T1 gadolinium-T1-weighted imaging, (**b**, **c**) 3DRA three-dimensional rotational angiography, (**d**) 3D three-dimensional, and (**e**, **f**) DSA digital subtraction angiography

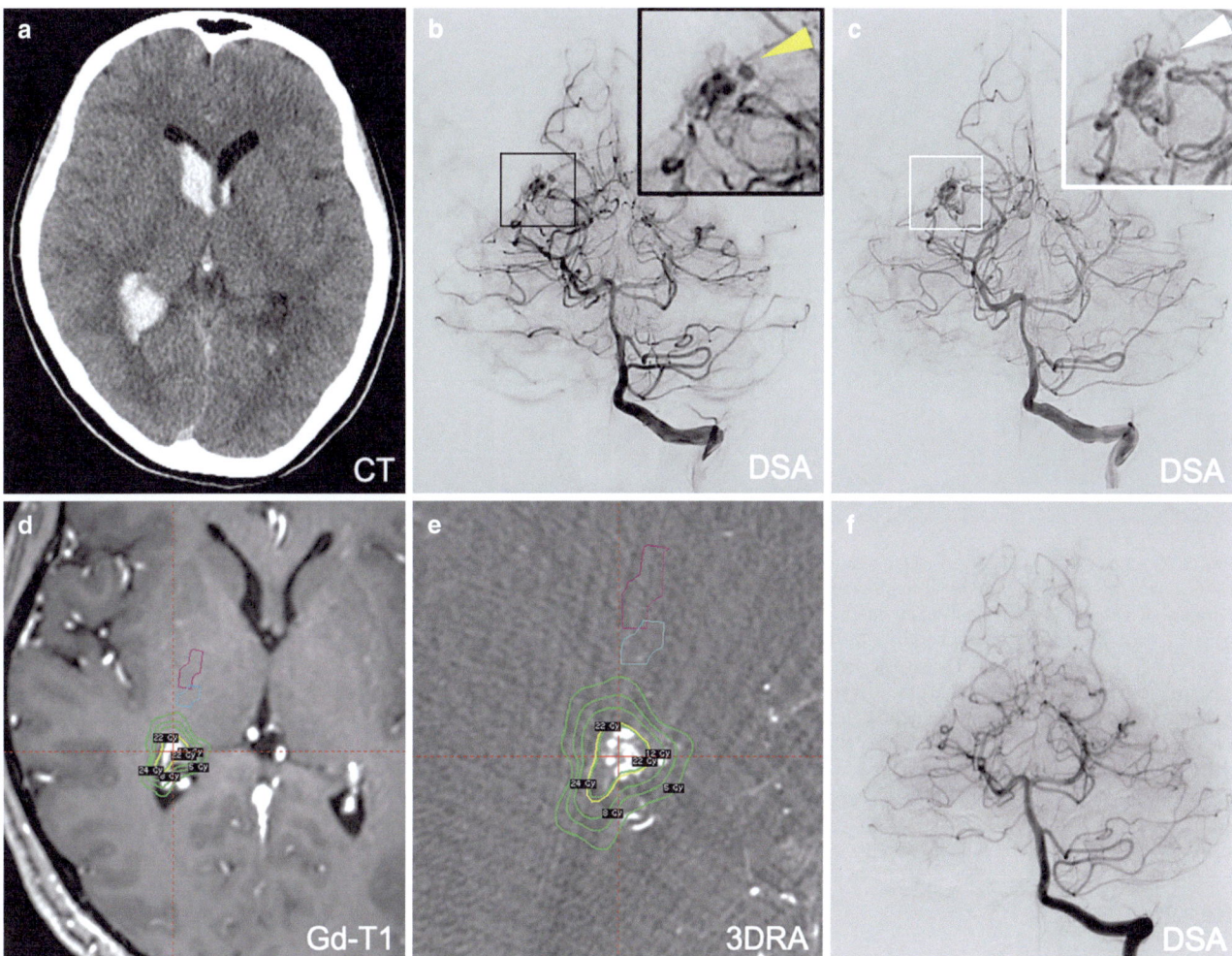

Fig. 2 Gamma knife radiosurgery after minimal target embolisation (MTE) and the integration of Q-ball tractography and rotational angiography (RA) for a 24-year-old woman with a ruptured right lateral ventricle inferior horn arteriovenous malformation (AVM). The nidus is 10 × 8 × 8 mm with intranidal aneurysm and close to the right corticospinal tract (CST) and spinothalamic tract (STT). The integration Q-ball tractography enables the distinct delineation of the CST and STT, while the integration RA can clearly visualise the faint nidus components. (**a**) shows an intraventricular haemorrhage from ruptured AVM on computed tomography (CT) imaging. (**b, c**) shows AVM before and after MTE in digital subtraction angiography (DSA). Yellow arrowhead indicates a ruptured intranidal aneurysm before MTE. White arrowhead indicates the disappearance of intranidal aneurysm after MTE. (**d, e**) shows a radiosurgical dose planning after the integration of Q-ball tractography and RA. Yellow line indicates the 50% isodose line for the prescribed treatment dose of 22 Gy, and green lines indicate marginal dose lines of 5, 8, 12, and 24 Gy, in order from the outside, respectively. The purple shape indicates the right CST, and the cyan shape indicates the right STT. (**e**) shows the AVM obliteration in DSA. (**a**) CT computed tomography, (**b, c, f**) DSA digital subtraction angiography, (**d**) Gd-T1 gadolinium-T1-weighted imaging, and (**e**) 3DRA three-dimensional rotational angiography

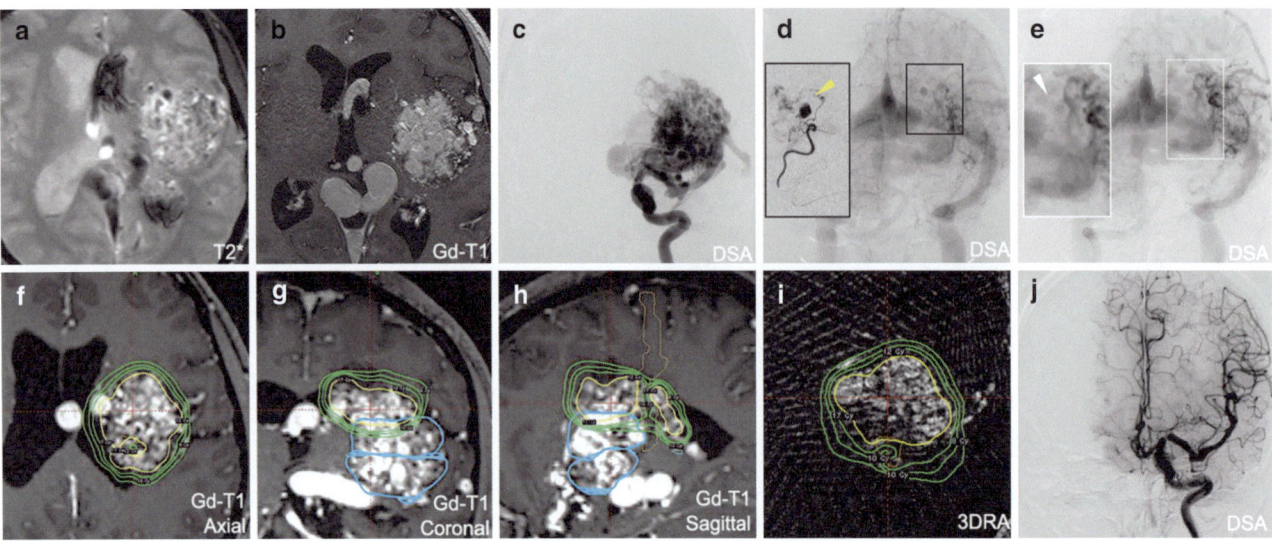

Fig. 3 Gamma knife radiosurgery after minimal target embolisation (MTE) and the integration of Q-ball tractography and rotational angiography (RA) for a 34-year-old woman with a large ruptured left basal ganglia arteriovenous malformation (AVM). The nidus is 36 × 37 × 57 mm with intranidal aneurysm and close to the right corticospinal tract (CST) and spinothalamic tract (STT). The integration Q-ball tractography enables the distinct delineation of the CST, while the integration RA can clearly visualise the detailed nidus components. (**a**) shows an intraventricular haemorrhage from ruptured AVM in a T2-star-weighted imaging. (**b**) shows a large ruptured deep-seated AVM in a gadolinium-T1-weighted imaging (Gd-T1). (**c–e**) shows AVM before and after MTE in digital subtraction angiography (DSA). Yellow arrowhead indicates a ruptured intranidal aneurysm before MTE. White arrowhead indicates a disappearance of intranidal aneurysm after MTE. (**f–i**) shows a volume-staged (three-staged) radiosurgical dose planning after the integration of Q-ball tractography and RA. Yellow line indicates the 50% isodose line for the prescribed treatment dose of 17 Gy, and green lines indicate marginal dose lines of 8, 10, and 12 Gy, in order from the outside, respectively. Light blue lines indicate previous target areas. The orange shape indicates the left CST. (**j**) shows the AVM obliteration in DSA. (**a**) T2* T2-star-weighted imaging, (**b, f–h**) Gd-T1 gadolinium-T1-weighted imaging, (**c–e, j**) DSA digital subtraction angiography, and (**i**) 3DRA three-dimensional rotational angiography

Results

Our Modern Radiosurgical Outcomes

Baseline Characteristics

Patients' background characteristics treated with our modern radiosurgical techniques are summarised in Table 1. RA-GKRS was applied to 88 patients (98%) without any reported iodine contrast agent allergy. Tractography was integrated into GKRS planning in 54 patients (60%), and MTE was utilised in five patients (6%) (Table 1).

Obliteration

Following initial GKRS, 57 AVMs (63%) showed nidus obliteration at a median interval of 30 months (range, 14–49 months). The cumulative obliteration rates were 61.0% at 3 years and 81.6% at 4 years (Fig. 4). Univariate analyses demonstrated that several factors were significantly associated with a better AVM obliteration rate, including planned target volume (continuous) (hazard ratio [HR] 0.88, 95% confidence interval [CI] 0.80–0.95; $p = 0.001$), planned target volume ≤2.0 cm^3 (HR 2.13, 95% CI 1.26–3.58; $p = 0.005$), maximum diameter (continuous) (HR 0.94, 95% CI 0.91–0.96; $p = 0.001$), maximum diameter ≤20 mm (HR 2.09, 95% CI 1.24–3.52; $p = 0.006$), margin dose (continuous) (HR 1.48, 95% CI 1.14–1.91; $p = 0.003$), margin dose ≥20 Gy (HR 2.19, 95% CI 1.19–4.02; $p = 0.012$), a modified Pittsburgh radiosurgical AVM score (continuous) (HR 0.50, 95% CI 0.27–0.84; $p = 0.019$), and Virginia radiosurgery AVM score 0–2 (HR 0.50, 95% CI 0.27–0.84; $p = 0.019$) (Table 2). Upon multivariable analyses, planned target volume ≤2.0 cm^3 (HR 1.82, 95% CI 1.06–3.11; $p = 0.029$) and margin dose ≥20 Gy (HR 1.94, 95% CI 1.04–3.62; $p = 0.036$) remained significant factors for a better AVM obliteration rate (Table 2).

Haemorrhagic Events and Survival

The annual haemorrhage rates of AVM decreased from 8.2% to 1.0% after GKRS and 0.0% after the confirmation of AVM obliteration. The cumulative post-GKRS haemorrhage rates were 2.2% at 2 years and 3.6% at 5 years, respectively (Fig. 5). Post-GKRS haemorrhage occurred in three patients (3.3%), resulting in dead in one patient (1.1%). Therefore, the 5-year cumulative DSS rate was 98.9% (Fig. 6). Of the remaining two patients who experienced post-GKRS haemorrhage, one underwent nidus resection, whereas the other was treated with conservative therapy, ultimately achieving AVM obliteration.

Table 1 Baseline characteristics of the patients treated with the most advanced gamma knife radiosurgery technique

Variable	All	Value, range (median) (%)
Patients' background		
Number of patients		90
Follow-up period, months		12–71 (41)
Age at treatment, years		3–76 (39)
Male sex		56 [62]
AVM characteristics		
Targeted nidus volume, mL		0.1–19.1 (2.1)
Maximum diameter, mm		6–47 (22)
History of haemorrhage		32 [36]
History of direct surgery		4 [4]
History of embolisation		15 [17]
Presence of deep drainer		45 [50]
Involving eloquent area		49 [54]
Location	Deep (BS/CPA, cerebellum, BGL/thalamus)	28 [31]
	Not deep (lobar, ventricle, callosal)	63 [69]
SMG	1	23 [25]
	2	29 [32]
	3	30 [33]
	4	8 [9]
	5	0 [0]
mPRAS		0.3–2.6 [1.2]
VRAS	0–2	66 [73]
	3–4	24 [27]
Radiosurgical parameters		
Margin dose, Gy		17–22 (20)
Central dose, Gy		21–51 (40)
3DRA		88 [98]
Tractography		54 [60]
Minimal targeting embolisation		5 [6]

Note: *3DRA* three-dimensional rotational angiography, *BS* brainstem, *BGL* basal ganglia, *CPA* cerebellopontine angle, *mPRAS* modified Pittsburgh radiosurgical AVM score, *SMG* Spetzler–Martin grade, and *VRAS* Virginia radiosurgical AVM score

Post-GKRS Early Signal Change and Neurological Outcomes

Post-GKRS signal change was observed in 31 patients (34%). The cumulative rates of post-GKRS signal change were 30.8% at 1 year and 35.3% at 3 years, respectively (Fig. 7). The post-GKRS signal change eventually resolved or significantly diminished in 22 patients (71%) without any treatment, while eight patients (26%) were administered oral steroid medication. Only one patient (3.2%) developed an asymptomatic small cyst. Of the entire cohort, only one patient (1.0%) developed a neurological complication as symptomatic epilepsy and was maintained with antiepileptic drugs. The 5-year cumulative rate of neurological preservation was 97.8% (Fig. 8).

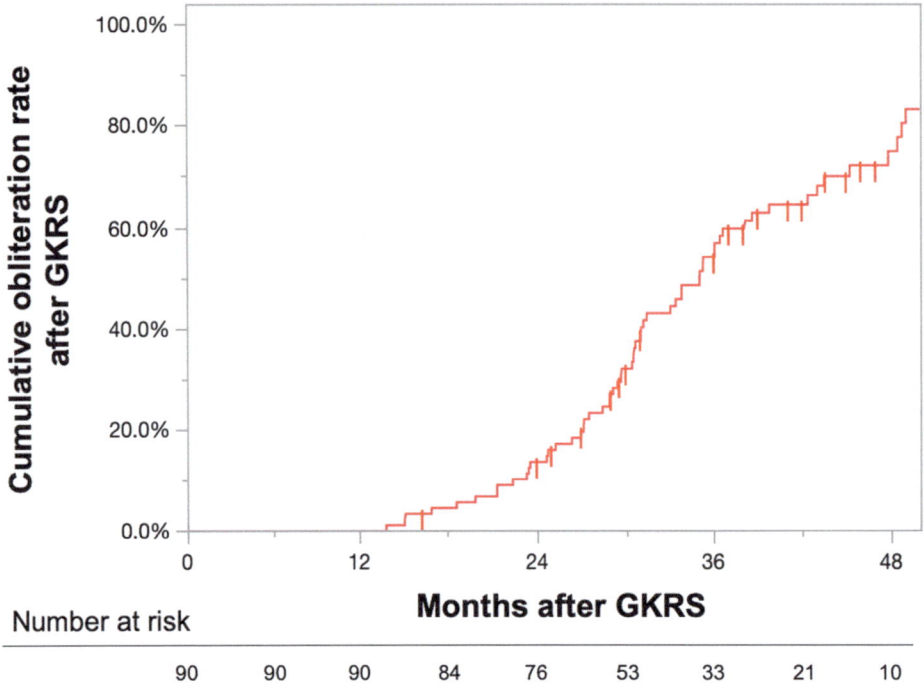

Fig. 4 Kaplan–Meier curve for the obliteration rate after GKRS treated with the most advanced techniques. GKRS gamma knife radiosurgery

Table 2 Bivariate and multivariable analyses of nidus obliteration

Variables	Bivariate p-value	HR (95% CI)	Forward stepwise selection p-value	Multivariable p-value	HR (95% CI)
Age at treatment (continuous)	0.443	1.01 (0.99–1.02)	/	/	/
Age at treatment >40 years	0.486	1.20 (0.71–2.03)	0.274	/	/
Planned target volume (continuous)	0.001*	0.88 (0.80–0.95)	/	/	/
Planned target volume ≤2.0 cm³	0.005*	2.13 (1.26–3.58)	0.063	0.029*	1.82 (1.06–3.11)
Maximum diameter (continuous)	0.001*	0.94 (0.91–0.96)	/	/	/
Maximum diameter ≤20 mm	0.006*	2.09 (1.24–3.52)	/	/	/
Margin dose (continuous)	0.003*	1.48 (1.14–1.91)	/	/	/
Margin dose ≥20 Gy	0.012*	2.19 (1.19–4.02)	0.033	0.036*	1.94 (1.04–3.62)
Central dose (continuous)	0.218	1.06 (0.97–1.17)	/	/	/
Central dose ≥40 Gy	0.277	1.34 (0.79–2.25)	/	/	/
History of direct surgery	0.318	1.68 (0.61–4.67)	0.375	/	/
History of embolisation	0.206	0.63 (0.31–1.29)	0.662	/	/
History of haemorrhage	0.061	1.65 (0.98–2.79)	0.152	0.080	1.60 (0.94–2.72)

(continued)

Table 2 (continued)

Variables	Bivariate p-value	HR (95% CI)	Forward stepwise selection p-value	Multivariable p-value	HR (95% CI)
Presence of deep drainer	0.738	1.09 (0.65–1.83)	0.358	/	/
Involving eloquent area	0.065	0.61 (0.36–1.03)	0.351	/	/
SMG ≤2	0.183	1.45 (0.84–2.49)	/	/	/
mPRAS (continuous)	0.019*	0.50 (0.27–0.84)	/	/	/
mPRAS ≤1.2	0.100	1.55 (0.92–2.60)	/	/	/
VRAS 0–2	0.001*	2.84 (1.43–5.65)	/	/	/

Note: *HR* hazard ratio, *CI* confidence interval, *SMG* Spetzler–Martin grade, *mPRAS* modified Pittsburgh radiosurgical AVM score, and *VRAS* Virginia radiosurgery AVM score
*Significant at $p < 0.05$

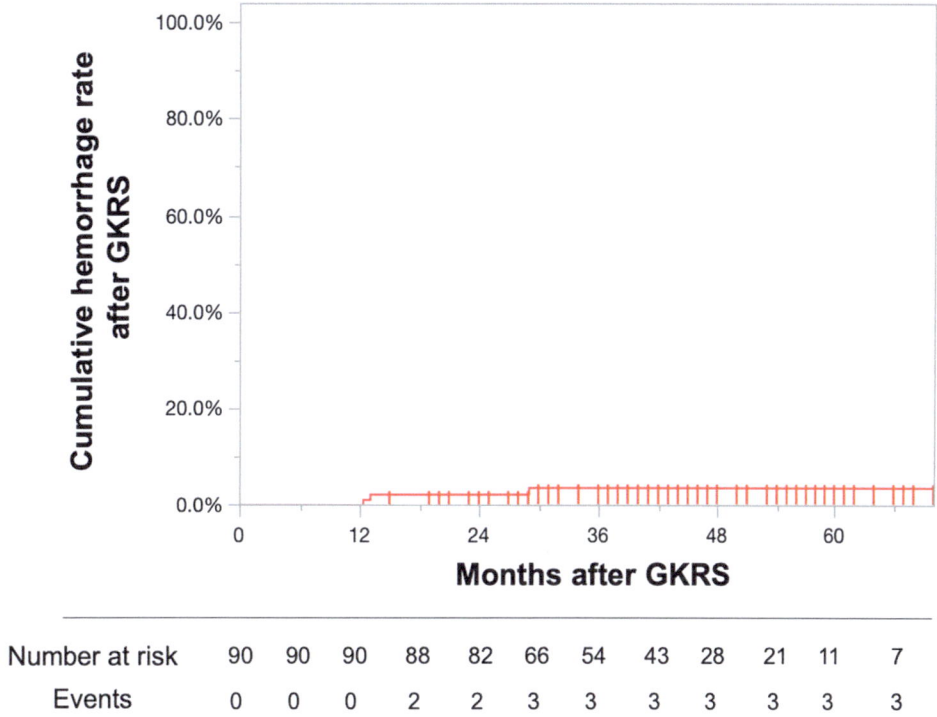

Fig. 5 Kaplan–Meier curve for the haemorrhage rate after GKRS treated with the most advanced techniques. GKRS gamma knife radiosurgery

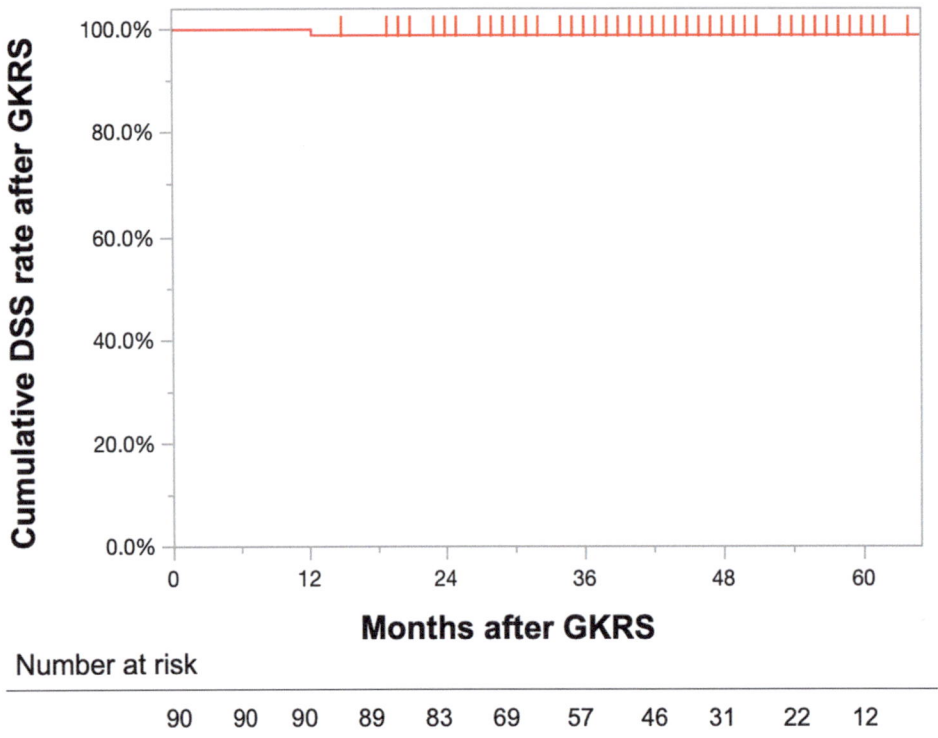

Fig. 6 Kaplan–Meier curve for the disease-specific survival rate after GKRS treated with the most advanced techniques. DSS disease-specific survival, GKRS gamma knife radiosurgery

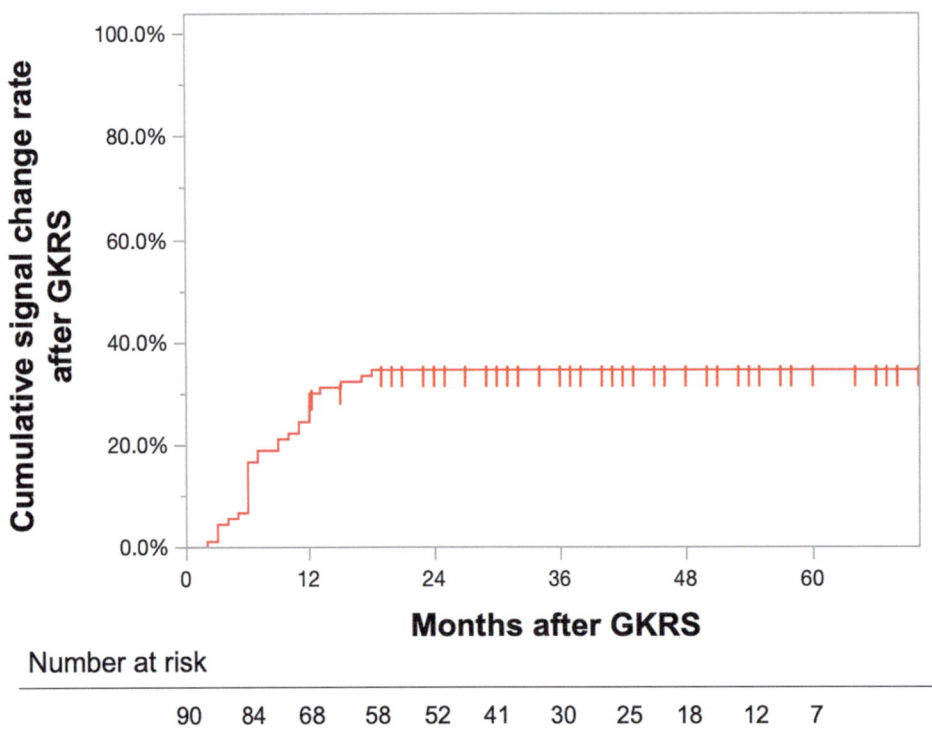

Fig. 7 Kaplan–Meier curve for the signal change rate after GKRS treated with the most advanced techniques. GKRS gamma knife radiosurgery

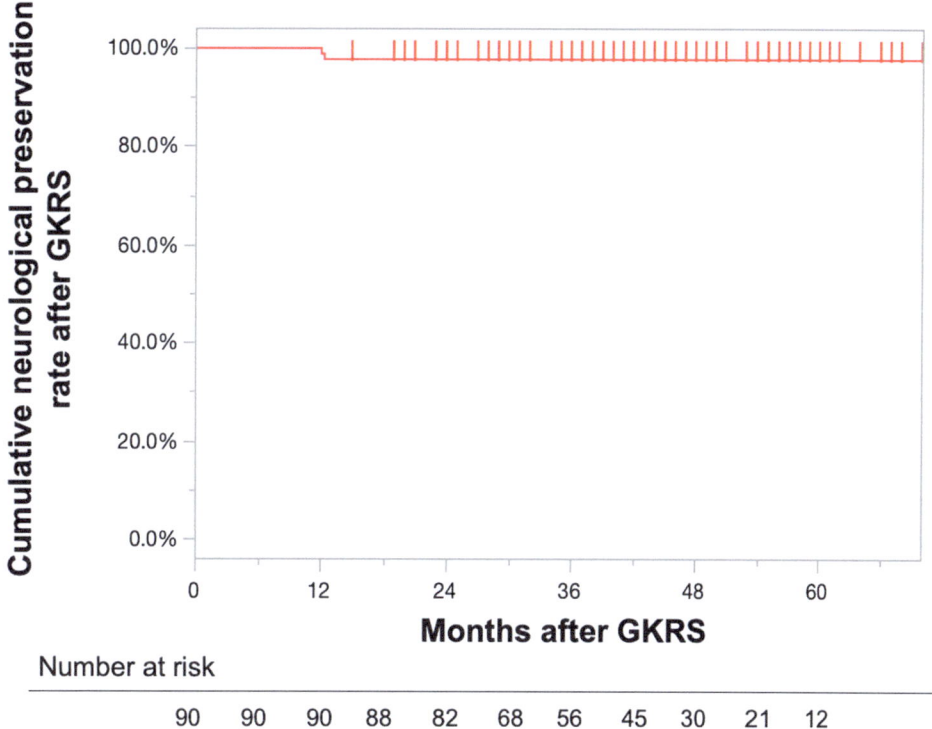

Fig. 8 Kaplan–Meier curve for the neurological preservation rate after GKRS treated with the most advanced techniques. GKRS gamma knife radiosurgery

Discussion

In this study, we present a comprehensive overview of the history of GKRS treatment for AVMs in our hospital over a period of more than 30 years. We have reported several articles analysing the outcomes of GKRS for AVMs, as well as new technologies and novel treatment strategies [8, 10, 13, 15, 16, 18, 20, 25–29, 31, 32]. Through more than 1100 GKRS treatments for AVMs, we have been aiming to improve therapeutic outcomes for AVM patients by utilising and integrating new radiographic imaging modalities and novel treatment strategies. Our study could provide an important contribution to the literature on GKRS for AVMs and highlight the significance of ongoing research and development in this field.

Improving the obliteration rate of the AVM is generally considered to be a critical factor in reducing post-GKRS haemorrhage rates and improving neurological function preservation [1, 7]. However, achieving a balance between a sufficient dose to the nidus and minimising excessive radiation dosing to surrounding normal brain tissue is essential. Therefore, accurately projecting the actual nidus structure onto the radiographic imaging is of paramount importance [9, 26, 29]. RA-GKRS has shown promise, with a median latency period of 30 months and a cumulative obliteration rate of over 80% at 4 years, as reported in our previous study [29]. In cases without complete obliteration, additional treatment options may be considered for remnant nidus. We believe that the final treatment outcome must be analysed after combining these additional treatments. Currently, we are continuing to explore the implementation of new treatment strategies to further enhance the obliteration rate.

Although improving AVM obliteration rates is expected to be able to reduce post-GKRS haemorrhage rates, this study and our previous article failed to demonstrate statistical significance in the difference between RA-GKRS and conventional GKRS [29]. The limitations of sample size and variability in background factors should also be taken into account. Although early achievement and improvement in the AVM obliteration were not directly associated with a reduced risk of AVM haemorrhage, we suggest that further analysis is necessary to identify additional related factors and develop new therapeutic strategies to improve the overall efficacy of AVM treatment.

The incidence of post-GKRS signal changes was higher than that in the previous report, which was consistent with RA-GKRS outcomes in our previous report [5, 6]. However, these events might be obliteration related, and 70% of those resolved spontaneously. In the remaining cases, signal changes almost disappeared following oral steroid treatment. Only one patient experienced persistent neurological adverse events, requiring continuous anticonvulsant medication for symptomatic epilepsy. However, if this patient and another patient who died from haemorrhage were excluded, then the overall neurological outcomes of patients were excellent. The reduction in the dose to critical nerve fibres achieved via the visualisation of nerve fibres and multiple shots and beam-blocking techniques may have contributed to this favourable neurological outcome. Further research is needed to investigate the effectiveness of these therapeutic strategies in reducing the incidence of late radiation-induced adverse events. We believe that the primary goal of radiosurgery for AVM is to achieve continuous neurological preservation in patients 20–30 years after GKRS.

This study has certain limitations. As this is a retrospective study, selection bias may potentially limit the generalisability of our findings, and further research with a larger sample size is desirable. Also, the significance of our advanced GKRS technique on late radiation-induced complications has yet to be established, and further analysis with a longer follow-up period will yield additional insight into the benefits of GKRS with tractography, RA, and MTE.

Conclusion

GKRS is a safe and effective treatment for AVMs. We represented our continuous development and advanced technique on GKRS for AVMs. Further studies with larger samples and longer follow-ups, as well as an analysis of late adverse events, are warranted.

Acknowledgements None.

Funding Information This work was supported by JSPS KAKENHI (grant number 20K17919 to Shinya).

Data availability Anonymized data in this article will be available upon request from any qualified investigator, and information about the method of analysis will be available from the corresponding author upon reasonable request.

Declarations
Conflicts of interest: The authors have no competing interests to declare that are relevant to the content of this chapter.

Compliance with ethical standards: The study was approved by the institutional review board of our institution (approval number 2231), and all patients provided written informed consent for study participation in accordance with the principles of the Declaration of Helsinki.

References

1. Choi JH, Mohr JP. Brain arteriovenous malformations in adults. Lancet Neurol. 2005;4:299–308.
2. Derdeyn CP, Zipfel GJ, Albuquerque FC, Cooke DL, Feldmann E, Sheehan JP, Torner JC, American Heart Association Stroke Council. Management of brain arteriovenous malformations: a scientific statement for healthcare professionals from the American Heart Association/American Stroke Association. Stroke. 2017;48:e200–24.
3. Ding D, Starke RM, Kano H, Mathieu D, Huang P, Kondziolka D, Feliciano C, Rodriguez-Mercado R, Almodovar L, Grills IS, Silva D, Abbassy M, Missios S, Barnett GH, Lunsford LD, Sheehan JP. Radiosurgery for cerebral arteriovenous malformations in a randomized trial of unruptured brain arteriovenous malformations (Aruba)-eligible patients: a multicenter study. Stroke. 2016;47:342–9.
4. Fleetwood IG, Steinberg GK. Arteriovenous malformations. Lancet. 2002;359:863–73.
5. Flickinger JC, Kondziolka D, Lunsford LD, Pollock BE, Yamamoto M, Gorman DA, Schomberg PJ, Sneed P, Larson D, Smith V, McDermott MW, Miyawaki L, Chilton J, Morantz RA, Young B, Jokura H, Liscak R. A multi-institutional analysis of complication outcomes after arteriovenous malformation radiosurgery. Int J Radiat Oncol Biol Phys. 1999;44:67–74.
6. Flickinger JC, Lunsford LD, Kondziolka D, Maitz AH, Epstein AH, Simons SR, Wu A. Radiosurgery and brain tolerance: an analysis of neurodiagnostic imaging changes after gamma knife radiosurgery for arteriovenous malformations. Int J Radiat Oncol Biol Phys. 1992;23:19–26.
7. Friedlander RM. Clinical practice. Arteriovenous malformations of the brain. N Engl J Med. 2007;356:2704–12.
8. Hanakita S, Koga T, Shin M, Igaki H, Saito N. Application of single-stage stereotactic radiosurgery for cerebral arteriovenous malformations >10 cm^3. Stroke. 2014;45:3543–8.
9. Hasegawa H, Hanakita S, Shin M, Kawashima M, Kin T, Takahashi W, Suzuki Y, Shinya Y, Ono H, Shojima M, Nakatomi H, Saito N. Integration of rotational angiography enables better dose planning in gamma knife radiosurgery for brain arteriovenous malformations. J Neurosurg. 2018;129 Supplement 1:17–25.
10. Hasegawa H, Kin T, Shin M, Suzuki Y, Kawashima M, Shinya Y, Shiode T, Nakatomi H, Saito N. Possible association between rupture and intranidal microhemodynamics in arteriovenous malformations: phase-contrast magnetic resonance angiography-based flow quantification. World Neurosurg. 2021;150:e427–35.
11. Hasegawa H, Yamamoto M, Shin M, Barfod BE. Gamma knife radiosurgery for brain vascular malformations: current evidence and future tasks. Ther Clin Risk Manag. 2019;15:1351–67.
12. Kano H, Lunsford LD, Flickinger JC, Yang HC, Flannery TJ, Awan NR, Niranjan A, Novotny J Jr, Kondziolka D. Stereotactic radiosurgery for arteriovenous malformations, part 1: management of Spetzler-Martin Grade I and II arteriovenous malformations. J Neurosurg. 2012;116:11–20.
13. Kawashima M, Hasegawa H, Shin M, Shinya Y, Ishikawa O, Koizumi S, Katano A, Nakatomi H, Saito N. Outcomes of stereotactic radiosurgery for hemorrhagic arteriovenous malformations with or without prior resection or embolization. J Neurol Surg. 2020;135:733–41.
14. Kim H, Al-Shahi Salman R, McCulloch CE, Stapf C, Young WL, MARS Coinvestigators. Untreated brain arteriovenous

malformation: patient-level meta-analysis of hemorrhage predictors. Neurology. 2014;83:590–7.
15. Koga T, Maruyama K, Kamada K, Ota T, Shin M, Itoh D, Kunii N, Ino K, Terahara A, Aoki S, Masutani Y, Saito N. Outcomes of diffusion tensor tractography-integrated stereotactic radiosurgery. Int J Radiat Oncol Biol Phys. 2012;82:799–802.
16. Koga T, Shin M, Maruyama K, Kamada K, Ota T, Itoh D, Kunii N, Ino K, Aoki S, Masutani Y, Igaki H, Onoe T, Saito N. Integration of corticospinal tractography reduces motor complications after radiosurgery. Int J Radiat Oncol Biol Phys. 2012;83:129–33.
17. Koizumi S, Shojima M, Shinya Y, Ishikawa O, Hasegawa H, Miyawaki S, Nakatomi H, Saito N. Risk factors of brain arteriovenous malformation embolization as adjunctive therapy: single-center 10-year experience. World Neurosurg. 2022;167:e1448–54.
18. Kurita H, Kawamoto S, Sasaki T, Shin M, Tago M, Terahara A, Ueki K, Kirino T. Results of radiosurgery for brain stem arteriovenous malformations. J Neurol Neurosurg Psychiatry. 2000;68:563–70.
19. Lawton MT, Kim H, McCulloch CE, Mikhak B, Young WL. A supplementary grading scale for selecting patients with brain arteriovenous malformations for surgery. Neurosurgery. 2010;66:702–13; discussion 713
20. Maruyama K, Kamada K, Shin M, Itoh D, Aoki S, Masutani Y, Tago M, Kirino T. Integration of three-dimensional corticospinal tractography into treatment planning for gamma knife surgery. J Neurosurg. 2005;102:673–7.
21. Maruyama K, Kawahara N, Shin M, Tago M, Kishimoto J, Kurita H, Kawamoto S, Morita A, Kirino T. The risk of hemorrhage after radiosurgery for cerebral arteriovenous malformations. N Engl J Med. 2005;352:146–53.
22. Mohr JP, Parides MK, Stapf C, Moquete E, Moy CS, Overbey JR, Salman RA, Vicaut E, Young WL, Houdart E, Cordonnier C, Stefani MA, Hartmann A, von Kummer R, Biondi A, Berkefeld J, Klijn CJM, Harkness K, Libman R, Barreau X, Moskowitz AJ. Medical management with or without interventional therapy for unruptured brain arteriovenous malformations (Aruba): a multicentre, non-blinded, randomised trial. Lancet. 2014;383:614–21.
23. Ogilvy CS, Stieg PE, Awad I, RD B Jr, Kondziolka D, Rosenwasser R, Young WL, Hademenos G, Special Writing Group of the Stroke Council, American Stroke Association. AHA scientific statement: recommendations for the management of intracranial arteriovenous malformations: a statement for healthcare professionals from a special writing group of the stroke council, American Stroke Association. Stroke J Cereb Circ. 2001;32:1458–71.
24. Pollock BE, Link MJ, Brown RD. The risk of stroke or clinical impairment after stereotactic radiosurgery for Aruba-eligible patients. Stroke. 2013;44:437–41.
25. Shin M, Kawahara N, Maruyama K, Tago M, Ueki K, Kirino T. Risk of hemorrhage from an arteriovenous malformation confirmed to have been obliterated on angiography after stereotactic radiosurgery. J Neurosurg. 2005;102:842–6.
26. Shinya Y, Hasegawa H, Kawashima M, Koizumi S, Katano A, Umekawa M, Saito N. Prognosis of rotational angiography-based stereotactic radiosurgery for dural arteriovenous fistulas: a retrospective analysis. Neurosurgery. 2023;92:167–78.
27. Shinya Y, Hasegawa H, Shin M, Kashiwabara K, Kawashima M, Hanakita S, Koga T, Koizumi S, Katano A, Suzuki Y, Saito N. Age-dependent hemorrhage risk and obliteration benefit after radiosurgery for brain arteriovenous malformation. Int J Radiat Oncol Biol Phys. 2023;116(5):1126–34.
28. Shinya Y, Hasegawa H, Shin M, Kawashima M, Koizumi S, Katano A, Suzuki Y, Kashiwabara K, Saito N. Stereotactic radiosurgery provides long-term safety for patients with arteriovenous malformations in the diencephalon and brainstem: the optimal dose selection and long-term outcomes. Neurosurgery. 2022;91:485–95.
29. Shinya Y, Hasegawa H, Shin M, Kawashima M, Sugiyama T, Ishikawa O, Koizumi S, Suzuki Y, Nakatomi H, Saito N. Rotational angiography-based gamma knife radiosurgery for brain arteriovenous malformations: preliminary therapeutic outcomes of the novel method. Neurosurgery. 2021;89:60–9.
30. Spetzler RF, Martin NA. A proposed grading system for arteriovenous malformations. J Neurosurg. 1986;65:476–83.
31. Takeda Y, Hasegawa H, Kin T, Shinya Y, Kawashima M, Furuta Y, Suzuki Y, Sekine T, Saito N. Hemodynamic changes during the obliteration process for cerebral arteriovenous malformations after radiosurgery. Neurosurg Focus. 2022;53:E7.
32. Takeda Y, Kin T, Sekine T, Hasegawa H, Suzuki Y, Uchikawa H, Koike T, Kiyofuji S, Shinya Y, Kawashima M, Saito N. Hemodynamic analysis of cerebral AVMs with 3D phase-contrast MR imaging. AJNR Am J Neuroradiol. 2021;42:2138–45.
33. van Beijnum J, van der Worp HB, Buis DR, Al-Shahi Salman R, Kappelle LJ, Rinkel GJ, van der Sprenkel JW, Vandertop WP, Algra A, Klijn CJ. Treatment of brain arteriovenous malformations: a systematic review and meta-analysis. JAMA. 2011;306:2011–9.
34. Wu EM, El Ahmadieh TY, McDougall CM, Aoun SG, Mehta N, Neeley OJ, Plitt A, Shen Ban V, Sillero R, White JA, Batjer HH, Welch BG. Embolization of brain arteriovenous malformations with intent to cure: a systematic review. J Neurosurg. 2019;132:388–99.

Open Access This chapter is licensed under the terms of the Creative Commons Attribution 4.0 International License (http://creativecommons.org/licenses/by/4.0/), which permits use, sharing, adaptation, distribution and reproduction in any medium or format, as long as you give appropriate credit to the original author(s) and the source, provide a link to the Creative Commons license and indicate if changes were made.

The images or other third party material in this chapter are included in the chapter's Creative Commons license, unless indicated otherwise in a credit line to the material. If material is not included in the chapter's Creative Commons license and your intended use is not permitted by statutory regulation or exceeds the permitted use, you will need to obtain permission directly from the copyright holder.

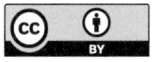

Role and Efficacy of Direct Surgery in the Management of Intracranial Dural Arteriovenous Fistulas

Taku Sugiyama, Toshiya Osanai, Masaki Ito, Haruto Uchino, and Miki Fujimura

Abbreviations

CVD   cortical venous drainage
CVJ   craniovertebral junction
dAVF dural arteriovenous fistula
EVT   endovascular treatment
ICH   intracranial hemorrhage
MRI   magnetic resonance imaging
mRS   modified Rankin scale
TAE   transarterial embolization
TSS   transverse-sigmoid sinus
TVE   transvenous embolization

Introduction

Intracranial dural arteriovenous fistulas (dAVFs) are uncommon vascular diseases characterized by pathological arteriovenous communication on the dura mater and/or venous sinuses. The clinical course of dAVF is associated with venous drainage, and dAVFs with cortical venous drainage (CVD) exhibit a high risk of intracranial hemorrhage (ICH) and neurological deficits [5, 16]. Thus, active and early interventional treatment should be considered for dAVF with CVD (Borden type II and III dAVF) [10, 21].

Endovascular treatment (EVT) is often used as the primary treatment, and the majority of dAVFs can be treated through transarterial embolization (TAE), transvenous embolization (TVE), or their combination [2, 10]. Stereotactic radiosurgery is another means; however, limitations such as a lower obliteration rate and a post-treatment latency period remain [3, 10].

A direct (or open) surgical procedure is also an established procedure with a long history. Despite its invasiveness, surgical procedures have an important role and an important effectiveness to a certain extent depending on the lesion location, angiographical architecture, pattern of onset, and eligibility or curability for EVT [1, 8, 21]. However, data regarding direct surgery in the management of intracranial dAVFs remain limited, possibly due to their rarity. This study aimed to clarify the role and efficacy of direct surgery in the management of intracranial dAVF by investigating the factors that influence the selection of direct surgery and surgical outcomes.

Methods

Patients

The institutional review board of the Hokkaido University Hospital, Sapporo, Japan, approved this study (No.017-0074). A multicenter retrospective survey was conducted by using a prospectively maintained institutional surgical registry of Hokkaido University Hospital and its affiliated hospitals, between April 2007 and March 2022. We identified 43 patients who had undergone direct surgery for dAVFs during the study period. Informed consent was obtained from all the patients included in this study.

Data Collection and Outcome Evaluation

We reviewed data concerning demographics, the location of the lesion, angiographical architecture, the pattern of onset, the preoperative modified Rankin scale (mRS) score, surgical procedures, and surgery-related complications. We also surveyed factors for the selection of direct surgery and prior treatment among the treatment modalities.

T. Sugiyama (✉) · T. Osanai · M. Ito · H. Uchino · M. Fujimura
Department of Neurosurgery, Hokkaido University Graduate School of Medicine, Sapporo, Japan
e-mail: takus1113@med.hokudai.ac.jp

Angiographic outcomes were postoperatively evaluated by using selective angiography within 7 days. Incomplete obliteration was defined as a treatment that resulted in residual CVD. Long-term outcomes were evaluated by using outpatient magnetic resonance imaging (MRI) follow-up data. Recurrence was defined as recanalization and progression to Borden type II or III during the period after shunt placement or CVD occlusion. A clinically favorable outcome was defined as an mRS score of 0–2 at the last evaluation [20, 21].

Indication and Selection of Treatment Modality

At our facilities, the presence of CVD, hemorrhagic presentation, and nonhemorrhagic neurological deficits are considered indicators of interventional treatment in dAVFs.

On the basis of the angiographical architecture of the lesion and patient condition, the treatment modality was decided through discussion by a multidisciplinary neurovascular team including a board-certified neurosurgeon, a neuroendovascular surgeon, and a radiologist. TVE was considered for the curative embolization of sinus-type dAVF, and TAE was also considered for all types of dAVFs as the primary option. When preoperative angiography indicated the existence of pial arterial feeders, TAE through the pial artery was first considered; however, when the pial arterial feeder was estimated to be unsafe for embolization, curative endovascular treatment was abandoned, even if TAE via the dural artery could be performed. Microsurgery was considered the next option.

Direct Surgical Procedure

Surgical approaches were determined mainly depending on the location of the CVD. Intradural obliteration of the arterialized CVD was performed at the exit point from the dura. Encountered or identifiable feeding arteries, including the pial arterial supply, were also coagulated. Intraoperative indocyanine green video-angiography and/or Doppler sonography were used routinely, while intraoperative selective angiography was used in patients with a complicated angioarchitecture or in those in whom combined endovascular and microsurgical treatment was considered.

Results

Patient Characteristics

The patient characteristics are summarized in Table 1. There were 31 male and 12 female patients, with a mean age of 64.1 (range, 39–86) years. More specifically, 21 (48.8%)

Table 1 Patient characteristics

Total number	$N = 43$
Age	64.1 (39–86)
Sex	
Male	31 (72.1%)
Female	12 (27.9%)
Presentation	
ICH	21 (48.8%)
NHND	6 (14.0%)
Minor symptom	5 (11.6%)
Asymptomatic	11 (25.6%)
Preoperative mRS	
0	15 (34.9%)
1–2	8 (18.6%)
3–5	20 (46.5%)
Location	
Ethmoid	11 (25.6%)
Tentorium	11 (25.6%)
Torcula	1
SPS	2
Vein of Galen	2
StrS	1
Tentorial sinus	5
CVJ	5 (11.6%)
TSS	11 (25.6%)
Others	5 (11.6%)
Middle fossa	1
Convexity	2
SSS	2
Borden type	
II	6 (14.0%)
III	37 (86.0%)

Note: *ICH* intracranial hemorrhage, *NHND* nonhemorrhagic neurological deficit, *mRS* modified Rankin scale, *SPS* superior petrosal sinus, *StrS* straight sinus, *CVJ* craniovertebral junction, *TSS* transverse-sigmoid sinus, and *SSS* superior sagittal sinus.

patients presented with ICH, which was characterized by various combinations of subdural, subarachnoid, intraparenchymal, and intraventricular hematomas. Six (14.0%) patients presented with nonhemorrhagic neurological deficits caused by intraparenchymal edema, spinal myelopathy, enlarged varix, and increased intracranial pressure. Five (11.6%) patients presented with minor symptoms, including headache, tinnitus, and vertigo. The remaining 11 (25.6%) patients were asymptomatic. The preoperative mRS scores were 0 in 15 (34.9%), 1–2 in 8 (18.6%), and 3–5 in 20 (46.5%) patients.

The lesions were located at the ethmoid in 11 (25.6%) patients, tentorium in 11 (25.6%), craniovertebral junction (CVJ) in 5 (11.6%), transverse-sigmoid sinus (TSS) in 11 (25.6%), middle fossa in 1, convexity in 2, and superior sagittal sinus in 2. Six (14.0%) and 37 (86.0%) patients had Borden type II and III lesions, respectively.

Factors for Selecting Surgery and Endovascular Attempts

The factors for selecting direct surgery and prior EVT are summarized in Table 2. EVT had never been attempted in patients with ethmoidal dAVF, and direct surgery was selected as the primary treatment in all cases. In addition, for patients with massive ICH presenting with signs of brain herniation, direct surgery was selected because of the necessity of hematoma evacuation. In the remaining patients, EVT was considered first; however, it was abandoned due to difficulty in catheter access or the high risk of embolization in the target artery.

EVT was performed in 15 patients. Four patients had high-flow shunts in whom intentional perioperative supportive embolization was performed to reduce intraoperative blood loss or to increase the curability of dAVFs. In ten patients, curative endovascular treatment resulted in incomplete obliteration, and additional EVT was deemed unfeasible or unsafe. In one patient, the catheter penetrated the transverse sinus during TVE, which required emergent open surgery. Notably, EVT resulted in incomplete obliteration in all CVJ dAVF patients and in the majority of tentorial dAVF patients with a pial arterial supply.

Surgical Details

Surgical procedural details are summarized in Table 3. The surgical approach was decided on the basis of the location of the CVD. The simple disconnection of CVD was performed in the majority of patients (97.7%); however, a radical resection of the transverse sinus was necessary in one patient, in whom catheter penetration occurred. The additional coagulation of the pial arterial branches was required in six patients (14.0%), and this was frequent in patients with tentorial dAVFs. Angiographically occult pial arterial supplies were intraoperatively found in three patients with tentorial dAVFs. Additional superior petrosal sinus packing through needle insertion into the transverse sinus was needed in one patient with TSS dAVF. In patients with massive ICH, the hematoma was evacuated first, and then the disconnection of CVD was conducted simultaneously. Intraoperative indocyanine green video-angiography and Doppler sonography were used routinely, whereas intraoperative selective angiography was used in five patients with complicated angioarchitecture.

Surgical Outcomes

One patient died postoperatively, although this was due to the initial ICH rather than the surgical procedure. Surgery-related permanent neurological deficits were observed in

Table 2 Factors for selection of direct surgery and prior endovascular treatment

Location	Ethmoid	Tentorium	CVJ	TSS	Others
N	11	11	5	11	5
No prior EVT attempt	11 (100%)	5 (45.5%)	2 (40.0%)	7 (63.6%)	3 (60.0%)
Massive ICH presentation	3	3	0	3	2
EVT deemed as unfeasible/unsafe	–	3	2	4	1
Prior EVT attempt	0 (0.0%)	6 (54.5%)	3 (60.0%)	4 (36.4%)	2 (40.0%)
Intentional supportive EVT	–	2	–	1	1
Incomplete obliteration	–	4	3	2	1
Presence of pial arterial supply	–	3	–	–	–
Complication during EVT	–	–	–	1	–

Note: *EVT* endovascular treatment, *CVJ* craniovertebral junction, *TSS* transverse-sigmoid sinus, *ICH* intracranial hemorrhage

Table 3 Surgical procedural details

Procedural Details	Ethmoid	Tentorium	CVJ	TSS	Others
N	11	11	5	11	5
Approach					
Bifrontal craniotomy	11				–
Subtemporal				1	1
Supratentorial–infraoccipital		5			
Posterior interhemispheric transtentorial		3			
Combined supra- and infratentorial				10	
Supracerebellar–infratentorial		1			
Retrosigmoid		2			
Far lateral			5		
Other craniotomies					4
Procedure					
Simple obliteration of CVD	11	11	5	10	5
Radical resection of the sinus				1	
Additional obliteration of pial arterial supplies		4		1	1
Additional sinus packing				1	
ICH removal	3	3	0	3	2
Intraoperative adjuncts					
ICG video-angiography	11	11	5	10	5
Catheter angiography		3		2	

Note: *CVD* cortical venous drainage, *ICH* intracranial hemorrhage, and *ICG* indocyanine green

Table 4 Short- and long-term results of surgery

Perioperative results	N = 43
Death	1 (2.3%)
Surgery-related complication	
Permanent deficit	3 (7.0%)
Brain edema	2
Postoperative hemorrhage	1
Transient complication	4 (9.3%)
Brain edema	2
CSF leakage	1
Hoarseness	1
Angiographical results	N = 42
Incomplete obliteration	1 (2.4%)
Complete obliteration	38 (90.5%)
Obliterated CVD	3 (7.1%)
Long-term results	N = 40
Mean follow-up period	33.4 (range 2–148)
Recurrence	0 (0.0%)
mRS score on last evaluation	
0	17 (42.5%)
1–2	16 (40.0%)
3–6	7 (17.5%)

Note: *CSF* cerebrospinal fluid, *CVD* cortical venous drainage, and *mRS* modified Rankin scale

three patients (7.0%), where two of these deficits originated from postoperative brain edema at the craniotomy site. Postoperative hemorrhage that required repeat surgery 3 days after the initial surgery was observed in one case. Transient complications, including brain edema, hoarseness of voice, and cerebrospinal fluid leakage, were observed in four patients (9.3%).

The short- and long-term surgical results are summarized in Table 4. All patients, except for the one who died, were evaluated angiographically within 7 days after surgery. Postoperative angiographies revealed that complete obliteration was achieved in 38 patients (90.5%), and the obliteration of the CVD was achieved in three (7.1%). Incomplete obliteration was observed in only one patient (2.4%) who required repeat surgery.

Long-term follow-up data, including MRI findings, were available for 40 patients. The mean follow-up period of our patient cohort was 33.4 months (range, 2–148 months). During this period, no recurrence of symptoms or dAVFs was observed. At the last evaluation, favorable outcomes were achieved in 33 patients (82.5%).

Discussion

This study reported on a relatively large series of patients with intracranial dAVFs who underwent direct surgery. All dAVFs were satisfactorily cured by using various surgical approaches, regardless of their location. Once the appropriate obliteration of CVD was achieved via direct surgery, dAVF recurrence became rare. Thus, direct surgery plays an important role in most dAVFs. Although EVT is often considered the predominant primary treatment, direct surgery was selected as the first-line treatment for ethmoidal dAVFs in our cohort. In addition, direct surgery was selected for patients who presented with massive ICH because direct surgery could remove ICH simultaneously in one session of the surgery.

Ethmoidal dAVF

Although EVT is often the first-line treatment modality for most dAVFs, ethmoidal dAVFs are exceptions. Because arterial feeders often arise from the ophthalmic artery, EVT poses a high risk of visual complications. However, it can be treated via direct surgery with a high obliteration rate and low complication rate. According to a recent meta-analysis of 84 patients who were treated with direct surgery, the cure and complication rates were 98.6% and 2.4%, respectively [21]. In contrast, the overall complication rate was 22.2% in a meta-analysis of 27 patients treated with EVT [7]. Another meta-analysis comparing EVT and direct surgery also revealed the superiority of direct surgery to EVT, in which the complete obliteration rate was 47% versus 100%, and the 30-day good outcome was 47% versus 98% [4]. Therefore, direct surgery may be the preferred first-line modality for ethmoidal dAVFs [11].

CVJ and Tentorial dAVF

The role of direct surgery is also important in CVJ and tentorial dAVFs because they may be difficult to obliterate by using EVT. Multiple arterial feeders arise from the internal carotid, vertebral, and radicular arteries, and they are usually very small and tortuous, making catheter access difficult and entailing a risk of ischemic complications. In addition, they often drain exclusively into the subarachnoid veins rather than into their associated sinus (fistula-type dAVF or Borden type III), preventing transvenous access [12, 24]. The overall complication rate of EVT is reportedly 15.8% in CVJ dAVFs and 15.3% in tentorial dAVFs [7]. Recently, a large series of CVJ dAVFs treated via direct surgery were documented as having an angiographic cure rate of 94.7%, a procedural complication rate of 2.6%, and favorable outcomes (mRS 0–2) of 81.6% [15]. According to a systematic review of 56 patients with CVJ dAVFs, direct surgery had a significantly higher initial complete obliteration rate than that of EVT (100% vs. 71.4%) [23]. Therefore, direct surgery may also be the predominant modality for CVJ dAVFs, although further accumulation of cases is needed.

Concerning tentorial dAVF, however, although the obliteration rate of direct surgery is as high as 91.9%, the total complication rate is also as high as 17.2%, according to a meta-analysis of 94 patients [21]. This is not surprising, because tentorial dAVFs are anatomically more complex and deeper than are dAVFs of other sites. Various surgical approaches are required to approach them depending on their location [9]. Additionally, pial arterial supplies are frequently observed in tentorial dAVFs requiring additional coagulation, even during direct surgery [13]. Therefore, a more sophisticated multimodal treatment might be needed for tentorial dAVF [2].

Pial Arterial Supply

Recent studies have revealed that the presence of pial arterial supply is not uncommon, approximately 11.3–23.8% of all dAVFs, and is detected frequently in tentorial and higher-grade dAVFs [6, 13, 14]. This has attracted increasing attention because several studies have revealed that it is a risk factor for both ischemic and hemorrhagic complications during EVT. Therefore, direct surgery may play an important role in the management of dAVFs with pial arterial supply. However, the additional coagulation of the pial arterial supplies after the simple disconnection of CVD is often needed to obliterate the dAVF. In addition, angiographically occult pial arterial supplies were detected through careful intraoperative observation. Therefore, even during direct surgery, the surgeon may have to pay attention to the existence of pial arterial supplies [13].

Massive ICH Presentation

Similar to the case of spontaneous ICH, emergent surgical evacuation is necessary in cases where ICH due to ruptured dAVF has a life-threatening mass effect [22]. However, in the case of arteriovenous malformations (AVMs), the immediate removal of AVMs in the acute phase of ICH onset is generally thought to be associated with higher morbidity and mortality due to brain swelling. Therefore, AVM resection is usually performed 2–6 weeks after the onset or emergent ICH evacuation surgery [17–19]. Although the majority of ruptured dAVFs could be occluded simultaneously during emergent ICH evacuation surgery in this series, further studies are needed to elucidate the optimal timing of surgery for hemorrhagic onset dAVF, as is the case with AVM.

Limitation

As this was a retrospective study including heterogeneous patient cohorts, the results should be interpreted with caution. The prospective accumulation of a large cohort for each dAVF location is expected to elucidate the outcomes of direct surgery for dAVF.

Conclusion

Direct microsurgery plays a crucial role in managing ethmoidal dAVFs and massive ICH. In addition, direct surgery tends to be selected for CVJ as well as tentorial dAVFs with a pial arterial supply. The outcomes of direct surgery are acceptable for various dAVFs; therefore, it can be a feasible option in the endovascular era.

Acknowledgments We thank Editage (www.editage.com) for English language editing.

Author contribution TS contributed to the study conception and design. Data collection was performed by TS, TO, MI, and HU. The first draft of the manuscript was written by TS. MF contributed to supervision of the study. All authors read and approved the final manuscript.

Funding Information None

Data availability The data that support the findings of this study are available from the corresponding author upon reasonable request.

Declarations

Conflict of interest: The authors declare that they have no conflict of interest.

Ethical approval: All procedures performed in studies involving human participants were in accordance with the ethical standards of the institutional and/or national research committee and with the 1964 Helsinki declaration and its later amendments or comparable ethical standards. This study was approved by the Institutional Review Board of Hokkaido University Hospital, Sapporo, Japan (No.017-0074).

Informed consent: Informed consent was obtained from all individual participants included in this study.

References

1. Baltsavias G, Valavanis A, Regli L. Cranial dural arteriovenous shunts: selection of the ideal lesion for surgical occlusion according to the classification system. Acta Neurochir. 2019;161(9):1775–81.
2. Cannizzaro D, Brinjikji W, Rammos S, Murad MH, Lanzino G. Changing clinical and therapeutic trends in tentorial dural arteriovenous fistulas: a systematic review. Am J Neuroradiol. 2015;36(10):1905–11.
3. Chen CJ, Lee CC, Ding D, Starke RM, Chivukula S, Yen CP, Moosa S, Xu Z, Pan DHC, Sheehan JP. Stereotactic radiosurgery for intracranial dural arteriovenous fistulas: a systematic review. J Neurosurg. 2015;122(2):353–62.
4. Giannopoulos S, Texakalidis P, Mohammad Alkhataybeh RA, Charisis N, Rangel-Castilla L, Jabbour P, Grossberg JA, Machinis T. Treatment of ethmoidal dural arteriovenous fistulas: a meta-analysis comparing endovascular versus surgical treatment. World Neurosurg. 2019;128:593–599.e1.
5. Gross BA, Du R. The natural history of cerebral dural arteriovenous fistulae. Neurosurgery. 2012;71(3):594–602.
6. Hetts SW, Yen A, Cooke DL, et al. Pial artery supply as an anatomic risk factor for ischemic stroke in the treatment of intracranial dural arteriovenous fistulas. Am J Neuroradiol. 2017;38(12):2315–20.
7. Hiramatsu M, Sugiu K, Hishikawa T, et al. Results of 1940 embolizations for dural arteriovenous fistulas: Japanese Registry of Neuroendovascular Therapy (JR-NET3). J Neurosurg. 2019;133(1):1–8.
8. Kakarla UK, Deshmukh VR, Zabramski JM, Albuquerque FC, McDougall CG, Spetzler RF. Surgical treatment of high-risk intracranial dural arteriovenous fistulae: clinical outcomes and avoidance of complications. Neurosurgery. 2007;61(3):447–57.
9. Lawton MT, Sanchez-Mejia RO, Pham D, Tan J, Halbach VV. Tentorial dural arteriovenous fistulae: operative strategies and microsurgical results for six types. Neurosurgery. 2008;62(3 Suppl 1):ONS110–25.
10. Lee SK, Hetts SW, Halbach V, et al. Standard and guidelines: intracranial dural arteriovenous shunts. J Neurointerv Surg. 2017;9(5):516–23.
11. Lefevre E, Lenck S, Navarro S, et al. Anterior interhemispheric approach for anterior fossa dural arteriovenous fistulas. Neurosurg Rev. 2022;45(2):1791–7.
12. Li Y, Chen SH, Guniganti R, et al. Onyx embolization for dural arteriovenous fistulas: a multi-institutional study. J Neurointerv Surg. 2021;14(1):57–62.
13. Okamoto M, Sugiyama T, Nakayama N, Ushikoshi S, Kazumata K, Osanai T, Tokairin K, Shimoda Y, Houkin K. Microsurgical findings of pial arterial feeders in intracranial dural arteriovenous fistulae: a case series. Oper Neurosurg. 2020;19(6):691–700.
14. Osada T, Krings T. Intracranial dural arteriovenous fistulas with pial arterial supply. Neurosurgery. 2019;84(1):104–14.
15. Salem MM, Srinivasan VM, Tonetti DA, et al. Microsurgical obliteration of craniocervical junction dural arteriovenous fistulas: Multicenter experience. Neurosurgery. 2023;92(1):205–12.
16. Sato K, Shimizu H, Fujimura M, Inoue T, Matsumoto Y, Tominaga T. Compromise of brain tissue caused by cortical venous reflux of intracranial dural arteriovenous fistulas: assessment with diffusion-weighted magnetic resonance imaging. Stroke. 2011;42(4):998–1003.
17. Sugiyama T, Clapp T, Nelson J, et al. Immersive 3-dimensional virtual reality modeling for case-specific presurgical discussions in cerebrovascular neurosurgery. Oper Neurosurg. 2021;20(3):289–99.
18. Sugiyama T, Gan LS, Zareinia K, Lama S, Sutherland GR. Tool-tissue interaction forces in brain arteriovenous malformation surgery. World Neurosurg. 2017;102:221–8.
19. Sugiyama T, Grasso G, Torregrossa F, Fujimura M. Current concepts and perspectives on brain arteriovenous malformations: a review of pathogenesis and multidisciplinary treatment. World Neurosurg. 2021;159:314–26.
20. Sugiyama T, Kazumata K, Asaoka K, Osanai T, Shimbo D, Uchida K, Yokoyama Y, Nakayama N, Itamoto K, Houkin K. Reappraisal of microsurgical revascularization for anterior circulation isch-

emia in patients with progressive stroke. World Neurosurg. 2015;84(6):1579–88.
21. Sugiyama T, Nakayama N, Ushikoshi S, et al. Complication rate, cure rate, and long-term outcomes of microsurgery for intracranial dural arteriovenous fistulae: a multicenter series and systematic review. Neurosurg Rev. 2021;44(1):435–50.
22. Sun W, Germans MR, Sebök M, Fierstra J, Kulcsar Z, Keller A, Regli L. Outcome comparison between surgically treated brain arteriovenous malformation hemorrhage and spontaneous intracerebral hemorrhage. World Neurosurg. 2020;139:e807–11.
23. Zhao J, Xu F, Ren J, Manjila S, Bambakidis NC. Dural arteriovenous fistulas at the craniocervical junction: a systematic review. J Neurointerv Surg. 2016;8(6):648–53.
24. Zhong W, Zhang J, Shen J, Su W, Wang D, Zhang P, Wang Y. Dural arteriovenous fistulas at the craniocervical junction: a series case report. World Neurosurg. 2019;122:e700–12.

Open Access This chapter is licensed under the terms of the Creative Commons Attribution 4.0 International License (http://creativecommons.org/licenses/by/4.0/), which permits use, sharing, adaptation, distribution and reproduction in any medium or format, as long as you give appropriate credit to the original author(s) and the source, provide a link to the Creative Commons license and indicate if changes were made.

The images or other third party material in this chapter are included in the chapter's Creative Commons license, unless indicated otherwise in a credit line to the material. If material is not included in the chapter's Creative Commons license and your intended use is not permitted by statutory regulation or exceeds the permitted use, you will need to obtain permission directly from the copyright holder.

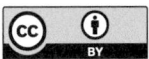

Paraspinal Arteriovenous Shunt Associated with PTEN Hamartoma Tumor Syndrome: A Case Report and Literature Review

Sayaka Ito and Naoki Hatsuda

Introduction

Having a paraspinal arteriovenous shunt (PAVS) located in the paraspinal region outside the spinal canal is rare [4, 8]. The incidence of PAVS is reported to be below 5% of spinal dural arteriovenous fistulas [9]. Germline mutations have been noted in specific PAVS cases [9]. Germline mutations in the phosphatase and tensin homolog (PTEN) gene cause PTEN hamartoma tumor syndrome (PHTS), which is characterized by various hamartomatous lesions in the skin, mucosa, gastrointestinal tract, breast, thyroid gland, endometrium, and brain. PHTS is an autosomal-dominant disorder. The majority of patients with PHTS might present with macrocephaly and multiple mucocutaneous lesions before their late 20s. Some pediatric patients with autism disorders or learning disabilities might be diagnosed with PHTS associated with other characteristic features, such as macrocephaly. Recently, multigene panel testing has allowed the differential diagnosis of PHTS in candidates without any syndrome other than cancers [6]. Herein, we report a case of an asymptomatic PAVS with multiple primary cancers, subsequently diagnosed with PHTS. The aim of this study was to elucidate strategies for identifying the features and comorbidities of PHTS and for diagnosing it.

Case Illustration

A 57-year-old woman was referred to our clinic with a mass in the parathoracic region. She was neurologically asymptomatic. Her mental state and visual appearance were also normal, and the laboratory data were unremarkable. Her parents had no apparently relevant medical history of cancer or vascular diseases. She had breast cancer for 17 years. Her breast cancer was surgically resected. Rib metastases were subsequently resolved via chemotherapy with an aromatase-inhibiting drug. She also had endometrial cancer for 14 years, which was totally resected with no recurrence. She had the comorbidities of an arteriovenous malformation on her lower leg, which had been partially embolized; hepatic cavernous malformation, which had been completely embolized; lung hamartoma; and a mass lesion in the thyroid gland, all of which were under observation. Computed tomography (CT) revealed a paraspinal mass lesion with a osteolytic appearance at the root of the right eighth costal bone and the right eighth lamina (Fig. 1a), which a CT obtained 1 year before presenting as normal. Magnetic resonance imaging (MRI) revealed a lesion with low intensity on T1- and T2-weighted images severely compressing the spinal cord (Fig. 1b). The lesions were homogenously enhanced (Fig. 1c). We suspected bone metastasis from the malignant tumor, and differential diagnoses included vascular lesions. We planned a laminectomy of the affected bone and a resection of the surrounding ligament and soft tissues. The surgical intervention might have been advantageous for confirming the pathological diagnosis compared to the associated perioperative risks. Under general anesthesia, a right T8 hemilaminectomy was performed. When we approached the right collapsed T8 lamina, a pulsatile mass with a tough fibrous membrane through the fenestrated lamina was observed. The surrounding ligaments, bones, and other soft tissues were resected as much as possible. Although these tissues bled easily, hemostasis could be achieved. We decided to withdraw further resection because a vascular lesion with a high-flow shunt was strongly suspected. If necessary, we could perform elective secondary surgery after confirming the diagnosis.

The postoperative course was uneventful. A spinal angiography and transarterial embolization was performed following the operation. A high-flow arteriovenous shunt in the paraspinal region was observed. The shunting point was located at the right T8 intervertebral foramen, and it was fed

S. Ito (✉) · N. Hatsuda
Department of Neurosurgery, Kohka Public Hospital, Minakuchi, Kohka, Shiga, Japan

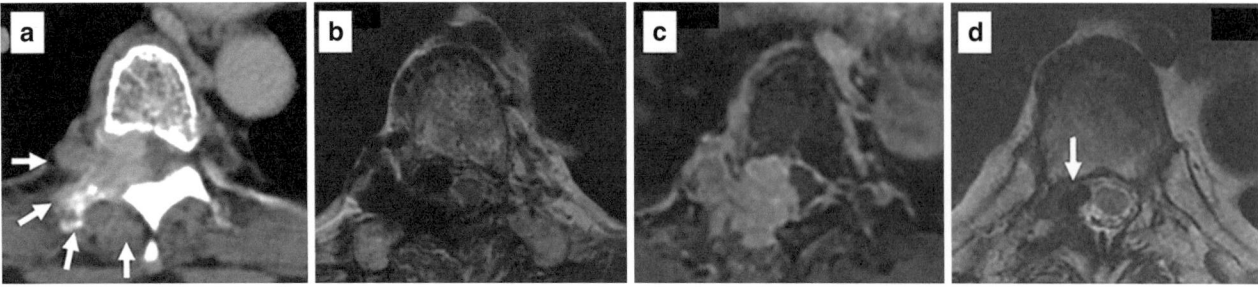

Fig. 1 (a) Contrast-enhanced CT scan obtained before surgery showing osteolytic contrast-enhanced mass lesion in the Th8 level (white arrows). (b) T2-weighted MRI obtained before surgery showing a low intensity mass in the right lateral paravertebral space in Th8 level. (c) Enhanced T1-weighted MRI before surgery showing an enhanced paravertebral mass severely compressing the spinal cord at the Th8 level. (d) T2-weighted MRI after surgery and transarterial embolization showing the shrinkage of the mass lesion (white arrow) and the reduction of the cord compression

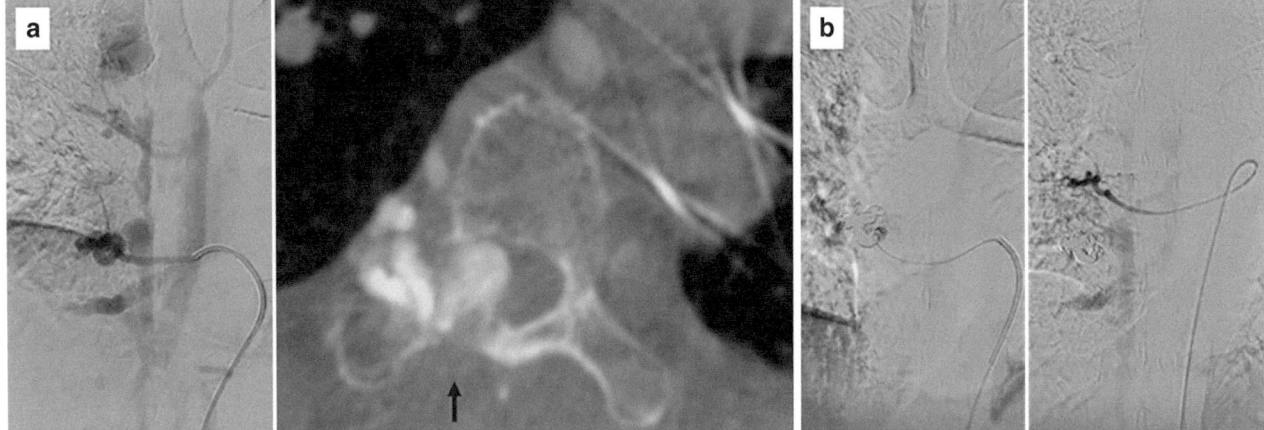

Fig. 2 (a) Right 8th intercostal arteriography showing an arteriovenous shunt at the right Th8 intervertebral foramen (left). A cone-beam CT demonstrating a dilated vein and epidural venous plexus (right/ black arrow). (b) Transarterial embolization using glue via the right 8th intercostal artery. The arteriovenous shunt was remarkably reduced following the embolization

mainly by the right eighth intercostal artery, draining into the epidural venous plexus and finally into the azygos vein through the right T5, 6, 7, 8, and 9 radicular veins. Distal to the shunting point, a large varix extended into the spinal canal (Fig. 2a). The shunt was also fed by the bilateral fifth, sixth, seventh, and ninth and the left eighth intercostal arteries. The transarterial embolization of the main feeding artery achieved flow reduction in the arteriovenous shunt (Fig. 2b). A postoperative MRI revealed that cord compression by the dilated vein was relieved (Fig. 1d). A germline PTEN mutation was detected in her blood sample, which led to a diagnosis of PHTS. The patient was involved in the cancer surveillance program.

Discussion

PAVS is a rare disease located outside the spinal canal and may be responsible for neurological symptoms due to cord compression by ectatic veins, venous congestion, or arterial stealing [8]. Clinical studies on PAVS are limited to case reports or case series. In 2021, Kim et al. conducted a systematic review and meta-analysis of the prognosis of PAVS patients [4], and Feng et al. carried out a cohort study on the natural history of PAVS [2]. In the meta-analysis of a systematic review of patients with traumatic or nontraumatic PAVS, Kim et al. reported systemic or genetic etiology and treatment. Multiple feeders worsened the prognosis of patients with PAVS, and the favored factor was traumatic etiology [4]. Feng et al. reported that PAVS patients with intradural reflux showed significantly worse neurological outcomes regarding gait independence and bladder function than their PAVS cohort without intradural reflux [2]. The etiology and clinical manifestations of PAVS remain unknown, and the treatment strategies are still unclear. A previous study reported that a nontraumatic PAVS with germline PTEN mutation associated with Lhermitte–Duclos disease was listed as a major "PHTS clinical diagnostic criteria." The National Comprehensive Cancer Network has established the testing criteria of PTEN testing on the basis of the clinical features of a patient [1]. The "revised PHTS clinical diagnostic criteria" aim to help clinicians make decisions [1, 6, 7]. Germline PTEN mutations result in cancers restricted to specific organs, including the breast, thyroid gland, endometrium, colon, and kidney [5]. Early diagnosis may enable the timely inclusion of patients in surveillance programs for early cancer diagnosis, and this can improve their prognosis and life expectancy [3]. Diagnoses of adult patients are occasionally not easy because of the broad range of clinical symptoms and various major and minor criteria. Drissen et al. attempted to reduce underdiagnosis for at-risk patients. They concluded that macrocephaly, multinodular goiter, and multiple oral features serve as red flags that should prompt further assessment for PHTS in adults [1]. The early onset of surveillance would greatly benefit strongly suspected candidates [3]. Recently, two types of PHTS have been elucidated: hereditary and de novo. De novo PHTSs might be more difficult to reach a diagnosis for, as seen in our patients, because of the lack of family history. The present case did not meet the revised clinical diagnostic criteria for PTEN hamartoma tumor syndrome; the existence of multiple primary cancers and arteriovenous shunt, however, strongly prompted us to test the patient for germline PTEN mutations. Finally, a pathogenic variant was detected in the patient's blood sample, confirming the diagnosis of PHTS. Genetic testing is recommended whenever possible to confirm a clinical diagnosis [6]. Because our patient showed germline PTEN mutations, PHTS could be confirmed. Even if the patient does not manifest any specific phenotypic presentation or has any abnormal development or family history, the coexistence of multiple primary cancers and vascular malformation would be red flags for PHTS. More PHTS cases need to be accumulated to gain a better understanding of the pathology and clinical manifestations of PHTS.

Acknowledgments We thank Editage (www.editage.com) for English language editing.

Author contributions All authors contributed to the study conception and design. Material preparation, data collection, and data analysis were performed by Sayaka Ito. The first draft of the manuscript was written by Sayaka Ito, and all authors commented on a previous version of the manuscript. All authors read and approved the final manuscript.

Funding Information No funds, grants, or other support was received.

Data availability Data can be provided by the corresponding author upon request.

Declarations

Competing interests: The authors declare that they have no conflicts of interest.

Consent: The patient signed informed consent regarding publishing her data and photographs.

References

1. Drissen MMCM, Schieving JH, Schuurs-Hoeijmakers JHM, Vos JR, Hoogerbrugge N. Red flags for early recognition of adult patients with PTEN Hamartoma Tumour Syndrome. Eur J Med Genet. 2021;64(12):104364.
2. Feng Y, Yu J, Xu J, He C, Bian L, Li G, Ye M, Hu P, Sun L, Jiang N, Ling F, Hong T, Zhang H. Natural history and clinical outcomes of paravertebral arteriovenous shunts. Stroke. 2021;52(12):3873–82.
3. Hendricks LAJ, Schuurs-Hoeijmakers J, Spier I, Haadsma ML, Eijkelenboom A, Cremer K, Mensenkamp AR, Aretz S, Vos JR, Hoogerbrugge N. Catch them if you are aware: PTEN postzygotic mosaicism in clinically suspicious patients with PTEN Hamartoma Tumour Syndrome and literature review. Eur J Med Genet. 2022;65(7):104533.
4. Kim JH, Yoon SH, Park SQ, Ban SP, Cho BK. Clinical features and treatment strategy of paraspinal arteriovenous shunt (PAVS): a systematic review with individual participants data meta-analysis. Eur Spine J. 2021;30(8):2385–400.
5. Ngeow J, Eng C. PTEN in hereditary and sporadic cancer. Cold Spring Harb Perspect Med. 2020;10(4):a036087.
6. Pilarski R, Burt R, Kohlman W, Pho L, Shannon KM, Swisher E. Cowden syndrome and the PTEN hamartoma tumor syndrome: systematic review and revised diagnostic criteria. J Natl Cancer Inst. 2013;105(21):1607–16.
7. Pilarski R, Stephens JA, Noss R, Fisher JL, Prior TW. Predicting PTEN mutations: an evaluation of Cowden syndrome and Bannayan-Riley-Ruvalcaba syndrome clinical features. J Med Genet. 2011;48(8):505–12.
8. Rodesch G, Lasjaunias P. Spinal cord arteriovenous shunts: from imaging to management. Eur J Radiol. 2003;46(3):221–32.
9. Wendl CM, Aguilar Pérez M, Felber S, Stroszczynski C, Bäzner H, Henkes H. Paraspinal arteriovenous fistula: Stuttgart classification based on experience and a review of the literature. Br J Radiol. 2018;91(1088):20170337.

Open Access This chapter is licensed under the terms of the Creative Commons Attribution 4.0 International License (http://creativecommons.org/licenses/by/4.0/), which permits use, sharing, adaptation, distribution and reproduction in any medium or format, as long as you give appropriate credit to the original author(s) and the source, provide a link to the Creative Commons license and indicate if changes were made.

The images or other third party material in this chapter are included in the chapter's Creative Commons license, unless indicated otherwise in a credit line to the material. If material is not included in the chapter's Creative Commons license and your intended use is not permitted by statutory regulation or exceeds the permitted use, you will need to obtain permission directly from the copyright holder.

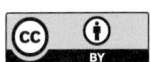

Efficacy of High-Resolution Cone-Beam CT for the Endovascular Treatment of Dural Arteriovenous Fistulas

Michihiro Tanaka, Keisuke Kadooka, Takafumi Mitsutake, Shimpei Tsuboki, and Kotaro Ueda

Abbreviations

DAVF dural arteriovenous fistula
CT computed tomography
DSA digital subtraction angiography
CBCT cone-beam CT

Introduction

A dural arteriovenous fistula (DAVF) is an abnormal connection between arteries and veins in the membrane covering the brain and spinal cord, called the dura mater [2, 4, 5, 8–10, 12, 13, 23]. Normally, blood flows from arteries to capillaries to veins, but in a DAVF, the direct connection between the artery and vein bypasses the capillary bed, leading to abnormal blood flow and pressure changes in the veins. With recent advancements in CBCT technology, the detailed microanatomy of complex shunt diseases with intricate vascular structures can now be depicted [15, 22, 24–26]. However, differences remain in the operation and imaging protocols of CBCT across facilities, and many facilities are not fully utilizing the potential performance of CBCT. In this study, we retrospectively examined the usefulness of CBCT in dural arteriovenous fistulas.

Case Materials and Methods

Case Materials

In this study, 83 cases of dural arteriovenous fistula performed between 2013 and 2021 were included. The mean age of the patients was 61.3 years, with 39 male and 44 female patients. The shunt sites included carotid cavernous fistula (26 cases), transverse-sigmoid junction (19 cases), olfactory groove (cribriform plate) (5 cases), tentorial sinus (5 cases), anterior condylar confluence (hypoglossal canal) (4 cases), falx (3 cases), spinal dural AVF (19 cases), and spinal epidural AVF (2 cases) (Table 1).

M. Tanaka (✉) · K. Kadooka · T. Mitsutake · S. Tsuboki · K. Ueda
Department of Neuroendovascular Surgery, Kameda Medical Center, Kamogawa City, Chiba Prefecture, Japan

Practice and Technical Points of Angiography

For transarterial contrast injection, a 4 French catheter was utilized via a femoral artery under local anesthesia or general anesthesia. The catheter was advanced to the targeted cervical segment through the internal carotid artery, external carotid artery, or the vertebral artery. In the case of an AV shunt predominantly supplied from ascending pharyngeal artery or occipital artery, the tip of the catheter was placed into each pedicle of these feeding arteries. The initial positioning of the C-arm and table was centered on the lesion. Contrast injections were performed with an automated contrast injector (Nemoto Kyorindo co., Ltd.) with a nonionic contrast medium (Iopamiron370; Iopamidol, Bayer-Schering, Berlin, Germany).

Table 1 The anatomical site of the shunt point

Location of shunt	
Carotid cavernous fistula	26
Transverse-sigmoid junction	19
Olfactory groove (cribriform plate)	5
Tentorial sinus	5
Anterior condylar confluence (hypoglossal canal)	4
Falx (SSS)	3
Spinal dural AVF	19
Spinal epidural AVF	2
Total	83

Protocol for CBCT

We utilized the Allura Xper FD20/20 system (Philips Healthcare, Best, the Netherlands) for X-ray angiography. The imaging modality, Xper CT, was achieved through the integration of a CBCT imaging system and a flat detector, with acquisition protocols and postprocessing algorithms being embedded within the system. Imaging via the Xper CT system involved the motorized rotational movement (propeller scan) of a C-arm perpendicular to the longitudinal table axis. The Xper CT system, featuring high-resolution 80-kV X-ray imaging capabilities, obtained 620 fluoroscopic frames through a circular motion over a total rotation time of 20 seconds and an angle of 240° (±120°), at a rotation speed of 22°/s, utilizing a 1024 × 1024 pixel matrix detector with an 8-inch field of view and a low 80 kV tube voltage. The patient's head was positioned at the isocenter of the system, and a propeller C-arm scan was performed. The dataset was automatically transferred, via a real-time digital link, to the three-dimensional (3D) workstation (Xtravision; Philips Healthcare) for processing during the propeller acquisition movement. The reconstructed 3D volume image, with a default reconstruction size of 256^3 pixels, was available in under 1 minute. Various types of image postprocessing techniques, including beam hardening and scatter corrections, were employed to achieve optimal spatial and contrast-resolution qualities. In CBCT imaging, knowing the arrival time of the contrast agent at the target lesion or shunt point that needs to be visualized is important. This arrival time can be measured by performing a conventional digital subtraction angiography (DSA) prior to CBCT imaging and then determining the timing at which the target lesion is best visualized. The time in seconds can then be set as a parameter on the contrast agent injection device to optimize the imaging conditions.

Results

In 83 cases, shunt point identification was possible in 68 cases (81.9%) via conventional cerebral angiography, whereas it was possible in 80 cases (96.3%) via CBCT. The shunt point could not be accurately identified in two cases of multiple shunts with clustered terminal feeders at the transverse-sigmoid junction and a case of falx dural AVF with expanded cortical veins near the shunt. CBCT imaging with contrast from a microcatheter clearly visualized the target lesions and surrounding venous sinuses, providing useful information for treatment strategies and the selection of embolic agents. Additionally, CBCT was superior in depicting terminal feeders running through the bone structure around the transverse-sigmoid junction and vascular structures within the hypoglossal canal.

Postoperative evaluation using a liquid embolic agent mixed with lipiodol and N-butyl cyanoacrylate (NBCA) showed a clear visualization of the distribution of the embolic agent and surrounding venous sinus structures.

Case Illustrations

Case 1

A 75-year-old woman presented with diplopia and chemosis on her left eye. Left common carotid angiography showed early venous filling in the cavernous sinus. The right superficial middle cerebral vein was also affected with venous hypertension, which falls into the category of Borden Type II or Cognard Type IIa+b dural AVF (Fig. 1a, b). A transvenous approach was performed. The shunt point was completely obliterated with a few platinum coils. The precise mapping of the target lesion based on the CBCT enabled the strategy of embolization to be effectively planned (Fig. 1c, d). A couple of days after embolization, her diplopia and chemosis improved markedly.

Case 2

A 56-year-old man was incidentally detected as having an olfactory groove dural AVF during the embolization of an anterior choroidal artery unruptured aneurysm (Fig. 2a, b).

CBCT showed the shunt point at the level of the cribriform plate (Fig. 2c, d). These high-resolution images provided the precise location and caliber of the initial foot of the draining vein. On the basis of this modality, successful superselective target embolization was achieved with the transvenous approach (Fig. 2e–g).

Case 3

A 64-year-old woman presented with the sudden onset of headache and vomiting. Emergency CT showed subarachnoid hemorrhage predominantly distributed in the craniocervical junction and posterior fossa (Fig. 3a). The right vertebral angiography showed early venous filling at the

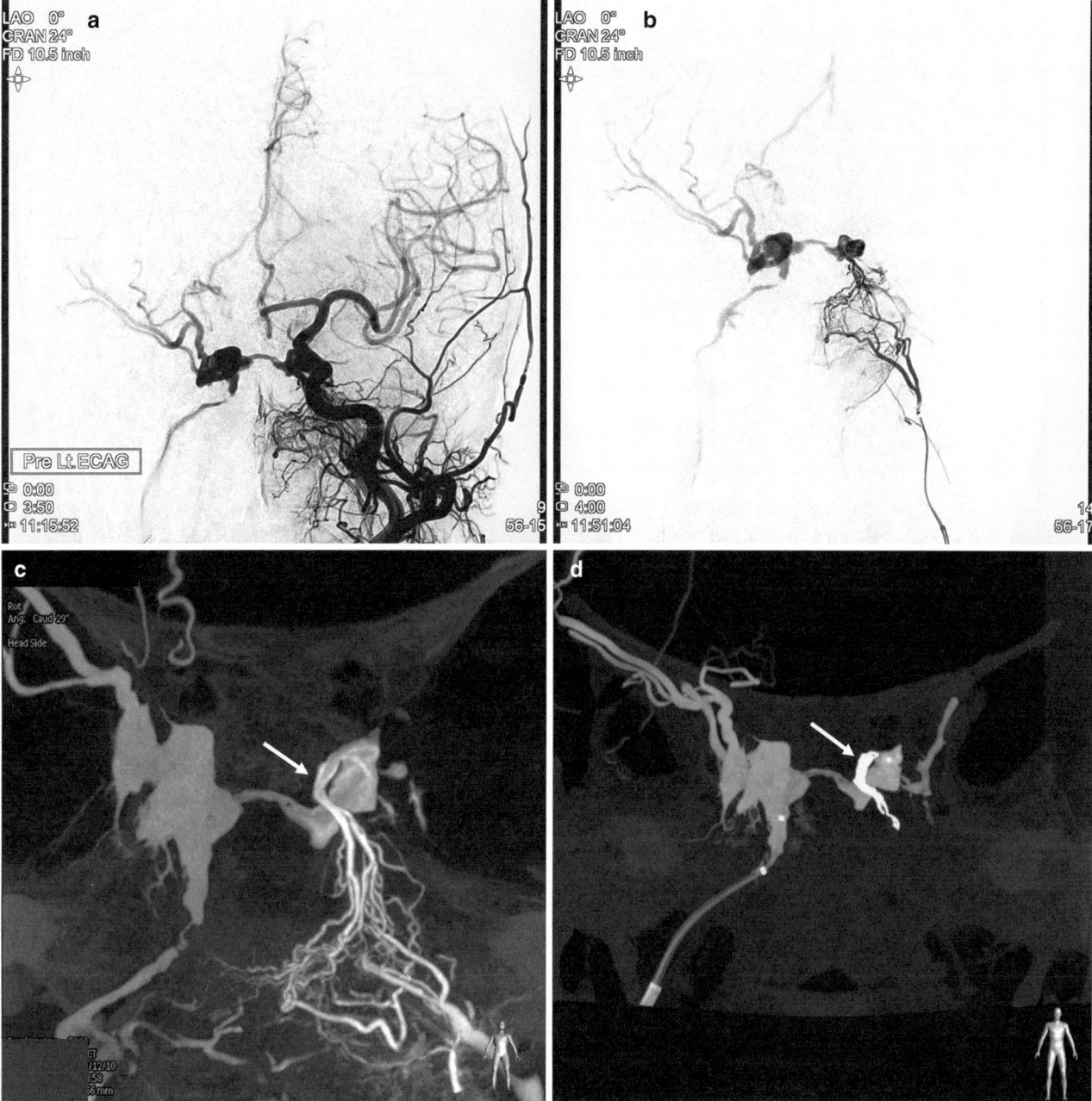

Fig. 1 (a) Angiography of the left common carotid artery demonstrating early venous filling in the cavernous sinus. Venous hypertension also affected the right superficial middle cerebral vein, indicating a dural AVF classified as Borden Type II or Cognard Type IIa+b. (b) Selective injection from the left ascending pharyngeal artery. The shunt was supplied mainly by the superior pharyngeal branch, and the cluster of terminal feeders was clearly visible. (c) CBCT with selective injection from the left ascending pharyngeal artery. The caliber change indicates the precise anatomical location of the shunt point (white arrow). (d) CBCT showing the deposition of platinum coils in the shunt point

level of the right C1 nerve root with a pathological dilatation of the anterior medullary vein (Fig. 3b). Superselective angiography from the right radiculo-medullary artery showed a small arteriovenous (AV) shunt draining to the anterior medullary vein and ponto-medullary vein (Fig. 3c). High-resolution CBCT showed the pathologically dilated vein locating the ventral aspect of the medulla oblongata (Fig. 3d, e).

Embolization with glue (12% concentration of NBCA mixture with lipiodol) was performed, and the CBCT after embolization showed the appropriate deposition of the glue including the initial foot of the bridging vein (Fig. 3f, g). The control angiography showed the complete obliteration of the AV shunt while preserving the entire anterior spinal artery (Fig. 3h). The patient recovered well without any neurological symptoms.

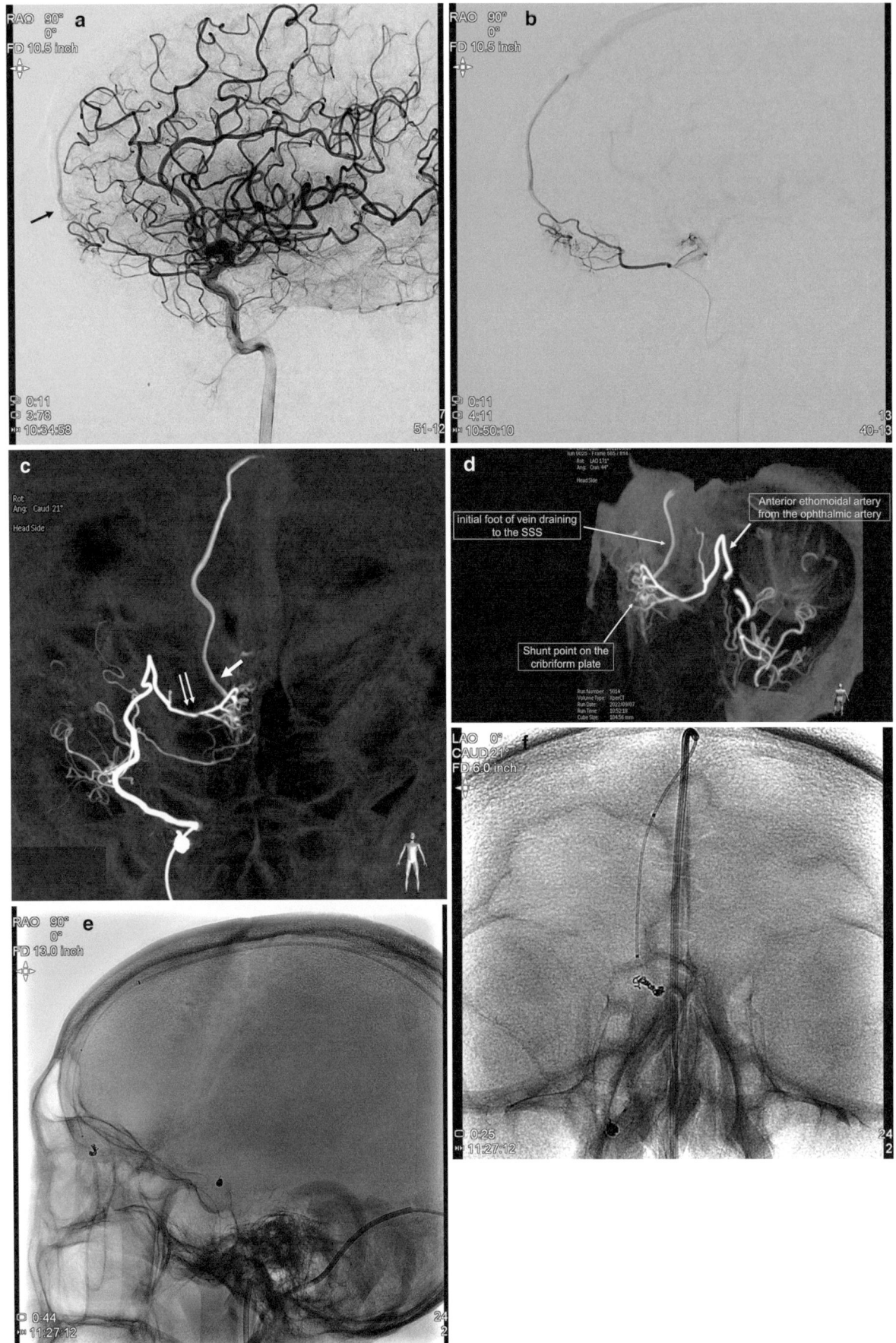

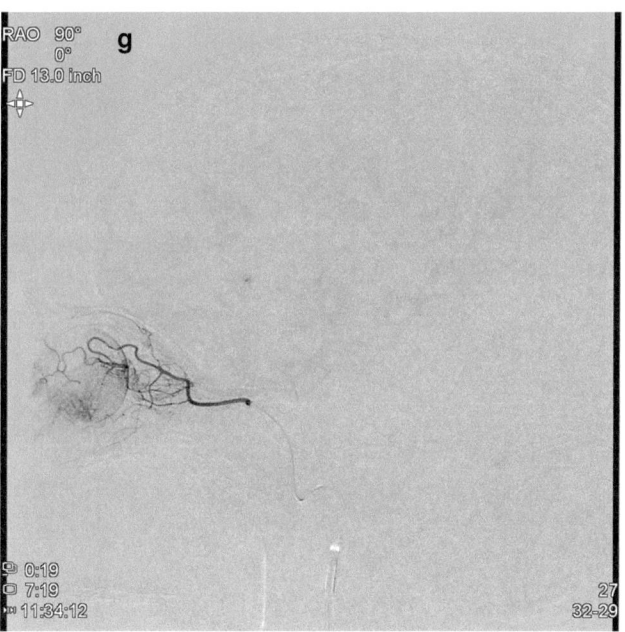

Fig. 2 (continued)

Fig. 2 (**a**) The lateral view of internal carotid angiography displayed the early venous filling at the level of the olfactory groove (arrow). (**b**) Superselective angiography from the right ophthalmic artery in a lateral view demonstrated the early venous filling at the olfactory groove. (**c**) CBCT in conjunction with superselective angiography from the right ophthalmic artery revealed the anterior ethmoidal artery supplying the dural AVF (double arrows) and the initial foot of the draining vein (arrow). (**d**) CBCT illustrated the anatomical structures surrounding the shunt point. (**e**) The transvenous approach with a distal access catheter was visible on the skull X-ray. The catheter reached the cribriform plate level via the superior sagittal sinus from the jugular vein. The microcatheter's tip reached the shunt point, and the white arrow indicates the deposition of platinum coils in the initial foot of the vein. (**f**) The platinum coils' deposition in the initial foot of the vein is displayed on the skull X-ray. (**g**) Postoperative superselective angiography from the ophthalmic artery demonstrates the complete obliteration of the shunt while preserving the entire central retinal artery

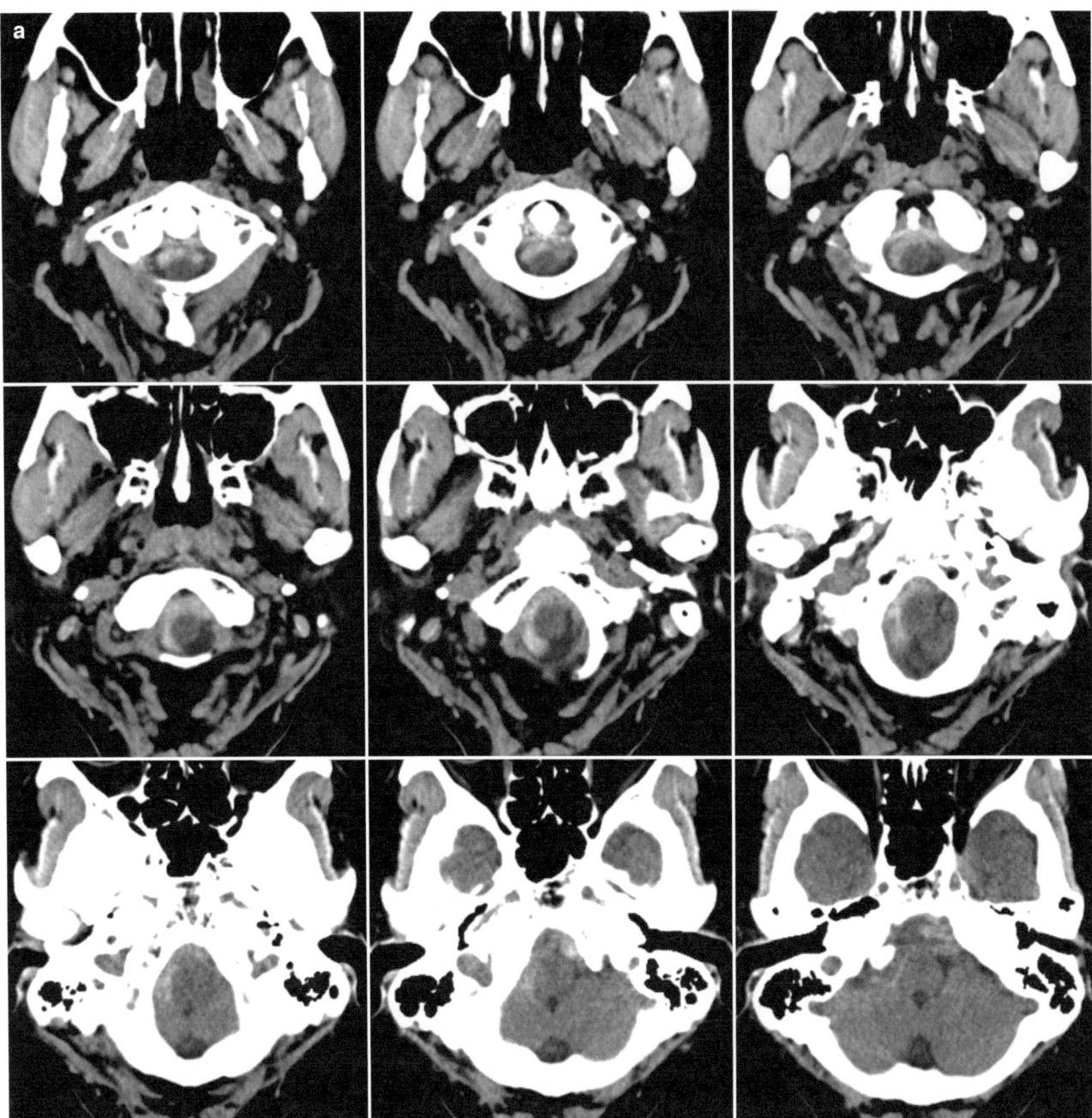

Fig. 3 (a) The plain CT scan revealed a high-density lesion primarily in the cisternal space at the level of the craniocervical junction, indicating a subarachnoid hemorrhage. (b) The right vertebral artery angiogram demonstrated early venous filling with a pathologically dilated perimedullary vein at the level of the craniocervical junction. (c) The superselective angiogram of the right radiculo-meningeal artery at the level of the C1 spinal cord displayed early venous filling into the perimedullary vein. Notably, there was pathological dilation of the anterior medullary vein, anterior pontine vein, and right petrosal vein (arrow). (d) The 3D rotational angiography illustrated the pathologically dilated vein located at the ventral aspect of the medulla oblongata. (e) The cone-beam computed tomography (CBCT) with superselective angiography from the radiculo-meningeal artery showed the arteriovenous (AV) shunt at the level of the right C1 nerve root (white arrow). (f) The axial view of the postoperative CBCT exhibited the cast of embolic material distributed at the shunt point, corresponding to the level of the right cervical spinal nerve C1 (white arrow). (g) The frontal view of the postoperative CBCT displayed the cast of embolic material distributed at the shunt point, as well as the initial foot of the vein (white arrow). (h) Postoperative right vertebral angiography showed the complete obliteration of the shunt while preserving the anterior spinal artery

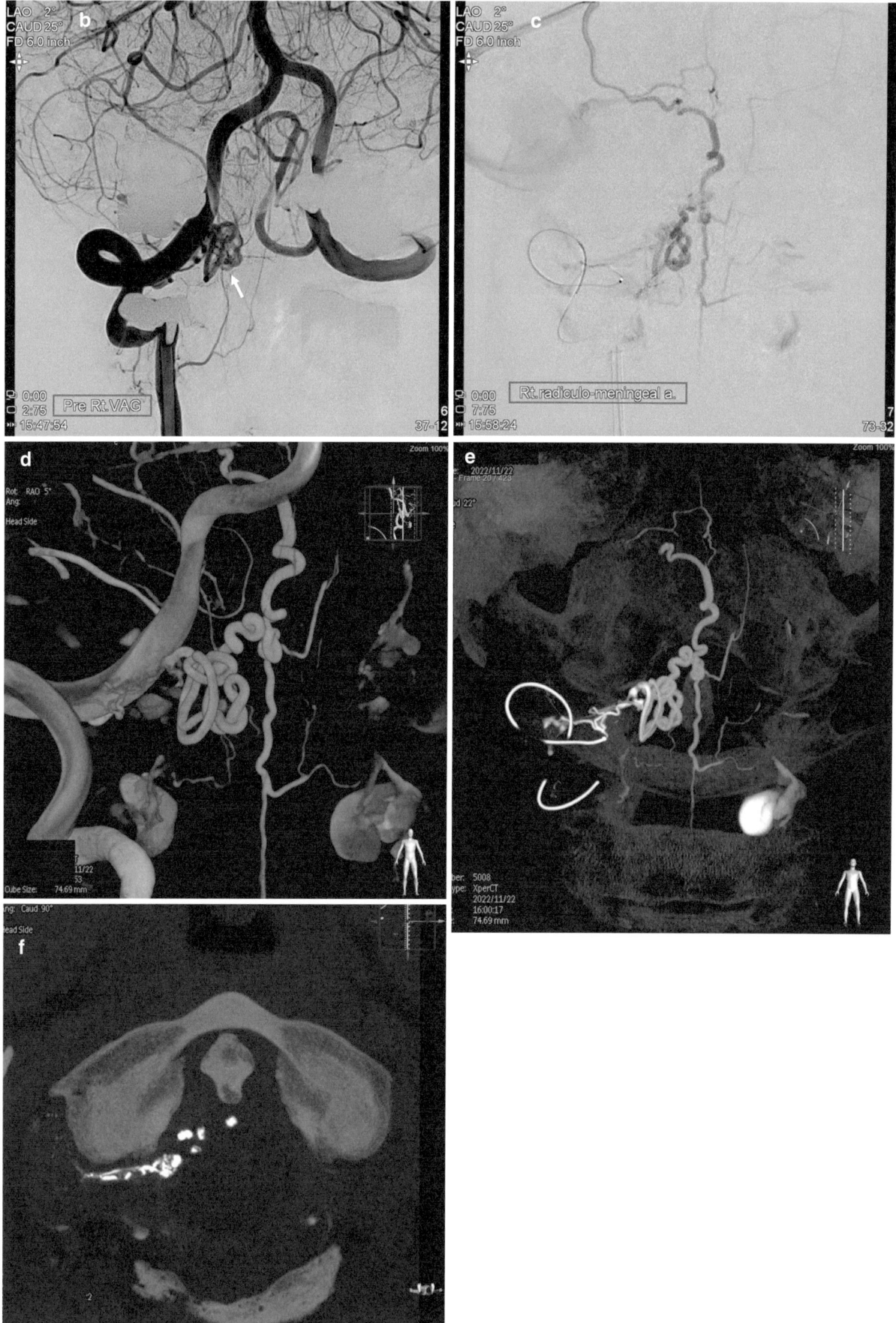

Fig. 3 (continued)

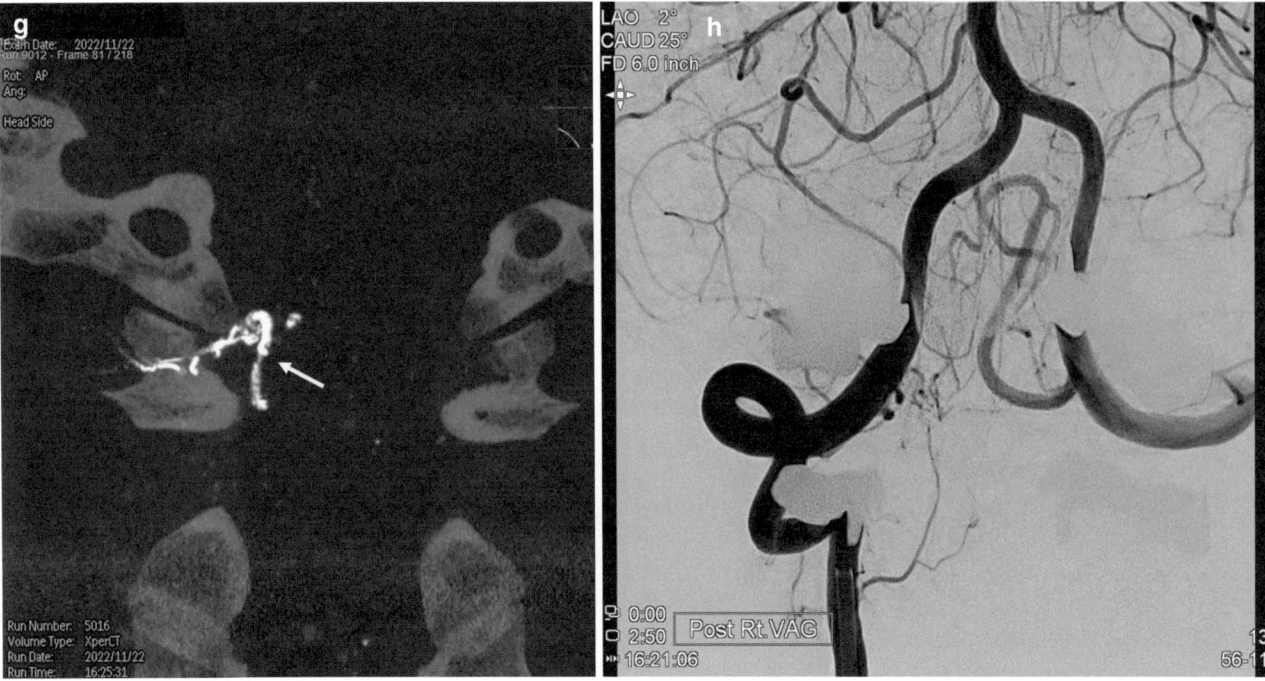

Fig. 3 (continued)

Discussion

CBCT technology differs from traditional computed tomography (CT) scans in several ways. Traditional CT scans use a fan-shaped X-ray beam that rotates around the body to create a series of two-dimensional (2D) images that are then assembled into a three-dimensional image [6, 11, 17, 18, 26]. In contrast, CBCT uses a cone-shaped X-ray beam that is rotated around the patient to capture images in a single rotation. This allows for the creation of a three-dimensional image with a single scan, resulting in faster imaging times and lower radiation exposure compared to traditional CT scans. CBCT imaging can be used to visualize structures such as bones, teeth, soft tissues, and blood vessels. It is particularly useful in dentistry for the diagnosis and treatment planning of dental implants, orthodontics, and oral surgery. In other medical fields, CBCT is used for preoperative planning, for postoperative assessment, and to guide minimally invasive procedures.

instruments and plates for spinal surgery, or clusters of platinum coils used in aneurysm treatment [7, 14, 16, 20, 21]. Although recent algorithm improvements and software advancements have introduced features such as metal artifact reduction to address these issues, they have yet to achieve practical effectiveness [1, 16]. Additionally, to obtain high-resolution images, a 20-second rotational imaging scan must be performed, which can lead to image degradation due to patient movement and difficulty in distinguishing between arterial and venous phases. The spatial resolution of CBCT currently used in clinical settings is limited by the number of pixels in the semiconductor elements that make up the flat panel detector and the algorithm used during image acquisition. Even with a voxel matrix of $512 \times 512 \times 512$ and an acquisition time of 20 seconds, the minimum spatial resolution is only about 0.15–0.43 isotropic mm as a voxel size, which may not be sufficient for delineating target lesions [3, 19, 27, 28]. The further development of and further improvements in flat panel detectors are necessary to depict microscopic anatomy at high resolution.

Limitations of Current CBCT Technology

The disadvantage of CBCT is the beam-hardening effect, which can cause artifacts in the imaging of the region of interest, particularly in the presence of venous varices near the shunt point or with the presence of dental implants,

Conclusion

Overall, CBCT is a valuable tool in medical imaging that provides high-quality three-dimensional images with minimal radiation exposure, allowing for accurate diagnosis and treatment planning for intracranial and spinal cord dural AVFs.

Declarations

Conflict of interest: The author has no potential conflict of interest to disclose.

Ethics and Patient Consent: We hereby declare that all human studies have received approval from the local Ethics Committee and were conducted in compliance with the ethical standards prescribed in the 1964 Declaration of Helsinki and its subsequent amendments. Informed consent from patients or their family members was obtained for CBCT studies; however, patient consent was waived for this retrospective study.

References

1. van der Bom IMJ, Hou SY, Puri AS, Spilberg G, Ruijters D, van de Haar P, Carelsen B, Vedantham S, Gounis MJ, Wakhloo AK. Reduction of coil mass artifacts in high-resolution flat detector conebeam CT of cerebral stent-assisted coiling. AJNR Am J Neuroradiol. 2013;34(11):2163–70.
2. Borden JA, Wu JK, Shucart WA. A proposed classification for spinal and cranial dural arteriovenous fistulous malformations and implications for treatment. J Neurosurg. 1995;82(2):166–79.
3. Brüllmann D, Schulze RKW. Spatial resolution in CBCT machines for dental/maxillofacial applications-what do we know today? Dentomaxillofac Radiol. 2015;44(1):20140204.
4. Cognard C, Casasco A, Toevi M, Houdart E, Chiras J, Merland JJ. Dural arteriovenous fistulas as a cause of intracranial hypertension due to impairment of cranial venous outflow. J Neurol Neurosurg Psychiatry. 1998;65(3):308–16.
5. Cognard C, Gobin YP, Pierot L, Bailly AL, Houdart E, Casasco A, Chiras J, Merland JJ. Cerebral dural arteriovenous fistulas: clinical and angiographic correlation with a revised classification of venous drainage. Radiology. 1995;194(3):671–80.
6. Crockett MT, Chiu AHY, Singh TP, McAuliffe W, Phillips TJ. Transvenous coil embolization with intra-operative cone beam CT assistance in the treatment of hypoglossal canal dural arteriovenous fistulae. J Neurointerv Surg. 2019;11(2):179–83.
7. Esmaeili F, Johari M, Haddadi P, Vatankhah M. Beam hardening Artifacts: comparison between two cone beam computed tomography scanners. J Dent Res Dent Clin Dent Prospects. 2012;6(2):49–53.
8. Gandhi D, Chen J, Pearl M, Huang J, Gemmete JJ, Kathuria S. Intracranial dural arteriovenous fistulas: classification, imaging findings, and treatment. AJNR Am J Neuroradiol. 2012;33(6):1007–13.
9. Gomez J, Amin AG, Gregg L, Gailloud P. Classification schemes of cranial dural arteriovenous fistulas. Neurosurg Clin N Am. 2012;23(1):55–62.
10. Gross BA, Du R. The natural history of cerebral dural arteriovenous fistulae. Neurosurgery. 2012;71(3):594–602.
11. Hayashi N, Tomura N, Okada H, Sasaki T, Tsuji E, Enomoto H, Kuwata T. Usefulness of preoperative cone beam computed tomography and intraoperative digital subtraction angiography for dural arteriovenous fistula at craniocervical junction: technical case report. Surg Neurol Int. 2019;10:5.
12. Hellstern V, Aguilar-Pérez M, Schob S, Bhogal P, AlMatter M, Kurucz P, Grimm A, Henkes H. Endovascular treatment of Dural arteriovenous fistulas of the anterior or posterior condylar vein: a cadaveric and clinical study and literature review. Clin Neuroradiol. 2019;29(2):341–9.
13. Herman JM, Spetzler RF, Bederson JB, Kurbat JM, Zabramski JM. Genesis of a dural arteriovenous malformation in a rat model. J Neurosurg. 1995;83(3):539–45.
14. Honarmand AR, Gemmete JJ, Hurley MC, Shaibani A, Chaudhary N, Pandey AS, Bendok BR, Ansari SA. Adjunctive value of intra-arterial cone beam CT angiography relative to DSA in the evaluation of cranial and spinal arteriovenous fistulas. J Neurointerv Surg. 2015;7:517. https://doi.org/10.1136/neurintsurg-2014-011139.
15. Kadooka K, Tanaka M, Sakata Y, Ideguchi M, Inaba M, Hadeishi H. Efficacy of cone beam computed tomography in treating cavernous sinus Dural arteriovenous fistula. World Neurosurg. 2018;109:328–32.
16. Kunz AS, Patzer TS, Grunz J-P, et al. Metal artifact reduction in ultra-high-resolution cone-beam CT imaging with a twin robotic X-ray system. Sci Rep. 2022;12(1):15549.
17. Mizutani K, Akiyama K, Minami Y, Toda M, Fujiwara H, Jinzaki M, Yoshida K. Intraosseous venous structures adjacent to the jugular tubercle associated with an anterior condylar dural arteriovenous fistula. Neuroradiology. 2018;60(5):487–96.
18. Morin O, Gillis A, Chen J, Aubin M, Bucci MK, Roach M, Pouliot J. Megavoltage cone-beam CT: system description and clinical applications. Med Dosim. 2006;31:51. https://doi.org/10.1016/j.meddos.2005.12.009.
19. Orth RC, Wallace MJ, Kuo MD, Technology Assessment Committee of the Society of Interventional Radiology. C-arm cone-beam CT: general principles and technical considerations for use in interventional radiology. J Vasc Interv Radiol. 2008;19(6):814–20.
20. Schulze R, Heil U, Gross D, Bruellmann DD, Dranischnikow E, Schwanecke U, Schoemer E. Artefacts in CBCT: a review. Dentomaxillofac Radiol. 2011;40(5):265–73.
21. Spin-Neto R, Gotfredsen E, Wenzel A. Impact of voxel size variation on CBCT-based diagnostic outcome in dentistry: a systematic review. J Digit Imaging. 2013;26(4):813–20.
22. Tanabe J, Tanaka M, Kadooka K, Hadeishi H. Efficacy of high-resolution cone-beam CT in the evaluation of carotid atheromatous plaque. J Neurointerv Surg. 2016;8(3):305–8.
23. Tanaka M. Embryological consideration of Dural arteriovenous fistulas. Neurol Med Chir. 2016;56(9):544–51.
24. Tanaka M. Embryological consideration of Dural AVF. Acta Neurochir Suppl. 2016;123(9):169–76.
25. Tanaka M. Spinal Dural AVFs: classifications and advanced imaging. Acta Neurochir Suppl. 2021;132:129–35.
26. Tsumoto T, Tsurusaki Y, Tokunaga S. Transvenous embolization using cone-beam CT and 3D roadmap function for Dural arteriovenous fistulas. J Neuroendovasc Ther. 2017;11(5):240–5.
27. Yu S, Shi C-C, Ma J, Wang Y, Zhu M, Bao-Ma RJ-Z, Han X-W, Li T-F. Clinical evaluation of high-resolution cone-beam computed tomography for the implantation of flow-diverter stents in intracranial aneurysms. J Clin Neurosci. 2022;103:14–9.
28. Yu L, Vrieze TJ, Bruesewitz MR, Kofler JM, DeLone DR, Pallanch JF, Lindell EP, McCollough CH. Dose and image quality evaluation of a dedicated cone-beam CT system for high-contrast neurologic applications. AJR Am J Roentgenol. 2010;194(2):W193–201.

Open Access This chapter is licensed under the terms of the Creative Commons Attribution 4.0 International License (http://creativecommons.org/licenses/by/4.0/), which permits use, sharing, adaptation, distribution and reproduction in any medium or format, as long as you give appropriate credit to the original author(s) and the source, provide a link to the Creative Commons license and indicate if changes were made.

The images or other third party material in this chapter are included in the chapter's Creative Commons license, unless indicated otherwise in a credit line to the material. If material is not included in the chapter's Creative Commons license and your intended use is not permitted by statutory regulation or exceeds the permitted use, you will need to obtain permission directly from the copyright holder.

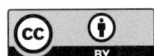

Part III

Bypass and Moyamoya

Cerebral Ischemic Complications of Surgical Treatment in Patients with Moyamoya Disease

Anna A. Shulgina, Vasily A. Lukshin, Anton A. Korshunov, and Dmitry Yu. Usachev

Introduction

Moyamoya disease is a rare cerebrovascular disease affecting the entire intracranial vascular system. The etiology of this disease is still unclear, but its genetic basis is assumed. Progressive stenoses in internal carotid (ICA), anterior (ACA), middle (MCA), and posterior cerebral (PCA) arteries typical for this disease result in the fundamental restructuring of the entire intracranial circulation with the development of complex collateral systems. The last ones are designed to maintain cerebral perfusion under a significant reduction in blood flow through the great cerebral arteries. Together with morphological changes in vascular walls, these processes lead to high cerebral sensitivity to systemic and local hemodynamic changes and a risk of stroke throughout the natural course of disease and during surgical treatment. Given the preventive nature of interventions in most patients with mild symptoms or the asymptomatic course of this disease, special attention should be paid to preventing perioperative complications.

According to the literature, perioperative ischemic complications make up 3.8–31% of all complications [1–4]. There are local (anastomosis function, restructuring of cerebral hemodynamics, and cerebral hyperperfusion syndrome) and systemic risk factors of complications. Systemic risk factors are represented primarily by the instability of systemic hemodynamics capable of triggering a cascade of ischemic events in the unilateral and contralateral hemispheres [5].

The purpose of this study was to identify the unfavorable prognostic factors of perioperative cerebral ischemic complications, to determine which group of patients is at high risk, and to develop guidelines for the perioperative management of these patients.

A. A. Shulgina (✉) · V. A. Lukshin · A. A. Korshunov
D. Y. Usachev
Burdenko Neurosurgical Center, Moscow, Russia
e-mail: AShulgina@nsi.ru

Material and Methods

There were 80 patients with various forms of moyamoya angiopathy between 2008 and April 2020 at the Burdenko Neurosurgery Center. The sample included 60 patients (75%) with moyamoya disease and 20 (25%) with moyamoya syndrome. An instrumental examination was carried out according to a single diagnostic protocol and included an assessment of the vascular system, morphological changes in brain tissue, and perfusion impairment [6].

We analyzed the following aspects during angiography: (1) the stage of the disease according to the Houkin magnetic resonance angiography grading system [7]; (2) the localization of ICA stenosis (proximal (precommunicant) and distal posterior communicating artery (PCoA)); (3) the state of the PCoA (intact/stenosis/occlusion/hypertrophy); (4) the stage of the disease according to the Suzuki staging system [8]; (5) the leptomeningeal collaterals according to the number of lobes (parietal, temporal, and frontal) supplied by the leptomeningeal vasculature from the PCA system [9]; (6) the transdural collaterals (spontaneous collaterals from the middle meningeal or the branches of external carotid arteries were assessed according to the number of lobes supplied by these vessels) [10].

An analysis of cerebrovascular insufficiency using arterial spin labeling (ASL) magnetic resonance imaging perfusion was carried out [11]. Given the data from this analysis, we distinguished 4 degrees of perfusion impairments on the basis of cerebral blood flow (CBF) and the presence of arterial transit artifact (ATA). The last one is a result of labeled blood congestion in vessels as a sign of collateral blood flow. The following are the degrees of perfusion impairment:

Degree 0—CBF 64.5 ± 16.2 ml/min/100 g, no ATA, compensation of CBF

Degree 1—CBF 61.5 ± 16.6 ml/min/100 g, ATA, subcompensation of CBF

Degree 2—CBF 26.5 ± 7.2 ml/min/100 g, ATA, initial decompensation of CBF

Degree 3—CBF 16.0 ± 4.7 ml/min/100 g, no ATA, decompensation of CBF

The indication for surgical treatment was symptomatic moyamoya disease Suzuki stage II–V and cerebrovascular insufficiency degree 2–3 (ASL) or with signs of disease progression. There were 134 revascularization procedures. The staged revascularization of both hemispheres was performed in 40 patients (80 surgeries). Most patients ($n = 55$) underwent combined brain revascularization (79 surgeries), including extra-intracranial microvascular anastomoses and indirect revascularization (flaps of the dura mater, temporal muscle, and periosteum). We have previously described this technique in detail [6]. Furthermore, 14 patients underwent 19 direct interventions (bypass only), and 17 patients underwent 36 indirect revascularization procedures. In the entire sample, favorable outcomes prevailed in the early postoperative period (7 postoperative days). Indeed, improvement in or the preservation of preoperative symptoms was noted in 67.7% of patients. Persistent postoperative complication (ischemic stroke) developed in seven cases (5.3%). Early postoperative transient neurological deficit with in-hospital regression was observed in 36 cases (27%). There were no lethal outcomes or hemorrhagic complications. We used regression analysis to identify the factors associated with perioperative transient and persistent complications and to predict the risk of surgical treatment. Differences were significant at $p < 0.05$.

Results

We revealed significant risk factors of transient and persistent postoperative neurological complications. They can be divided into clinical, angiographic, and perfusion ones (Table 1). One significant risk factor of transient and persistent ischemic events was early surgery (within 3 months) after the last stroke or transient ischemic attack (TIA) ($\chi^2 = 6.146$; $p < 0.013$; Fisher's exact test, $p = 0.016$) with a modified Rankin score (mRS) of 1–2 points.

Angiographic factors were ICA stenosis proximal to the PCoA or PCA ($\chi^2 = 20.085$, $p < 0.0001$) and the involvement of the PCA pool ($\chi^2 = 29.127$, $p < 0.0001$). One of the most significant factors influencing the development of ischemic complications was the severity of baseline perfusion impairment (ASL grade 2—3; $\chi^2 = 11.212$, $p < 0.001$; Fisher's exact test, $p = 0.001$) indirectly reflecting its "ivy sign" ($\chi^2 = 4.078, p = 0.043$).

Regarding various surgical options, complications were significantly more common after indirect revascularization (42.7%, $\chi^2 = 10.892$, $p = 0.028$) compared to combined (26.6%) and direct (0%) revascularization. This is also true for persistent adverse events (8.3% compared to 5.1 and 0%, respectively). Despite insignificant differences, 80% of complications occurred in patients younger than 16 years old. The mean age of patients with complications was 11.17 ± 9.1 years compared to 14.08 ± 10.8 years in patients without complications. Younger age was a significant factor influencing the risk of persistent complications. For example, the risk of ischemic stroke increased by almost 3.5 times in patients younger than 6 years old ($B = 1.235$; $\mathrm{Exp}(B) = 14.546$; $p = 0.019$).

According to regression analysis, the most significant risk factors were unilateral PCoA stenosis or occlusion, signs of the decompensation of cerebral perfusion (degree 2–3), and unstable clinical symptoms (TIA) or stroke within 3 months prior to surgical treatment. Stenosis or occlusion of the PCoA increased the risk of postoperative stroke by almost 10 times (OR = 9.7), signs of cerebral blood flow decompensation by more than 5 times (OR = 5.393), and TIA or stroke within 3 months prior to surgery by more than 6 times (OR = 6.433). According to logistic regression model, the high-risk group consisted of patients with ≥ 2 factors. The sensitivity and the specificity of the models in predicting the development of transient and persistent neurological deficit were 80.7 and 88.6%, respectively (AUC 84.6%, ROC analysis). Outside this group, severe postoperative complications did not occur, and the incidence of transient perfusion impairment was 5.6%. A clinical example of severe postoperative ischemic stroke reflecting the importance of carrying out a preoperative assessment of risk factors is shown in Fig. 1.

Table 1 Risk factors of transient and persistent postoperative cerebrovascular accidents

Factor	Group without complications, % (number of patients, n = 35)	Group with complications (n = 83)	Significance
Clinical factors			
TIA/stroke within 3 months	77.2% (n = 64)	54.3% (n = 19)	$\chi^2 = 6.146, p < 0.013$
No	22.9% (n = 19)	**45.7% (n = 16)**	Fisher's exact test, $p = 0.016$
Yes			
mRS			
Grade 1	34.4% (n = 33)	16.7% (n = 6)	$\chi^2 = 7.918, p = 0.048$
Grade 2	21.9% (n = 21)	44.4% (n = 16)	
Grade 3	21.9% (n = 38)	33.3% (n = 12)	
Grade 4	21.9% (n = 4)	5.6% (n = 2)	
Angiographic factors			
ICA stenosis			
Proximal to PCoA	30.1% (n = 25)	**77.1% (n = 27)**	$\chi^2 = 20.085, p < 0.0001$
Distal to PCoA	69.9% (n = 58)	22.9% (n = 8)	
PCA stenosis			
No	78.3% (n = 65)	21.7% (n = 18)	$\chi^2 = 29.127, p < 0.0001$
Yes	25.7% (n = 9)	**74.3% (n = 26)**	
Perfusion factors			
Perfusion impairment			
Degree 0	3.6% (n = 3)	0% (n = 0)	$\chi^2 = 9.399, p = 0.024$
Degree 1	34.9% (n = 29)	11.4% (n = 4)	
Degree 2	44.6% (n = 37)	**57.1% (n = 20)**	
Degree 3	16.9% (n = 14)	**31.4% (n = 11)**	
"Ivy sign"			
No	92.8% (n = 77)	80.0% (n = 28)	$\chi^2 = 4.078, p = 0.043$
Yes	7.2% (n = 6)	**20.0% (n = 7)**	
Surgical factors			
Surgical option			
Direct	110% (n = 19)	0% (n = 0)	$\chi^2 = 10.892, p = 0.028$
Indirect	58.3% (n = 21)	42.7% (n = 15)	
Combined	73.4% (n = 58)	26.6% (n = 21)	
Additional factors			
Age, years			
Mean age	14.08 ± 10.8 (n = 49)	11.17 ± 9.109	ANOVA $F_{1,116} = 1.943, p = 0.166$
Children (younger 16 years old)	67.5% (n = 56 from 83)	80.0% (n = 28 from 35)	$\chi^2 = 11,184, p = 0,170$ younger 6 years old—$p = 0.019$

Note: *TIA* transient ischemic attack, *mRS* modified Rankin scale, *ICA* internal carotid artery, *PCA* posterior cerebral artery, *PCoA* posterior communicating artery

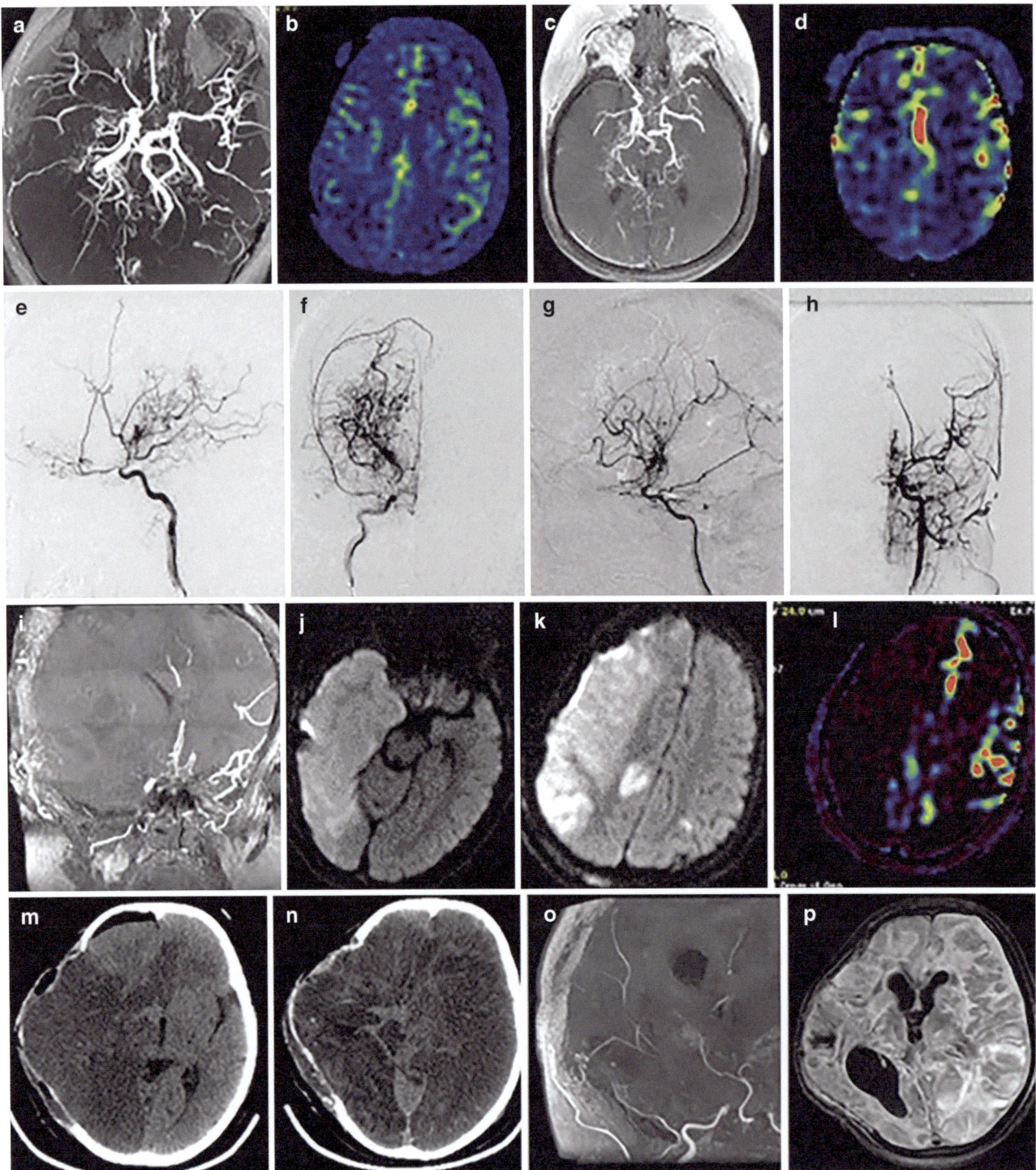

Fig. 1 Severe postoperative ischemic stroke in a 9-year-old patient with moyamoya disease. There were several previous strokes in both hemispheres. MR angiography revealed moyamoya disease (**a**). ASL perfusion revealed a reduction in blood flow in both hemispheres with single ATA (perfusion impairment degree 2) (**b**). Surgery was postponed due to a cold. Throughout this period, transient ischemic attacks in the right middle cerebral artery pool became more common. Also, 2 weeks before admission, the central paresis of the left facial nerve and slurred speech persisted. An MRI revealed the progression of the disease with stenoses of ICA, MCA, and ACA (**c**). Stenosis of the right ICA spread proximally to the posterior communicating artery. ASL perfusion confirmed further bilateral reduction in CBF (**d**). Direct angiography of the right ICA in lateral projection revealed its stenosis below the orifice of the posterior communicating artery and signs of trifurcation in the right internal carotid artery (discharge of the right PCA from ICA) (**e**); signs of moyamoya disease Suzuki grade III are visualized (**f**); left ICA in lateral (**g**) and direct projections (**h**)—signs of moyamoya disease Suzuki grade II, precommunicant stenosis of ICA. The right hemisphere with more-severe lesion was preferred for the first stage of treatment (double bypass between superficial temporal artery and cortical branches of the M4 segment of MCA, encephaloduromyoperiosteosynangiosis). The intraoperative period was uneventful. On the first day, clinical deterioration and left-side hemiplegia occurred. An MRI revealed extensive ischemic damage to the right temporal, parietal, and occipital lobes and single small ischemic foci in the right cerebellar hemisphere, the right occipital and frontal lobes, and the left frontal and parietal lobes (**i–l**). Despite intensive therapy, progressive edema of the right hemisphere required extensive decompressive craniotomy (**m**). The clinical condition progressively worsened with progressive edema of both hemispheres (**n**). A few days later, the patient's condition was stabilized. MR angiography confirmed patent bypass (**o**). Nevertheless, the consequences of edema and brainstem dislocation determined the patient's subsequent vegetative status (**p**)

Discussion

Postoperative complications are obstacles in the development and wider spread of brain revascularization procedures in the treatment of chronic cerebral ischemia. Thus, the multiple-center cooperative trial devoted to the role of bypass in the treatment of patients with ICA occlusion (Carotid Occlusion Surgery Study, 2009) revealed that the incidence of early postoperative ischemic stroke was up to 16.5%. It was the main cause of failed treatment [12]. Similar problems are typical for the treatment of patients with moyamoya disease. The risk of perioperative stroke is significantly higher in these patients compared to patients with other cerebrovascular diseases (up to 30%) [1–4]. In our sample, persistent postoperative complications (ischemic stroke) developed in seven cases (5.3%). Another 36 patients (27%) had transient neurological deficit in the early postoperative period with a complete in-hospital regression of symptoms. According to modern concepts, the causes of such episodes can include various circulatory disorders in cortical arteries following both hypoperfusion and local hyperperfusion, as well as nonspecific early postoperative symptoms following surgical trauma. Our findings are consistent with the world literature data. Guzman et al. [1] analyzed 450 surgical revascularizations, and the incidence of ischemic stroke was 3.5% [1]. Choi et al. [13] found stroke in 5.1% of patients and Kazumata et al. [14] in 7.9% of cases, and the incidence of TND was up to 32.7% [15].

An analysis of our own results and literature data suggests that the likelihood of postoperative complications among all patients with moyamoya disease is heterogeneous and depends on numerous baseline factors determining different degrees of clinical decompensation [13, 16]. In our sample, stenosis or occlusion of unilateral PCA increased the risk of stroke by almost 10 times (9.7, $p < 0.0001$) compared to patients without PCA stenosis or occlusion (*angiographic factor*). There was a similar tendency in critical stenosis of ICA proximal to the PCoA orifice, especially in the fetal type of the circle of Willis (OR = 9.065; $p = 0.001$). These results are consistent with the meta-analysis data on the significantly higher risk of ischemic stroke in patients with PCA stenosis (OR = 4.60; $p = 0.000$) [17]. Indeed, PCA lesion in patients with moyamoya disease occurs in the last turn after previous damage to the ICA, MCA, and ACA [18]. Therefore, this artery is especially important in compensatory circulation through the network of leptomeningeal collaterals. Severe perfusion impairment was a result of insufficient collateral circulation and posed a high risk of postoperative ischemic events (*perfusion factor*). In our sample, severe cerebrovascular insufficiency ASL grade 2–3 [11] increased the risk of intra- and postoperative stroke by more than 5 times (OR = 5.393, $p = 0.023$). Other large international studies have also identified the influence of signs of decompensated cerebral circulation on the risk of postoperative complications. In particular, the study of the Berlin grading system for moyamoya disease found this effect in 16% of cases [19] and the COSS cooperative multiple-center study in 16.5% of patients [12].

Surgical treatment was especially dangerous in patients with an unstable clinical course (regular TIA) or in a subacute (within 3 months) period of ischemic stroke (*clinical factor*). Moreover, Kim et al. [20] found a significant increase in the incidence of postoperative complications after bypass within 6 weeks after the last ischemic stroke. A similar clinical picture was common in depleted reserves of collateral circulation and severe perfusion impairment. Under such conditions, even minimal hemodynamic changes can trigger a cascade of ischemic events in both the unilateral and contralateral hemispheres [5].

Treatment strategy for high-risk patients is still unclear, and further study is required. Given the high risk of ischemic complications, we cannot unambiguously choose a surgical approach, and comprehensive an interdisciplinary approach may be advisable. In case of surgical revascularization, preoperatively preventing brain perfusion impairment by excluding the factors provoking cerebral ischemia is essential. Thus, therapy is required in the acute period of stroke until clinical improvement. Later, surgical treatment can be performed. The situations potentially provoking cerebral ischemia should be avoided in the perioperative period. Iwama et al. [21] found ischemic stroke as a result of unstable intraoperative hemodynamics or inadequate perioperative management in 16.9% of patients.

In this regard, anesthetic support for surgeries is essential and should be performed by well-experienced specialists. The following four abnormal perioperative conditions should be excluded in patients with signs of decompensated cerebral circulation:

1. *Dehydration and hypovolemia* can contribute to cerebral ischemia due to impaired blood rheology and reduced perfusion pressure. Dehydration may be a result of preoperative fasting, poor appetite, and insufficient fluid intake within a few days after surgery, vomiting, or fever. The careful pre- and postoperative replenishment of fluid loss using infusion therapy is necessary.
2. *Hyperventilation* provokes hypocapnia and cerebral vasoconstriction [22] under mechanical ventilation and during crying and anxiety associated with painful medical procedures. Younger children requiring premedication in a ward, accurate awakening without anxiety, and adequate pain relief during dressings and other procedures need special attention [23]. Tests with hyperventilation during electroencephalography are contraindicated.
3. *Hypotension* should be excluded, as hypertension is common in patients with moyamoya disease. Hypertension usually has a central compensatory character and is aimed at maintaining cerebral perfusion. It is necessary to maintain normal blood pressure. Aggressive reduction of blood pressure is inappropriate.
4. *Severe anemia* in the early postoperative period under reduced perfusion can provoke cerebral ischemia. Therefore, careful monitoring and timely compensation for possible blood loss are necessary. Hemoglobin level > 10 g/dL should be maintained [23].

Younger children are especially sensitive to these conditions. Therefore, they are primarily at risk of ischemic complications [13]. In our study, the incidence of postoperative ischemic stroke was higher by almost 3.5 times in children younger than 6 years old ($B = 1.235$; $Exp(B) = 14.546$; $p = 0.019$), especially if they had several risk factors.

Of course, the choice of surgical approach also matters. In our study, combined methods involving direct anastomoses were accompanied by a significantly lower incidence of complications (5.1%) compared to indirect brain revascularization (8.3%, $\chi^2 = 10.892$, $p = 0.028$). Indeed, the development of synangiosis with cortical arteries takes a certain amount of time (up to 3 months), whereas the imposition of bypass is followed by early improvement in cerebral perfusion and compensation of the disease [24].

Conclusion

(1) The risk of perioperative complications in patients with moyamoya disease is heterogeneous and determined, first of all, by critical stenosis or occlusion of PCA, severe perfusion deficit, and subacute (within 3 months after cerebrovascular accident (CVA)) or unstable (serial TIAs) clinical symptoms. These factors increase the risk of complications by 10, 5, and 6 times, respectively. (2) The combination of ≥ 2 risk factors increases the risk of perioperative ischemic cerebral events, with a sensitivity and specificity of 80.7 and 88.6%, respectively. (3) Early surgical treatment is advisable to reduce the risk of ischemic and hemorrhagic lesions following the natural course of the disease and severe perioperative complications. (4) Combined brain revascularization is preferable for high-risk patients. Surgery should be provided with qualified anesthetic support and the timely correction of dehydration, hyperventilation, arterial hypotension, hypovolemia, and anemia.

Declarations
Conflict of interest: No conflict of interests to declare.

Informed consent: For this type of study, formal consent is not required.

Informed consent: Informed consent was obtained from all individual participants included in the study.

Human and animal rights: This chapter does not contain any studies with animals performed by any of the authors.

References

1. Guzman R, Lee M, Achrol A, Bell-Stephens T, Kelly M, Do HM, Marks MP, Steinberg GK. Clinical outcome after 450 revascularization procedures for moyamoya disease. J Neurosurg. 2009;111(5):927–35. https://doi.org/10.3171/2009.4.JNS081649.
2. Iwama T, Hashimoto N, Tsukahara T, Murai B. Peri-operative complications in adult moyamoya disease. Acta Neurochir. 1995;132(1–3):26–31. https://doi.org/10.1007/BF01404844.
3. Sakamoto T, Kawaguchi M, Kurehara K, Kitaguchi K, Furuya H, Karasawa J. Risk factors for neurologic deterioration after revascularization surgery in patients with moyamoya disease. Anesth Analg. 1997;85(5):1060–5. https://doi.org/10.1097/00000539-199711000-00018.

4. Starke RM, Komotar RJ, Connolly ES. Optimal surgical treatment for moyamoya disease in adults: direct versus indirect bypass. Neurosurg Focus. 2009;26(4):E8. https://doi.org/10.3171/2009.01.FOCUS08309.
5. Jung YJ, Ahn JS, Kwon DH, Kwun BD. Ischemic complications occurring in the contralateral hemisphere after surgical treatment of adults with moyamoya disease. J Korean Neurosurg Soc. 2011;50(6):492–6. https://doi.org/10.3340/jkns.2011.50.6.492.
6. Shulgina AA, Lukshin VA, Usachev DY, Korshunov AE, Belousova OB, Pronin IN. Combined brain revascularization in the treatment of moyamoya disease. Voprosy nejrohirurgii im NN Burdenko. 2021;85(2):47–59. (In Russ.). 10.17116/neiro20218502147
7. Houkin K, Nakayama N, Kuroda S, Nonaka T, Shonai T, Yoshimoto T. Novel magnetic resonance angiography stage grading for Moyamoya disease. Cerebrovasc Dis. 2005;20(5):347–54. https://doi.org/10.1159/000087935.
8. Suzuki J, Takaku A. Cerebrovascular «moyamoya» disease. Disease showing abnormal net-like vessels in base of brain. Arch Neurol. 1969;20(3):288–99. https://doi.org/10.1001/archneur.1969.00480090076012.
9. Togao O, Mihara F, Yoshiura T, Tanaka A, Noguchi T, Kuwabara Y, Kaneko K, Matsushima T, Honda H. Cerebral hemodynamics in Moyamoya disease: correlation between perfusion-weighted MR imaging and cerebral angiography. AJNR Am J Neuroradiol. 2006;27(2):391–7.
10. Baltsavias G, Khan N, Valavanis A. The collateral circulation in pediatric moyamoya disease. Child's Nervous Syst. 2015;31(3):389–98. https://doi.org/10.1007/s00381-014-2582-5.
11. Shulgina AA, Lukshin VA, Shultz EI, Batalov AI, Pronin IN, Usachev DY. Methods for assessing cerebrovascular insufficiency in patients with moyamoya angiopathy by MR-ASL perfusion. Medicinskaya vizualizaciya. 2021;25(2):102–15. (In Russ.). 10.24835/1607-0763-883
12. Grubb RL, Powers WJ, Derdeyn CP, Adams HP, Clarke WR. The carotid occlusion surgery study. Neurosurg Focus. 2003;14(3):1–7. https://doi.org/10.3171/foc.2003.14.3.10.
13. Choi JW, Chong S, Phi JH, Lee JY, Kim H-S, Chae JH, Lee J, Kim SK. Postoperative symptomatic cerebral infarction in pediatric moyamoya disease: risk factors and clinical outcome. World Neurosurg. 2020;136:158–64. https://doi.org/10.1016/j.wneu.2019.12.072.
14. Kazumata K, Ito M, Tokairin K, Ito Y, Houkin K, Nakayama N, Kuroda S, Ishikawa T, Kamiyama H. The frequency of postoperative stroke in moyamoya disease following combined revascularization: a single-university series and systematic review. J Neurosurg. 2014;121(2):432–40. https://doi.org/10.3171/2014.1.JNS13946.
15. Uchino H, Nakayama N, Kazumata K, Kuroda S, Houkin K. Edaravone reduces hyperperfusion-related neurological deficits in adult moyamoya disease: historical control study. Stroke. 2016;47(7):1930–2. https://doi.org/10.1161/STROKEAHA.116.013304.
16. Funaki T, Takahashi JC, Takagi Y, Kikuchi T, Yoshida K, Mitsuhara T, Kataoka H, Okada T, Fushimi Y, Miyamoto S. Unstable moyamoya disease: clinical features and impact on perioperative ischemic complications. J Neurosurg. 2015;122(2):400–7. https://doi.org/10.3171/2014.10.JNS14231.
17. Wei W, Chen X, Yu J, Li XQ. Risk factors for postoperative stroke in adults patients with moyamoya disease: a systematic review with meta-analysis. BMC Neurol. 2019;19(1):1–8. https://doi.org/10.1186/s12883-019-1327-1.
18. Huang APH, Liu HM, Lai DM, Yang CC, Tsai YH, Wang KC, Yang SH, Kuo MF, Tu YK. Clinical significance of posterior circulation changes after revascularization in patients with moyamoya disease. Cerebrovasc Dis. 2009;28(3):247–57. https://doi.org/10.1159/000228254.
19. Czabanka M, Boschi A, Acker G, Pena-Tapia P, Schubert GA, Schmiedek P, Vajkoczy P. Grading of moyamoya disease allows stratification for postoperative ischemia in bilateral revascularization surgery. Acta Neurochir. 2016;158(10):1895–900. https://doi.org/10.1007/s00701-016-2941-y.
20. Kim SH, Choi JU, Yang KH, Kim TG, Kim DS. Risk factors for postoperative ischemic complications in patients with moyamoya disease. J Neurosurg. 2005;103(5):433–8. https://doi.org/10.3171/ped.2005.103.5.0433.
21. Iwama T, Hashimoto N, Yonekawa Y. The relevance of hemodynamic factors to perioperative ischemic complications in childhood moyamoya disease. Neurosurgery. 1996;38(6):1120–5.; discussion 1125-11256. https://doi.org/10.1097/00006123-199606000-00011.
22. Yusa T, Yamashiro K. Local cortical cerebral blood flow and response to carbon dioxide during anesthesia in patients with moyamoya disease. J Anesthesiah. 1999;13(3):131–5. https://doi.org/10.1007/s005400050043.
23. Nomura S, Kashiwagi S, Uetsuka S, Uchida T, Kubota H, Ito H. Perioperative management protocols for children with moyamoya disease. Child's Nervous Syst. 2001;17(4–5):270–4. https://doi.org/10.1007/s003810000407.
24. Sun H, Wilson C, Ozpinar A, Safavi-Abbasi S, Zhao Y, Nakaji P, Wanebo JE, Spetzler RF. Perioperative complications and long-term outcomes after bypasses in adults with Moyamoya disease: a systematic review and meta-analysis. World Neurosurg. 2016;92:179–88. https://doi.org/10.1016/j.wneu.2016.04.083.

Open Access This chapter is licensed under the terms of the Creative Commons Attribution 4.0 International License (http://creativecommons.org/licenses/by/4.0/), which permits use, sharing, adaptation, distribution and reproduction in any medium or format, as long as you give appropriate credit to the original author(s) and the source, provide a link to the Creative Commons license and indicate if changes were made.

The images or other third party material in this chapter are included in the chapter's Creative Commons license, unless indicated otherwise in a credit line to the material. If material is not included in the chapter's Creative Commons license and your intended use is not permitted by statutory regulation or exceeds the permitted use, you will need to obtain permission directly from the copyright holder.

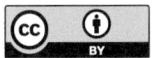

Long-Term Outcome of Moyamoya Disease

Peter Birkeland, Victoria Hansen, Vinosha Tharmabalan, Jens Lauritsen, Troels Nielsen, Thomas Truelsen, Sverre Rosenbaum, and Paul von Weitzel-Mudersbach

Introduction

Moyamoya disease (MMD) is a rare idiopathic steno-occlusive cerebrovascular disease affecting the distal intracranial internal carotid artery or its proximal branches with a network of basal collaterals [1]. The disease was first described in Japan [2] and was formerly almost exclusively associated with East Asia, but it is now known to occur worldwide [3]. Characteristically, the disease presents in either childhood or young middle age [4]. Clinical events include ischemic stroke caused by narrowed vessels and hemorrhage from the rupture of fragile collaterals. MMD is considered a progressive disease, but there is a lack of data on long-term outcomes to substantiate this [5, 6].

Bypass surgery is performed to prevent stroke and alter the disease course [1], but its long-term durability and its overall impact in preventing ischemic stroke has never been demonstrated [7]. In the subgroup of patients presenting with brain hemorrhage (i.e., hemorrhagic MMD), a randomized trial showed a marginally statistically significant effect of bypass surgery on reducing stroke risk [8]. Still, it was not able to show an impact on the clinical outcome.

Previously, we described a Danish cohort of 50 patients with MMD diagnosed between 1994 and 2017 [9]. Reflecting the era, our cohort is a case mix of operated and conservatively treated patients with an extended follow-up—of which most patients would likely have been offered surgery by today's standard. This has given us a unique opportunity to look into the natural history of the disease and investigate the long-term course and outcome after bypass surgery. Retrospective observational data from our cohort [10] provided evidence for the hitherto assumption of a continued risk of recurrent stroke in MMD. For this study, we conducted a structured telephone interview with cohort patients to determine how this would affect the long-term outcome.

Methods

The Cohort Population

The cohort was established as previously described [9, 10]. Briefly, all patients diagnosed with MMD (I67.5) between 1994 and 2017 were identified in the Danish National Patient Register, which covers all hospital discharges and visits to outpatient clinics in Denmark [11]. Clinical notes, clinic letters, and radiology reports from 13 clinical departments from six Danish hospitals were reviewed. The diagnosis was validated according to the definition of *MMD* stated by the Research Committee on Spontaneous Occlusion of the Circle of Willis (moyamoya disease) in Japan [12]. We conducted a

P. Birkeland (✉) · V. Tharmabalan
Department of Neurosurgery, Copenhagen University Hospital, Copenhagen, Denmark
e-mail: Peter@Birkeland.dk

V. Hansen
Department of Neurology, Aalborg University Hospital, Aalborg, Denmark

J. Lauritsen
Department of Orthopaedic Surgery, Odense University Hospital, Odense, Denmark

Department of Clinical Research, University of Southern Denmark, Odense, Denmark

T. Nielsen
Department of Neurosurgery, Odense University Hospital, Odense, Denmark

T. Truelsen
Department of Neurology, Copenhagen University Hospital, Copenhagen, Denmark

S. Rosenbaum
Department of Neurology, Bispebjerg Hospital, Copenhagen, Denmark

P. von Weitzel-Mudersbach
Department of Neurology, Gødstrup Hospital, Herning, Denmark

pooled analysis of patients with probable (pMMD) and definite MMD (dMMD). We reviewed all collected data up to March 15, 2021, to ensure that the previous diagnosis of MMD could be maintained. The following features were recorded: age at diagnosis, sex, race, and initial clinical presentation (transient ischemic attack (TIA), ischemic stroke, brain hemorrhage, seizures, headache, other presentation, asymptomatic). *TIA* was defined as neurological deficits of presumed vascular origin resolving within 24 h.

Study Timeline

Subjects were included at the date of the first angiography when they met the diagnostic criteria for MMD and were followed up until March 15, 2021, or death.

Medical Management and Revascularization Surgery

We recorded the date, type (direct or indirect), and side of the surgical revascularization procedure if applicable. We also noted whether patients were on antiplatelet medication.

Outcomes

Vital status was assessed from patients' electronic records. Alive adult patients—or, if appropriate, their next of kin—were approached and requested to participate in a telephone interview. VH (Victoria Hansen) and VT (Vinosha Tharmabalan) conducted the telephone interviews. Patients were assigned a modified Rankin Scale (mRS) score on the basis of a structured phone interview. We used a simplified modified Rankin Scale questionnaire with excellent reliability [13]. An mRS < 3 was considered a favorable outcome. We also asked about the patient's source of income and whether the patient lived independently, in sheltered housing, or at a nursing home. We also approached pediatric patients' parents and asked about special educational needs. In adult patients diagnosed before the age of 18 years, we asked about the highest academic level attained.

Statistical Analysis

Data were collected on data sheets by using EpiData Entry software (www.epidata.dk; the EpiData Association). Analyses were performed by using EpiData Analysis software (www.epidata.dk; the EpiData Association) and OpenEpi software (www.openepi.com). We used chi-squared tests with a significance level of 0.05 for statistics.

Standard Protocol Approvals, Registration, and Patient Consent

The Danish Patient Safety Authority (ref. no. 3-3013-1699/1 and ref. no. 3-3013-1699/2) and the Capital Region of Denmark (ref. no. R-21016187) approved the study. Patient consent was not required.

Data Availability Statement

The data supporting this study's findings are available from the corresponding author upon reasonable request.

Results

Characteristics of the Cohort

The cohort consisted of 50 patients, of whom 33 were female. 16 patients were diagnosed before the age of 18 years. Eight patients had an East Asian background. Also, 17 patients had an ischemic stroke; 11 had a brain hemorrhage, eight had headaches, seven had TIA, two had seizures, four had other presentations, and one was asymptomatic at diagnosis.

Medical and Surgical Management

16 patients were treated conservatively, while 34 underwent bypass surgery. Sex and clinical presentation were not significantly different between groups. Still, more pediatric patients had bypass surgery ($p = 0.04$), and a trend toward more patients of East Asian origin in the bypass group was also noticed. Among those conservatively treated, bypass surgery was not found to be indicated in six patients, due to a lack of ongoing symptoms; in one case, after the vascular neurosurgeon reviewed the angiogram; and in another case, because of a normal positron emission tomography with acetazolamide challenge. For four other patients, we did not find clinical notes indicating that bypass surgery was even considered. Four patients declined surgery. The most common indication for surgery was a previous cerebrovascular event. In one of 34 surgically treated patients, a bypass was considered only after a second stroke. The median time from

diagnosis to first bypass was 116 days (range 5–8401 days). Furthermore, 26 cases (76%) were direct or combined bypasses, and eight (24%) were indirect; 25 patients had additional bypass(es) performed. 26 patients were on aspirin, five on clopidogrel, and six on both. Among surgically treated patients, 22 patients were on aspirin, three on clopidogrel, and three on both. Aspirin and clopidogrel were generally administrated at a dose of 75 mg o.d.

Structured Telephone Interviews

Five patients had died after a follow-up of 507 person-years (median: 9 years; range: 0.10–29.0 years). Only one of the deaths was related to a cerebrovascular event. Thus, 45 patients, or their next of kin, were approached for a telephone interview. Two patients could not be reached, and two declined to participate. Six patients were still younger than 18 years old, while ten pediatric patients had reached adulthood and could be assigned an mRS score (mRSs) based on the structured telephone interview.

Outcomes

The overall mRSs and the mRSs for patients reaching a follow-up of 5, 10, and 15 years are depicted in Fig. 1. Overall, 24 of 40 patients (60%) who could be assigned an mRSs had a favorable outcome. This proportion was 63%, 65%, and 46% after 5, 10, and 15 years of follow-up, respectively.

Notably, none of the deaths occurred between 10 and 15 years of follow-up. At the end of the study, four patients (aged 27 years, 45 years, 56 years, and 70 years) lived in a nursing home.

Income Source

Figure 2 shows the income source for live adult patients at the end of the study. Here, 20 of 37 patients were outside the workforce or educational system, whereas only six worked full time.

Academic Level in Pediatric Patients

Two of the six children had special educational needs. Two of the ten grown-up pediatric patients had graduated from high school, whereas seven had no education beyond primary school. In the last case, information could not be obtained.

Subgroup Analyses

Since our previous data suggested that conservatively treated and female patients might have a higher stroke risk, we performed subgroup analyses based on bypass status and sex. Overall, five of the 13 patients (39%) who were conserva-

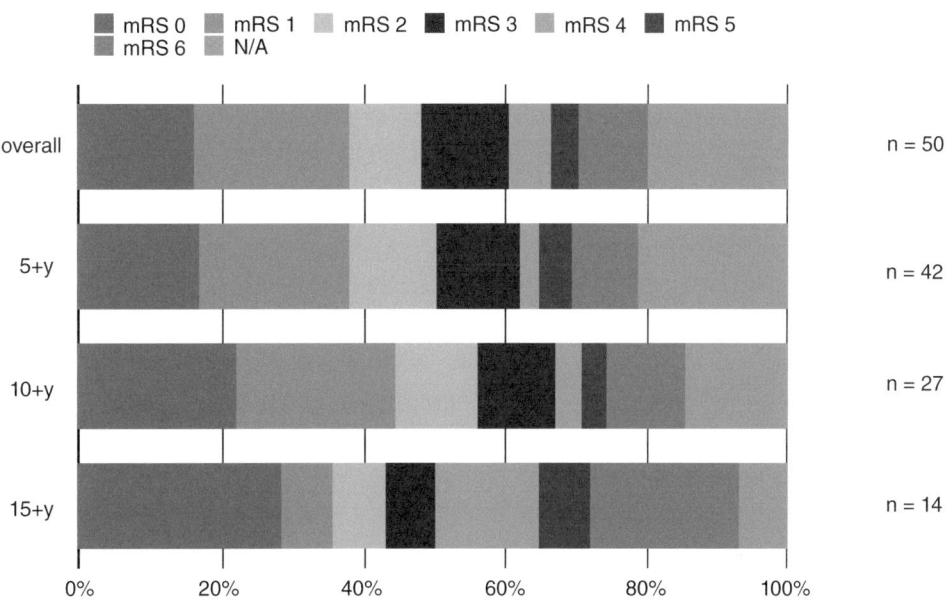

Fig. 1 Overall outcome and outcome in patients who reached 5, 10, and 15 years of follow-up

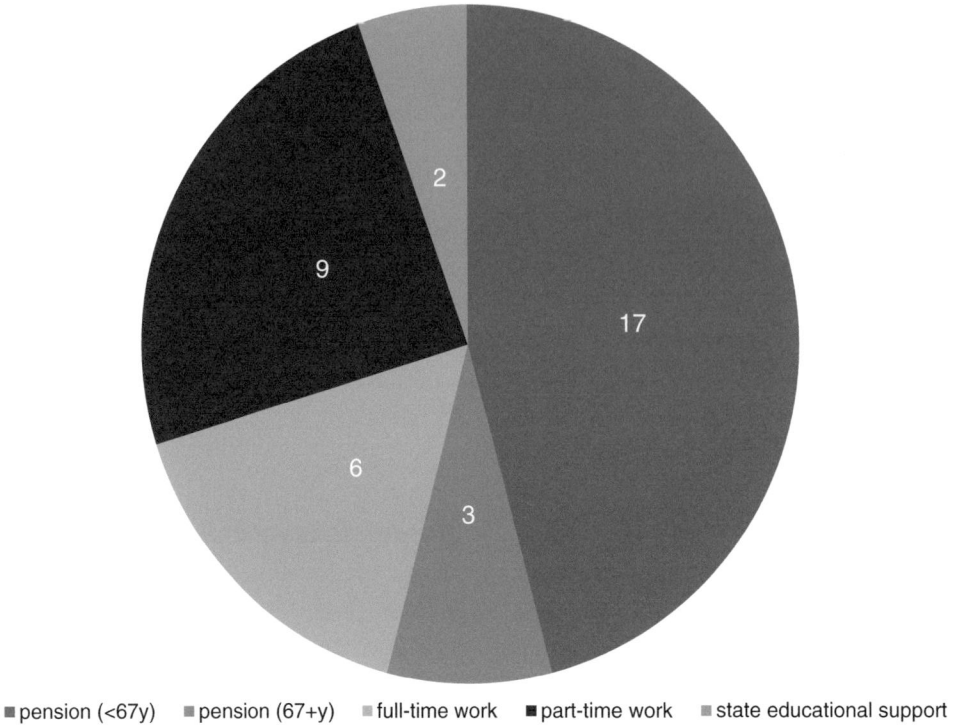

Fig. 2 Income source in adult patients

tively treated and could be assigned an mRSs had a favorable outcome after 5 years, whereas this applied to 19 of 27 patients (70%) in the bypass group ($p > 0.05$). Also, 16 of the 27 female patients (59%) who could be assigned an mRSs had a favorable outcome after 5 years, as compared to eight of the 13 male patients (61%, $p > 0.05$). We refrained from making comparisons at later time points because the groups were small.

Discussion

The long-term outcome of MMD in Europe and, for that matter, elsewhere is not well known. This, in particular, applies to conservatively treated patients. In our cohort, a case mix of operated and conservatively treated patients followed for a median of 9 years, we found that 60% of patients had a favorable outcome, with only 16% of adult patients working full time. In other words, our data suggest that MMD considerably impacts daily life in a substantial number of those affected, with only a minority being able to provide for themselves. There was also a trend toward a greater degree of disability after 15 years of follow-up. Based on our data, we cannot establish whether this is explained by strokes seen during follow-up or whether it is otherwise related to MMD; that would require a matched control group. Many studies, including ours [10], have sug-

gested that revascularization reduces the stroke risk. One would expect that reducing this risk would improve outcomes, but this may prove challenging to determine. Our data showed a trend toward better outcomes in the bypass group. In a Finnish study of 61 patients, the median mRS was 1 after a mean follow-up period of 9.5 years, with no difference between surgically and conservatively treated patients [14]. A study from the United Kingdom demonstrated favorable outcomes (mRS < 3) in 63.5% and 60.6% after a median follow-up of 43 months of surgically treated pediatric patients and conservatively treated pediatric patients, respectively [14].

Another finding worth noting was that two of the six children in our cohort had special educational needs, and only two of 10 grown-up pediatric patients had graduated from high school. A possible explanation is cognitive impairment caused by stroke and hypoperfusion, to which children are particularly vulnerable [7].

Strengths and Limitations

The strength of this study rests on providing complete long-term follow-ups in a nationwide cohort of 50 MMD patients with strict inclusion criteria, including 16 patients treated conservatively. Being a national cohort eliminates the referral bias associated with case series from large tertiary centers. There are also some limitations. First, our cohort is a real-world case mix of operated and conservatively treated patients. This introduces a selection bias as the selection for surgery may be confounded by severity. The reasons for choosing a conservative approach may point to lesser disease severity, but interestingly, all but one conservatively treated patient had been symptomatic, and 62.5% had had a previous stroke. The study period was a transitional phase from MMD being relatively unknown in Denmark to an increased understanding of indications for surgery.

Many conservatively treated patients would likely have been referred for surgery by today's standards. Also, the groups were balanced except for more East Asians and pediatric patients in the bypass group. This reduces but does not eliminate the selection bias. Ultimately, there was a trend toward a worse outcome in the conservatively treated patients compared to that in the bypass group. However, the study did not aim to prove bypass surgery's efficacy. Second, observations in conservatively treated patients can be only a substitute for natural history. They are subjected to the same selection bias as above, as disease severity may distinguish conservatively treated patients from those referred for surgery. However, long-term natural history studies are not feasible, because some patients will invariably be referred for surgery. Third, retrospective data have inherent limitations, but comparable prospective data over so many years will not likely be collated. Fourth, the cohort size is limited to 50 patients, but assembling a large cohort in a primarily non-Asian population is challenging. In particular, the subgroup analyses should be interpreted cautiously. In conclusion, our data suggest that MMD considerably impacts daily life in a substantial number of those affected, with only a minority able to provide for themselves.

Declarations
Conflicts of interest: The authors have no conflicts of interest to disclose.

References

1. Scott RM, Smith ER. Moyamoya disease and moyamoya syndrome. N Engl J Med. 2009;360:1226–37.
2. Suzuki J, Takaku A. Cerebrovascular "moyamoya" disease. Disease showing abnormal net-like vessels in base of brain. Arch Neurol. 1969;20:288–99.
3. Kleinloog R, Regli L, Rinkel GJE, Klijn CJM. Regional differences in incidence and patient characteristics of moyamoya disease: a systematic review. J Neurol Neurosurg Psychiatry. 2012;83:531–6.
4. Baba T, Houkin K, Kuroda S. Novel epidemiological features of moyamoya disease. J Neurol Neurosurg Psychiatry. 2008;79:900–4.
5. Ahmed SU, Steinberg GK. Long-term outcomes in the USA. In: Kuroda S, editor. Moyamoya disease: current knowledge and future perspectives. Springer; 2021. p. 253–64.
6. Ganesan V, Smith ER. Moyamoya: defining current knowledge gaps. Dev Med Child Neurol. 2015;57(9):786–7.
7. Kuroda S, Houkin K. Moyamoya disease: current concepts and future perspectives. Lancet Neurol. 2008;7(11):1056–66.
8. Miyamoto S, Yoshimoto T, Hashimoto N, Okada Y, Tsuji I, Tominaga T, et al. Effects of extracranial–intracranial bypass for patients with hemorrhagic Moyamoya disease. Stroke. 2014;45:1415–21.
9. Birkeland P, Tharmabalan V, Lauritsen J, Bjarkam C, Ganesan V, von Weitzel-Mudersbach P. Moyamoya disease in a European setting: a Danish population-based study. Eur J Neurol. 2020;12:2446–52.
10. Birkeland P, Hansen V, Tharmabalan V, Lauritsen J, Nielsen TH, Truelsen T, Rosenbaum S, von Weitzel-Mudersbach P. Long-term stroke risk in moyamoya disease. Int J Stroke. 2024;19(4):452–9.
11. Schmidt M, Schmidt SA, Sandegaard JL, Ehrenstein V, Pedersen L, Sørensen HT. The Danish national patient registry: a review of content, data quality, and research potential. Clin Epidemiol. 2015;7:449–90.
12. Guidelines for diagnosis and treatment of moyamoya disease (spontaneous occlusion of the circle of Willis). Neurol Med Chir (Tokyo). 2012;52:245–66.
13. Bruno A, Akinwuntan AE, Lin C, Close B, Davis K, Baute V, Aryal T, Brooks D, Hess DC, Switzer JA, Nichols FT. Simplified modified Rankin Scale questionnaire reproducibility over the telephone and validation with quality of life. Stroke. 2011;42:2276–9.
14. Savolainen M, Mustanoja S, Pekkola J, Tyni T, Uusitalo A-M, Ruotsalainen S, Poutiainen E, Hernesniemi J, Kivipelto L, Tatlisumak T. Moyamoya angiopathy: long-term follow-up study in a Finnish population. J Neurol. 2019;266:574–81.

Open Access This chapter is licensed under the terms of the Creative Commons Attribution 4.0 International License (http://creativecommons.org/licenses/by/4.0/), which permits use, sharing, adaptation, distribution and reproduction in any medium or format, as long as you give appropriate credit to the original author(s) and the source, provide a link to the Creative Commons license and indicate if changes were made.

The images or other third party material in this chapter are included in the chapter's Creative Commons license, unless indicated otherwise in a credit line to the material. If material is not included in the chapter's Creative Commons license and your intended use is not permitted by statutory regulation or exceeds the permitted use, you will need to obtain permission directly from the copyright holder.

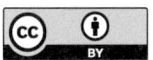

Efficacy and Safety of Combined Revascularization Surgery for Moyamoya Disease: Standard Procedure and Perioperative Management

Miki Fujimura, Masaki Ito, Haruto Uchino, Masahito Kawabori, and Taku Sugiyama

Introduction

Moyamoya disease (MMD) is a chronic, occlusive cerebrovascular disease with an unknown etiology characterized by the progressive stenosis of the internal carotid artery (ICA) terminus and abnormal vascular network formation at the base of the brain [17, 19]. Surgical revascularization via superficial temporal artery (STA)–middle cerebral artery (MCA) anastomosis is generally accepted as the standard surgical procedure for symptomatic MMD patients, especially in adults [9, 11, 13, 14]. The STA-MCA anastomosis has been known to prevent cerebral ischemic attack by improving cerebral hemodynamics in the affected hemisphere [9, 11, 14]. Recent results from the Japan Adult Moyamoya (JAM) trial, a randomized controlled clinical trial that investigated the efficacy of direct revascularization on the prevention of rebleeding in hemorrhagic MMD patients, further indicated that STA-MCA anastomosis is a powerful management choice to reduce the risk of rebleeding in MMD patients with posterior hemorrhage, in which annual rebleeding risk was as high as 17.1% under conservative management [18, 20]. According to such evidence, an increasing number of symptomatic MMD patients undergo STA-MCA anastomosis as a standard management in East Asia. Regarding the details of the surgical procedure, a recent study indicates the superiority of direct-indirect combined revascularization surgery such as STA-MCA anastomosis with indirect pial synangiosis [1, 2].

Despite the long-term favorable outcome of combined revascularization surgery, however, local cerebral hyperperfusion syndrome and simultaneous occurrence of cerebral ischemia caused by watershed shift phenomenon are potential complications of this surgery [3–5, 7, 11–13, 21–23].

Cerebral hyperperfusion syndrome could result in transient neurological deterioration, in seizure, and rarely also in delayed intracerebral hemorrhage [4, 5, 23]. Therefore, complication avoidance in the acute stage after revascularization surgery is critical while managing MMD patients surgically. In the present study, we sought to clarify the efficacy and safety of our standardized combined revascularization procedure and perioperative management.

Materials and Methods

Inclusion Criteria of Patients and the Surgical Procedure

The present study included 37 consecutive patients with MMD (2–60 years old, 42.0 on average) surgically treated in 42 affected hemispheres by the same surgeon (M.F.) between January 2021 and March 2023. The indication for revascularization surgery for MMD included all of the following items: the presence of ischemic symptoms (minor completed stroke and/or transient ischemic attack (TIA)) and/or posterior hemorrhage, the presence of hemodynamic compromise, independent activity in daily living (modified Rankin Scale scores 0–2), and the absence of major brain damage that exceeded the vascular territory of one major branch of MCA. Direct-indirect combined revascularization surgery was performed on most hemispheres (41/42, 97.6%), including STA-MCA bypass (39 hemispheres) and occipital artery (OA)–posterior cerebral artery (PCA) bypass (two hemispheres). Preoperative cerebral blood flow (CBF) was assessed via the autoradiographic method using N-isopropyl-p-[^{123}I] iodoamphetamine single-photon emission computed tomography (^{123}I-IMP-SPECT) [3, 7]. All patients underwent strict perioperative management with strict blood pressure control (110–130 mmHg) based on ^{123}I-IMP-SPECT findings. Most patients underwent STA-MCA (M4) anastomosis

M. Fujimura (✉) · M. Ito · H. Uchino · M. Kawabori · T. Sugiyama
Department of Neurosurgery, Hokkaido University Graduate School of Medicine, Sapporo, Japan
e-mail: fujimur@med.hokudai.ac.jp

with encephaloduromyosynangiosis (EDMS) [8, 10]. Craniotomy was performed around the Sylvian fissure end, and the stump of STA was anastomosed to the M4 segment of MCA, which was followed by EDMS. All patients satisfied the diagnostic criteria of the Research Committee on the Spontaneous Occlusion of the Circle of Willis, of the Ministry of Health, Labor, and Welfare in Japan [17].

Postoperative CBF Measurement and Perioperative Management Protocol

CBF was routinely measured via ^{123}I-IMP-SPECT at postoperative day (POD) 1 and 7 after surgery in all patients [4, 7]. The criteria for local cerebral hyperperfusion included all the following items: (1) the presence of a significant local CBF increase at the site of the anastomosis that exceeds the CBF value of the other supratentorial region of the bilateral hemispheres; (2) the apparent visualization of STA-MCA bypass via magnetic resonance angiography (MRA); (3) the absence of other pathologies, such as compression of the brain surface by the temporal muscle inserted for indirect pial synangiosis and CBF increase secondary to seizure. The criteria for the watershed shift phenomenon included the following items: (1) the presence of local cerebral hyperperfusion and (2) a paradoxical CBF decrease in the cerebral cortex adjacent to local cerebral hyperperfusion [21, 22].

All 36 patients undergoing combined revascularization surgeries on 41 hemispheres were prospectively subjected to prophylactic blood pressure lowering (110–130 mmHg of systolic blood pressure) according to standardized postoperative management protocol using 1–10 mg/hour of a continuous intravenous drip infusion of nicardipine hydrochrolide to prevent cerebral hyperperfusion syndrome, as previously described [8]. In all patients, antiplatelet agents (100 mg aspirin/day or 200 mg cilostazol/day) were preoperatively used until 3 days before surgery. All patients were managed via the intraoperative and postoperative intravenous administration of minocycline hydrochloride (200 mg/day) until 7 days after surgery [9]. Most patients were also managed via the postoperative intravenous administration of lacosamide (100 mg/day). We routinely administered antiplatelet agents (100 mg aspirin/day) starting the day after surgery in all cases [8, 10]. On the basis of the temporal profile of ^{123}I-IMP-SPECT and magnetic resonance imaging (MRI)/magnetic resonance angiography (MRA) findings, we gradually allowed a return to normotensive conditions within 7–10 days after combined revascularization [8, 10]. Then we investigated the postoperative neurological status, the neuroradiological outcomes, and the incidence of surgical complications after the revascularization surgery for MMD.

Results

Outcome of Revascularization Surgery for MMD

The outcome of 42 surgeries was favorable in all cases except for one (2.3%), where that one manifested as cerebral hyperperfusion syndrome after STA-MCA anastomosis combined with EDMS, leading to neurological worsening. The result of the 41 surgeries of combined revascularization is summarized

Table 1 Summary of revascularization surgeries for 42 affected hemispheres of moyamoya disease

	Items	Number of hemispheres (%)
Patient's age	Adults (16 years old ~)	33 (78.6 %)
	Children (~15 years old)	9 (21.4 %)
Sex	Men	9 (21.4 %)
	Women	33 (78.6 %)
Onset type	TIA	24 (57.1 %)
	Cerebral infarction	13 (31.0 %)
	Hemorrhage	5 (11.9 %)
Surgical procedure	Combined bypass	
	STA-MCA bypass with EDMS	39 (92.9 %)
	OA-PCA bypass with EDMS	2 (4.8%)
	Indirect bypass	
	EDAS	1 (2.3%)
Surgical complication	CHP syndrome	1 (2.3%)
	Would healing delay	2 (4.7%)

Note: *TIA* transient ischemic attack, *STA-MCA* superficial temporal artery–middle cerebral artery, *OA-PCA* occipital artery–posterior cerebral artery, *EDAS* encephaloduroarteriosynangiosis, *CHP* cerebral hyperperfusion

in Table 1. None of the patients developed perioperative cerebral infarction (0/42; 0%), and the patency of the direct bypass was confirmed via MRA in all cases undergoing the combined procedure (41/41, 100%). Two patients suffered wound-healing delay, one of which required resuture.

Representative Case

A 41-year-old man, presenting with the newly formed minor hemorrhage demonstrated by the development of microbleed along the periventricular anastomosis in the left hemisphere, was admitted to our hospital. He had a history of intracerebral hemorrhage in the right hemisphere due to MMD, which had been managed via combined revascularization surgery and the superselective embolization of the pseudoaneurysm previously located at the choroidal channel. Neurological examination was unremarkable, but T2*weighted imaging MRI demonstrated the hemorrhage at the posterior part of the left lateral ventricle (arrow in Fig. 1a). While considering the surgical indication on the left hemisphere with posterior hemorrhage, we chose to have the patient undergo catheter angiography, which demonstrated the significant narrowing of left ICAs at their terminal portion as well as the marked development of the basal vascular network formation including the extended choroidal artery, the so-called choroidal channel (Fig. 1b). On the basis of these findings, we planned flow-augmentation bypass on the left hemisphere.

Under general anesthesia, the head was positioned at 80° via a three-point fixture. We made a skin incision along with the donor STA approximately 10 cm in length. Craniotomy was performed around the Sylvian fissure end, approximately 10 cm in diameter (Fig. 2a), and the stump of the STA was prepared as a semi-fish mouth shape with a stump of 2.0 mm. Then the stump of the STA is anastomosed via a 10-0 nylon monofilament suture to the M4 segment of the MCA, 1.0 mm in diameter (Fig. 2b, c). After reperfusion, the patency of STA-MCA anastomosis was confirmed via intraoperative indocyanine green (ICG) video-angiography and Doppler ultrasonography (Fig. 2d). The direct anastomosis procedure was followed by EDMS. To avoid postoperative compression of the brain surface by the temporal muscle, we drilled out the inner layer of the bone flap and made a wide bone window on the side of EDMS, and we also split the temporal muscle into two layers not only to reduce the thickness of EDMS flap but also to preserve the outer layer for cosmetic coverage around the preauricular area. The bone flap was fixed both by two pieces of titanium plates and a bioabsorbable plate named LactoSorb (82% poly-L-lactic acid and 18% polyglycolic acid).

The postoperative course was uneventful, and the patient did not suffer neurological deterioration. ^{123}I-IMP-SPECT on the day after surgery showed significant CBF increase on the operated hemisphere (Fig. 3a), and the STA-MCA anastomosis was clearly visualized as thick high signal intensity via MRA 2 days after surgery (arrow in Fig. 3b). The patient was discharged without neurological worsening 14 days after revascularization surgery. There was no cerebrovascular event during the follow-up period of 1 year.

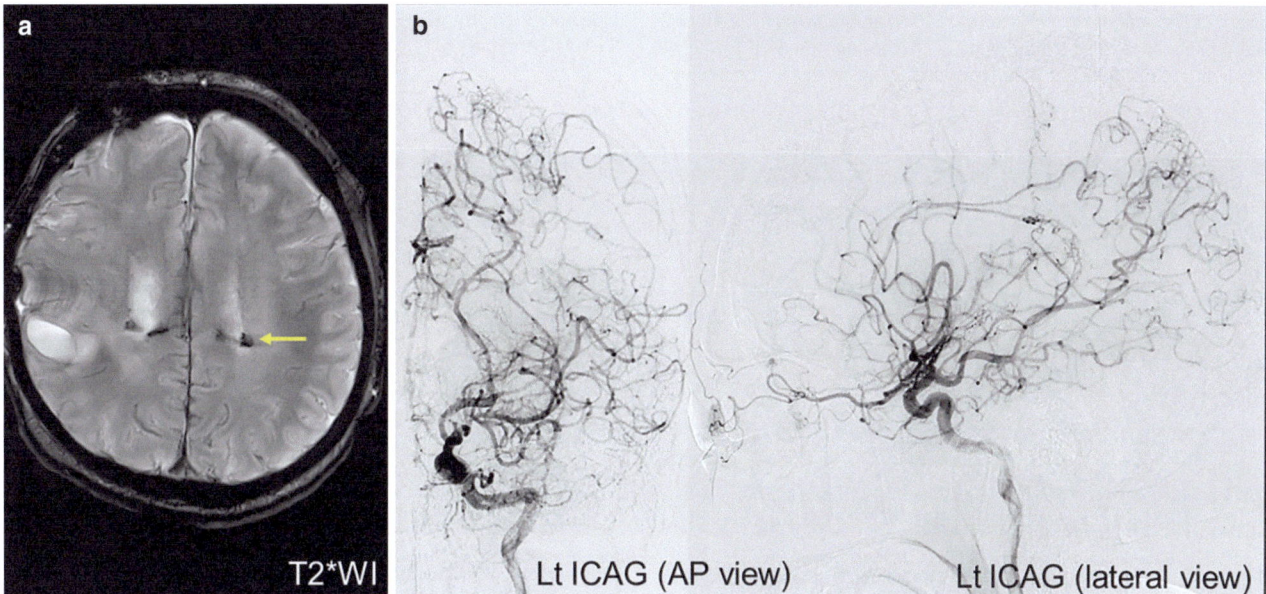

Fig. 1 (a) The magnetic resonance images of T2*weighted imaging (WI) demonstrated the hemorrhage at the posterior part of the left lateral ventricle (arrow in **a**). (**b**) Left internal carotid artery (ICA) angiogram showed the significant narrowing of left ICA terminus with the marked development of the basal vascular network formation

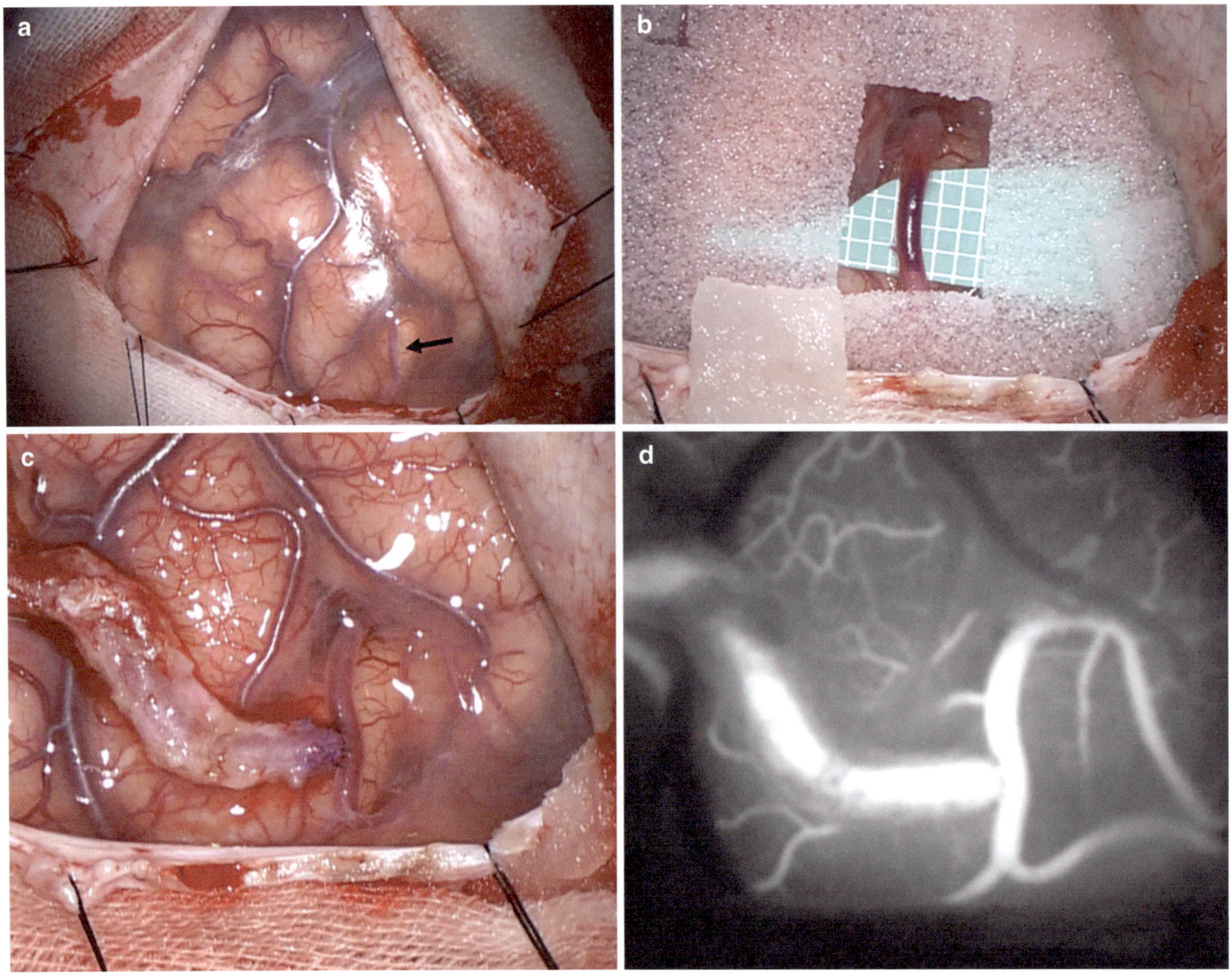

Fig. 2 Intraoperative microscopic view of left superficial temporal artery (STA)–middle cerebral artery (MCA) anastomosis for a 41-year-old patient. (**a–c**) The stump of the STA was anastomosed to the M4 segment of left MCA at 1.0 mm in diameter (arrow in **a**), with a temporary occlusion time of 21 min. (**c**) Intraoperative indocyanine green video-angiography after the anastomosis showing apparently patent STA-MCA bypass (**d**)

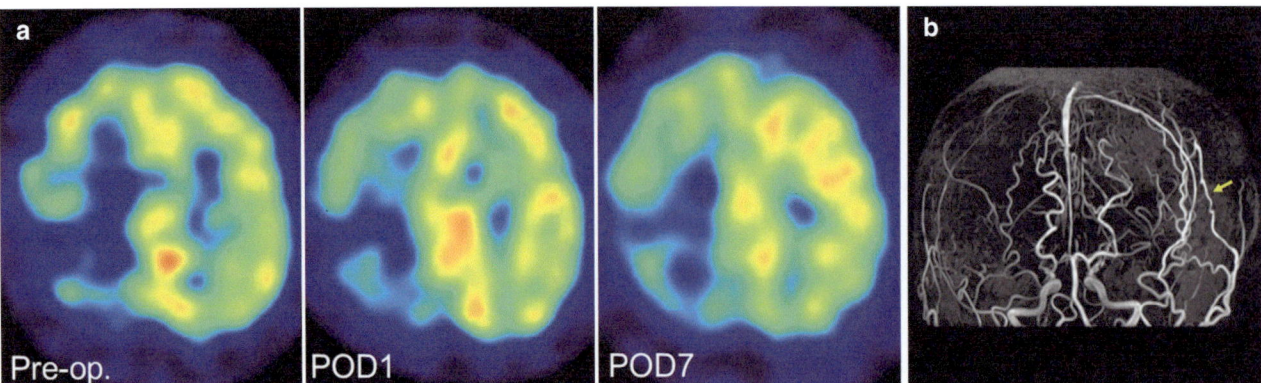

Fig. 3 (**a**) N-isopropyl-p-[^{123}I] iodoamphetamine single-photon emission computed tomography before and after surgery, showing a significant increase in cerebral blood flow in the left frontal lobe 1 and 7 days after surgery. (**b**) Magnetic resonance angiography 2 days after surgery demonstrated apparently patent bypass as thick high signal intensity (arrow)

Discussion

The present study indicated that combined revascularization surgery, such as STA-MCA bypass with EDMS, is a safe and effective management choice if it is promptly followed by the standardized perioperative management protocol. On the basis of our previous reports, indicating the transient local CBF increase pattern in the acute stage after STA-MCA anastomosis with indirect pial synangiosis for MMD patients [7, 10], we argue that conducting the standardized perioperative management via mild blood pressure lowering combined with neuroprotective/anti-inflammatory agents to avoid surgical complications such as cerebral hyperperfusion syndrome appears reasonable [10]. Due to the potentially higher risk of postoperative cerebral hyperperfusion syndrome in adult MMD patients [4, 23], we recommend the application of this perioperative management protocol, especially for adult MMD patients. In fact, the pattern of postoperative cerebral hemodynamics after combined revascularization surgery is different in pediatric MMD patients than in adult patients [15]. Approximately 40% of pediatric MMD patients were found to paradoxically present transient global hypoperfusion on the operated hemisphere after successful STA-MCA anastomosis [15]. The high incidence of global hypoperfusion phenomenon in pediatric patients is apparently different from the hemodynamic pattern in adult patients, who commonly exhibit the transient local hyperperfusion pattern [10, 23].

The surgical complications of the revascularization surgery for MMD include perioperative cerebral infarction and cerebral hyperperfusion syndrome [6, 11, 13, 15]. Perioperative cerebral ischemia can be caused by a variety of pathophysiologies, such as hemodynamic ischemia due to the intraoperative hypotension, anemia/dehydration, thromboembolism at the site of the anastomosis [7, 13], and the watershed shift phenomenon [21, 22]. In case of indirect or combined revascularization, mechanical compression of the brain surface by a swollen temporal muscle used for the indirect bypass procedure could also cause cerebral ischemia [6]. Prompt anesthesia by maintaining normocapnia, sufficient hydration, and proper hemoglobin concentration is essential to avoid ischemic complication [11]. Besides perioperative cerebral infarction, a rapid increase in local CBF at the site of the direct revascularization is known to cause local vasogenic edema and/or hemorrhagic conversion in adult MMD [3–5, 7, 16, 23]. We initially reported that the incidence of cerebral hyperperfusion syndrome after STA-MCA bypass was significantly higher in MMD patients than that in patients with atherosclerotic occlusive cerebrovascular diseases [7]. The risk factors of cerebral hyperperfusion syndrome in MMD patients include older patient age (adult onset) [4, 23], preoperative CBF decrease [21], a preoperative increase in cerebral blood volume [23], the onset of hemorrhage [4], operation on the dominant hemisphere [10], and a smaller-diameter recipient artery [10]. Therefore, adult MMD patients with these factors must be promptly managed to avoid the deleterious effect of cerebral hyperperfusion during the early perioperative period. Because the cerebral hyperperfusion phenomenon is resolved within 7–10 days in most cases, we recommend intensive perioperative management under the standardized perioperative protocol within 7 days after combined revascularization surgery.

In conclusion, the combined revascularization surgery is a safe and effective treatment for MMD, while local cerebral hyperperfusion is a potential complication that should be avoided by administering intensive perioperative care.

Funding Information This work was supported by JSPS KAKENHI Grant Number 20K09362.

Declarations

Conflicts of interest The authors declare that they have no conflicts of interest. All authors certify that they have no affiliations with or involvement in any organization or entity with any financial interest (such as honoraria; educational grants; participation in speakers' bureaus; membership, employment, consultancies, stock ownership, or other equity interest; and expert testimony or patent-licensing arrangements) and no nonfinancial interest (such as personal or professional relationships, affiliations, knowledge, or beliefs) in the subject matter or materials discussed in this manuscript.

Ethical approval All procedures performed in this study were carried out in accordance with the ethical standards of the institution and with the 1964 Helsinki declaration and its later amendments or comparable ethical standards. For this type of study, formal consent is not required.

Informed consent Informed consent was obtained from the individual participants included in the study.

References

1. Bang JS, Kwon OK, Kim JE, Kang HS, Park H, Cho SY, Oh CW. Quantitative angiographic comparison with the OSIRIS program between the direct and indirect revascularization modalities in adult moyamoya disease. Neurosurgery. 2012;70:625–32.
2. Cho WS, Kim JE, Kim CH, Ban SP, Kang HS, Son YJ, Bang JS, Sohn CH, Paeng JC, Oh CW. Long-term outcomes after combined revascularization surgery in adult moyamoya disease. Stroke. 2014;45:3025–31.
3. Fujimura M, Kaneta T, Mugikura S, Shimizu H, Tominaga T. Temporary neurologic deterioration due to cerebral hyperperfusion after superficial temporal artery-middle cerebral artery anastomosis in patients with adult-onset moyamoya disease. Surg Neurol. 2007;67:273–82.
4. Fujimura M, Mugikura S, Kaneta T, Shimizu H, Tominaga T. Incidence and risk factors for symptomatic cerebral hyperperfusion after superficial temporal artery-middle cerebral artery anastomosis in patients with moyamoya disease. Surg Neurol. 2009;71:442–7.

5. Fujimura M, Shimizu H, Mugikura S, Tominaga T. Delayed intracerebral hemorrhage after superficial temporal artery-middle cerebral artery anastomosis in a patient with moyamoya disease: possible involvement of cerebral hyperperfusion and increased vascular permeability. Surg Neurol. 2009;71:223–7.
6. Fujimura M, Kaneta T, Shimizu H, Tominaga T. Cerebral ischemia owing to compression of the brain by swollen temporal muscle used for encephalo-myo-synangiosis in moyamoya disease. Neurosurg Rev. 2009;32:245–9.
7. Fujimura M, Shimizu H, Inoue T, Mugikura S, Saito A, Tominaga T. Significance of focal cerebral hyperperfusion as a cause of transient neurologic deterioration after EC-IC bypass for moyamoya disease: comparative study with non-moyamoya patients using n-isopropyl-p-[(123)i]iodoamphetamine single-photon emission computed tomography. Neurosurgery. 2011;68:957–65.
8. Fujimura M, Inoue T, Shimizu H, Saito A, Mugikura S, Tominaga T. Efficacy of prophylactic blood pressure lowering according to a standardized postoperative management protocol to prevent symptomatic cerebral hyperperfusion after direct revascularization surgery for moyamoya disease. Cerebrovasc Dis. 2012;33:436–45.
9. Fujimura M, Tominaga T. Lessons learned from moyamoya disease: outcome of direct/indirect revascularization surgery for 150 affected hemispheres. Neurol Med Chir (Tokyo). 2012;52:327–32.
10. Fujimura M, Niizuma K, Inoue T, Sato K, Endo H, Shimizu H, Tominaga T. Minocycline prevents focal neurologic deterioration due to cerebral hyperperfusion after extracranial-intracranial bypass for moyamoya disease. Neurosurgery. 2014;74:163–70.
11. Fujimura M, Tominaga T, Kuroda S, Takahashi JC, Endo H, Ogasawara K, Miyamoto S. 2021 Japanese guidelines for the Management of Moyamoya Disease: guidelines from the research committee on Moyamoya disease and Japan Stroke Society. Neurol Med Chir (Tokyo). 2022;62:165–70.
12. Hayashi T, Shirane R, Fujimura M, Tominaga T. Postoperative neurological deterioration in pediatric moyamoya disease. Watershed shift and hyperperfusion. J Neurosurg Pediatr. 2010;6:73–81.
13. Houkin K, Ishikawa T, Yoshimoto T, Abe H. Direct and indirect revascularization for moyamoya disease: surgical techniques and peri-operative complications. Clin Neurol Neurosurg. 1997;99(Suppl 2):S142–5.
14. Jeon JP, Kim JE, Cho WS, Bang JS, Son YJ, Oh CW. Meta-analysis of the surgical outcomes of symptomatic moyamoya disease in adults. J Neurosurg. 2018;128:793–9.
15. Kanoke A, Fujimura M, Tashiro R, Ozaki D, Tominaga T. Transient global cerebral hypoperfusion as a characteristic cerebral hemodynamic pattern in the acute stage after combined revascularization surgery for pediatric moyamoya disease: N-isopropyl-p-[123I] iodoamphetamine single-photon emission computed tomography study. Cerebrovasc Dis. 2022;51:453–60.
16. Kim JE, Oh CW, Kwon OK, Park SQ, Kim SE, Kim YK. Transient hyperperfusion after superficial temporal artery/middle cerebral artery bypass surgery as a possible cause of postoperative transient neurological deterioration. Cerebrovasc Dis. 2008;25:580–6.
17. Kuroda S, Fujimura M, Takahashi JC, Kataoka H, Ogasawara K, Iwama T, Tominaga T, Miyamoto S. Diagnostic criteria for Moyamoya disease—2021 revised version. Neurol Med Chir (Tokyo). 2022;62:307–12.
18. Miyamoto S, Yoshimoto T, Hashimoto N, Okada Y, Tsuji I, Tominaga T, Nakagawara J, Takahashi JC. Effects of extracranial-intracranial bypass for patients with Hemorrhagic Moyamoya disease: results of the Japan adult Moyamoya trial. Stroke. 2014;45:1415–21.
19. Suzuki J, Takaku A. Cerebrovascular 'moyamoya' disease. Disease showing abnormal net-like vessels in base of brain. Arch Neurol. 1969;20:288–99.
20. Takahashi JC, Funaki T, Houkin K, Inoue T, Ogasawara K, Nakagawara J, Kuroda S, Yamada K, Miyamoto S. Significance of the Hemorrhagic site for recurrent bleeding: Prespecified analysis in the Japan adult Moyamoya trial. Stroke. 2016;47:37–43.
21. Tashiro R, Fujimura M, Kameyama M, Mugikura S, Endo H, Takeuchi Y, Tomata Y, Niizuma K, Tominaga T. Incidence and risk factors of the watershed shift phenomenon after superficial temporal artery-middle cerebral artery anastomosis for adult moyamoya disease. Cerebrovasc Dis. 2019;47:178–87.
22. Tu XC, Fujimura M, Rashad S, Mugikura S, Sakata H, Niizuma K, Tominaga T. Uneven cerebral hemodynamic change as a cause of neurological deterioration in the acute stage after direct revascularization for moyamoya disease: cerebral hyperperfusion and remote ischemia caused by the 'watershed shift'. Neurosurg Rev. 2017;40:507–12.
23. Uchino H, Kuroda S, Hirata K, Shiga T, Houkin K, Tamaki N. Predictors and clinical features of postoperative hyperperfusion after surgical revascularization for moyamoya disease: a serial single photon emission CT/positron emission tomography study. Stroke. 2012;43:2610–6.

Open Access This chapter is licensed under the terms of the Creative Commons Attribution 4.0 International License (http://creativecommons.org/licenses/by/4.0/), which permits use, sharing, adaptation, distribution and reproduction in any medium or format, as long as you give appropriate credit to the original author(s) and the source, provide a link to the Creative Commons license and indicate if changes were made.

The images or other third party material in this chapter are included in the chapter's Creative Commons license, unless indicated otherwise in a credit line to the material. If material is not included in the chapter's Creative Commons license and your intended use is not permitted by statutory regulation or exceeds the permitted use, you will need to obtain permission directly from the copyright holder.

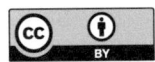

Comparison of Exoscopic and Microscopic Superficial Temporal Artery to Middle Cerebral Artery Bypass

Takuma Maeda, Hidetoshi Ooigawa, Koki Onodera, Yushiro Take, Hiroki Sato, Kaima Suzuki, and Hiroki Kurita

Introduction

Exoscopes have been used as reliable surgical tools in the neurosurgical field [11]. They can improve surgical field visibility with 4K three-dimensional (4K-3D) monitors and provide alleviation for the physical strain associated with a surgeon's neutral posture [1]. Although exoscopes have demonstrated utility in a variety of neurosurgical procedures, their use has not been standardized, and as of 2023, no studies have compared them with the conventional microscope in bypass surgery.

In this study, we present the clinical outcomes for patients who underwent superficial temporal artery (STA) to middle cerebral artery (MCA) bypass with an exoscope compared with a conventional microscope. The aim of this study is to investigate the pros and cons of exoscopic STA-MCA bypass, including its setting in early experience.

Methods

We retrospectively reviewed the medical records and intraoperative videos of all patients ($n = 58$) who had undergone STA-MCA bypass at our institution between January 2021 and August 2022. Patients who underwent the STA-MCA bypass that uses an exoscope (ORBEYE, Olympus, $n = 36$) were compared with those who underwent the procedure that uses a conventional microscope (OME-9000, Olympus, $n = 22$). Both groups were assessed for the following factors: age, sex, medical history, operative details (surgeon; setup time, defined as the time from the entry into the operating room to the start of surgery; the duration of MCA occlusion; operative time; bypass patency; and surgical complications, such as bypass occlusion, hyperperfusion, intracranial hemorrhage, infarction, thromboembolic problem, contusion, neurological event, and wound infection), and modified Rankin Scale (mRS) score at 3 months after surgery. The patients were divided into two groups on the basis of their mRS score at 3 months after surgery: favorable (0–3) and unfavorable (4–6). Additionally, a total of 19 surgeons (five attending staff members, seven staff members, and seven residents) evaluated the effects of exoscope on the cerebrovascular procedure by using a questionnaire (Fig. 1).

The diagnoses of the included patients were as follows: ischemic status including internal carotid artery (ICA) stenosis, ICA occlusion, MCA stenosis, MCA occlusion, and moyamoya disease with ischemic onset. All patients underwent three-dimensional computed tomography (3D-CT) angiography or digital subtraction angiography so that their detailed vascular anatomy could be analyzed and single-photon emission computed tomography so that the hemodynamics of their ischemic hemispheres could be investigated. All aspects of this study were approved by the Ethics Committee of Saitama Medical University International Medical Center (2021–230). The need for written informed consent was waived due to the study's retrospective design.

T. Maeda (✉) · H. Ooigawa · K. Onodera · Y. Take · H. Sato
K. Suzuki · H. Kurita
Department of Cerebrovascular Surgery, Saitama Medical University International Medical Center, Hidaka, Japan
e-mail: maeda412@saitama-med.ac.jp

Questionnaire (Fig. 1)

The evaluation questionnaire consisted of 10 questions, of which eight were rating 5-level-based questions. Questions 1–8 aimed to compare the provision of the basic requirements for cerebrovascular procedures between the exoscope and conventional microscope, whereas questions 9 and 10 investigated the shortcomings and future perspective of the exoscope.

Surgical Procedure

All procedures were performed under general anesthesia. A parietal branch of the STA was routinely anastomosed to a cortical branch of the MCA. The central or precentral artery was usually chosen as a recipient. In the moyamoya cases, combined revascularization consisted of anastomosis between the STA and MCA with encephaloduromyosynangiosis. We used indocyanine green video angiography and

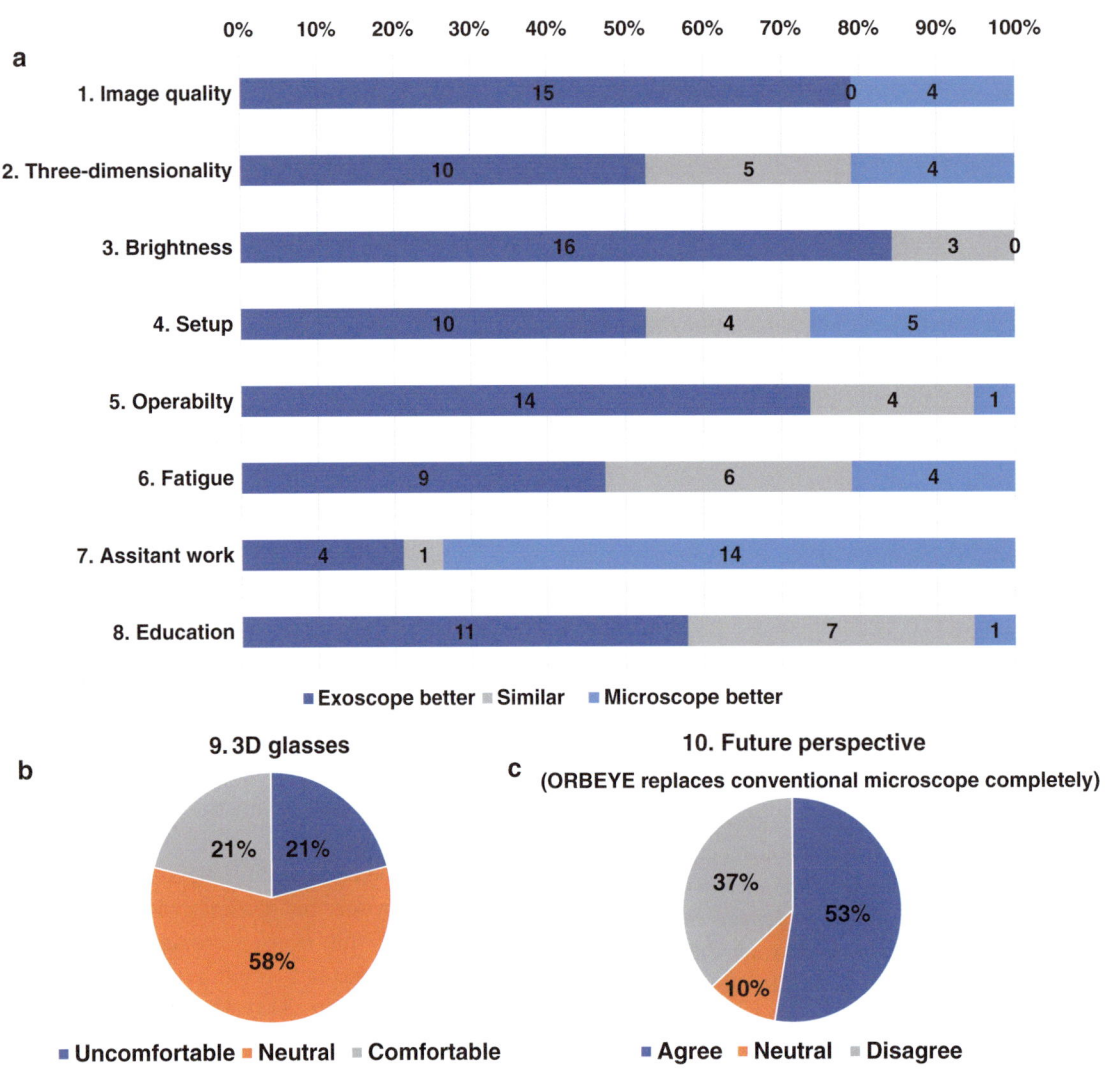

Fig. 1 The results of the postoperative questionnaire evaluation for exoscopes

pulse Doppler to evaluate the intraoperative hemodynamics. We also used motor-evoked potentials for neuromonitoring during the procedure to prevent postoperative hemiparesis. Heparin administration was started if a thrombus was observed at the anastomosis to achieve an activated clotting time of >250 s. Antiplatelet agents for ischemic status were continued on the day of the procedure to prevent procedure-related ischemic complications.

The Setup and Setting of the Exoscope

Figure 2 and Table 1 show the setup and setting of the exoscope used in our institute. We set up the 55-inch main monitor on the opposite side of the lesion as close to the patients as possible. The assistants were positioned on the right side of the surgeons. In the left-side lesions, the main monitor was positioned on the right side of the patients for the surgeon, and a submonitor was also positioned on the left side for the assistant (Fig. 2a). In cases of right-side lesions, the main monitor was positioned on the left side of the patients, wherein the surgeon and assistant share the same main monitor in proximity (Fig. 2b). The anesthesia machine was placed close to the patient's feet so as not to interfere with the monitor.

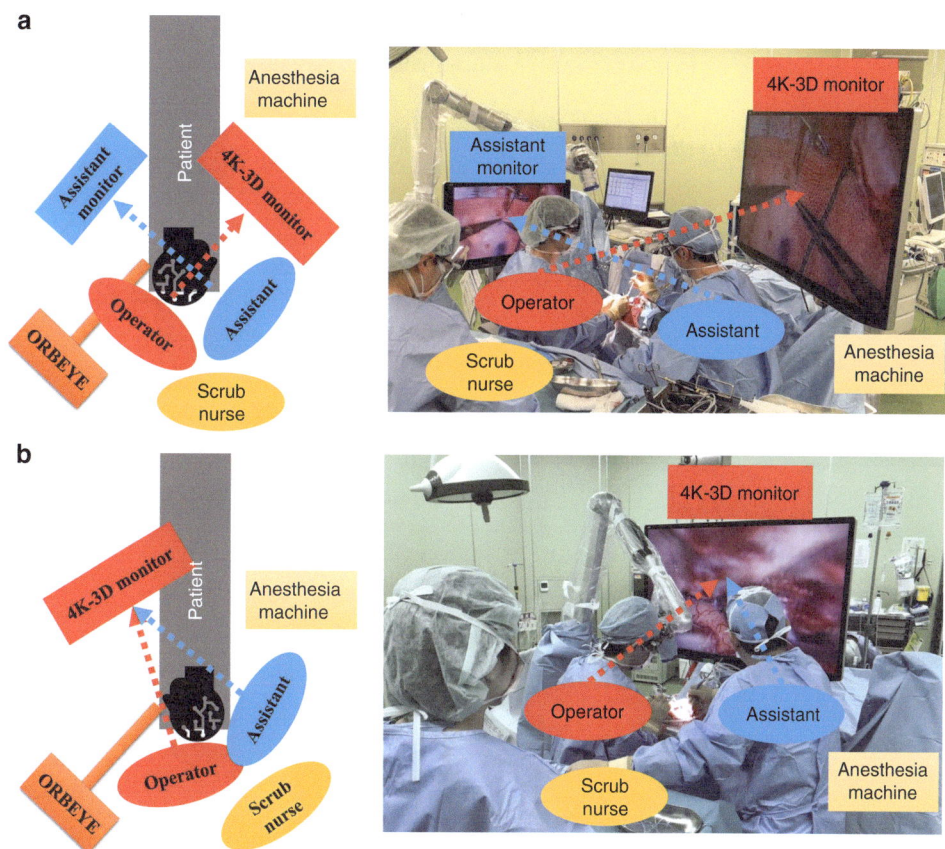

Fig. 2 Intraoperative exoscope setup: (**a**) In the case of left-side lesions, the surgeon and assistant use their own monitors, and the visual axes are orthogonal; (**b**) in the case of right-side or median lesions, the surgeon and assistant share the same 4K-3D monitor in proximity

Table 1 Configuration details for ORBEYE at our institute

Item	Setting
Common image adjustment	
Dimming area	All
Dimming sensitivity	Low
Normal image setting	
Brightness	0
AGC maximum gain	18 dB
Shutter speed	Auto
Color mode	**Mode 4 (red-color suppression)**
Contrast	Normal
Image enhancement	Mode 2
Structure enhancement A	A3
Structure enhancement B	B3
Contour enhancement E	E5
Focus setting	
Focus speed	3
Focus depth	**1 (shallow depth of field and strong 3D effect)**
AF setting	
AF	**Continuous AF: OFF, single AF: ON**
AF frame	ON
Synchronized AF	–
Zoom +	ON
Arm-free	ON
Motorized view	ON

Note: **Bold** denotes importance, *AGC* automatic gain control, and *AF* auto focus

Statistical Analysis

Quantitative variables were expressed as mean ± standard deviation. The chi-square or Fisher's exact test was used to identify the covariates that could be used as binary categorical dependent variables. Unpaired sample tests using Welch's correction were used for parametric data, and the Mann–Whitney U tests were used for nonparametric data. Statistical significance was set to a *p*-value of <0.05. SPSS version 24 (IBM Corp., Armonk, New York, USA) was used for all statistical analyses.

Results

Table 2 shows the patient characteristics. The mean age of the patients was 51.1 (range, 16–75) years old. There were more female (69.0%) than male patients (31.0%) in the present study. Of all patients, 23 (39.7%) had developed moyamoya disease, and all patients presented with ischemic onset. A total of 36 patients (62.0%) underwent the procedure that uses an exoscope, and 22 patients (38.0%) underwent the procedure that uses a microscope. No significant differences were observed in any parameters between the two groups.

Figure 3 shows the intraoperative images of the conventional microscope and exoscope with digital zoom during STA-MCA bypass.

Table 3 shows the clinical outcomes for each therapeutic modality. Residents served as the primary operator significantly more often in the exoscopic group (n = 25; 69.4%) than in the microscopic group (n = 5; 22.7%) (p < 0.001).

Table 2 Characteristics of 58 patients who underwent STA-MCA bypass

	Exoscope	Microscope	*p*-Value
Number of patients	36 (62.0)	22 (38.0)	
Age (years), median [IQR]	49 [41, 59]	53 [47, 65]	0.102
Female sex	28 (77.8)	12 (54.5)	0.083
Left side	15 (41.7)	9 (40.9)	1.000
Diagnosis			0.098
Atherosclerotic disease	25 (69.4)	10 (45.5)	
Moyamoya disease	11 (30.6)	12 (54.5)	

Note: Values are numbers (%) except where indicated otherwise

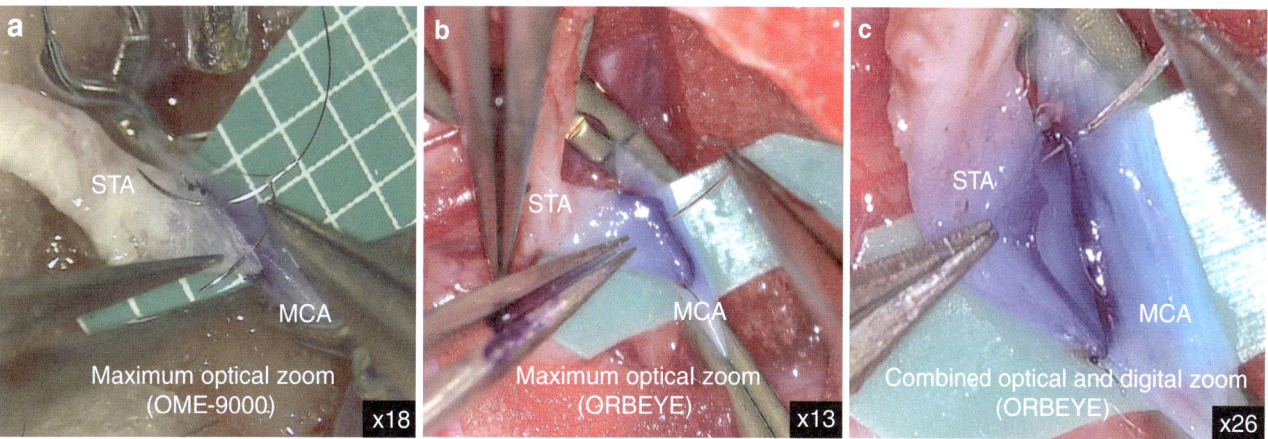

Fig. 3 Intraoperative pictures of superficial temporal artery–middle cerebral artery bypass using the conventional microscope and exoscope: (**a**) intraoperative capture with a maximum optical zoom using the conventional microscope (OME-9000) and (**b**, **c**) intraoperative captures with maximum optical zoom and combined zoom using an exoscope

Table 3 Clinical outcomes of patients who underwent STA-MCA bypass

	Exoscope ($n = 36$)	Microscope ($n = 22$)	p-Value
Surgeon			
Attending staff	1 (2.8)	5 (22.7)	0.025
Staff	10 (27.8)	12 (54.5)	0.054
Resident	25 (69.4)	5 (22.7)	<0.001
Setup time (min), median [IQR]	74 [66, 83]	73 [67, 80]	0.974
Ischemic time (min), median [IQR]	55 [44, 67]	45 [33, 58]	0.053
Operative time (min), median [IQR]	382 [347, 440]	385 [329, 432]	0.665
Patency at postoperative day 1	35 (97.2)	21 (95.5)	1.000
Surgical complication	1 (2.8)	1 (4.5)	1.000
Favorable outcome	36 (100)	21 (95.5)	0.379

Note: Values are numbers (%) except where indicated otherwise. *IQR* interquartile range

No cases with an exoscope required switching to a conventional microscope. The setup time (74 vs. 73 min, $p = 0.974$) and operative time (382 vs. 385 min, $p = 0.665$) were similar for the two therapeutic modalities. On the other hand, the duration of MCA occlusion was slightly longer in the exoscopic group (55 min) than in the microscopic group (45 min), although no significant differences were observed ($p = 0.053$). Regarding the bypass patency, 35 (97.2%) and 21 (95.5%) patients had patency at postoperative day 1 in the exoscope and microscope groups, respectively ($p = 1.000$). Similarly, 36 (100%) and 21 (95.5%) patients had favorable outcomes in the exoscope and microscope groups, respectively ($p = 0.379$). In the present study, only two patients (3.4% of all patients) showed postprocedural complications. One patient experienced wound infection after discharge and required readmission and antibiotic treatment in the exoscopic group, and one patient experienced osteonecrosis, which was not associated with the procedure itself in the microscopic group.

Questionnaire (Fig. 1)

The exoscope scored highly on image quality, brightness, operability, and education, whereas the conventional microscope scored highly on assistant work. Regarding the shortcomings and future perspective of the exoscope, four surgeons (21.1%) felt uncomfortable wearing 3D glasses. Also, ten surgeons (52.6%) agreed that exoscopes will completely replace the conventional microscope, whereas seven surgeons (36.8%) disagreed. Additionally, some surgeons described specific problems, such as the red-enhanced images of the exoscope, in addition to image vibration with maximum magnification and the misalignment of the assistant monitor.

Discussion

Neurosurgery assisted by the operating microscope was first introduced in the 1960s by Yasargil [14]. In 1967, the first STA-MCA bypass under an operating microscope was also reported by Yasargil et al. [15]. Although the microscope has been the gold standard in neurosurgery, surgeons had been forced into uncomfortable positions to be in proximity to the lens of the microscope [14]. The exoscope is a new visualization device consisting of compact lens barrel placed over the surgical field, which was first reported in the neurosurgical field in 2008 by Mamelak et al. [6]. ORBEYE (OLYMPUS, Tokyo, Japan) is the exoscope that launched in Japan in October 2017 [8]. It provides 4K, high-quality, three-dimensional imaging on a 55-inch monitor, which was also introduced in our institute in 2021 [5]. Since then, we have aimed to incorporate the exoscope into all our cerebrovascular surgeries.

As shown in Fig. 3, the first reported advantages of the exoscope were its mobility with a small camera and its visual axis, which can be adjusted by the surgeon. Because the exoscope has no eye piece, it provides alleviation for the physical strain by maintaining the surgeon's neutral posture. In previous surgeries with the conventional microscope, some surgeons, especially female surgeons, have been forced to unnaturally stretch their arms due to the focus length and eye piece of the optical unit [10]. In exoscopic surgery, the elimination of the eye piece solved this problem. The exoscope enables surgeons to get any visual axis without forcing the patient into an untenable position, reducing the risk of cervical spine injury or air embolization, although there were none of these complications in either of the therapeutic modalities in this study. In exoscopic surgery, surgeons must get used to head-up surgery. However, it took just a few surgeries to get used to exoscopic surgery because many neurosurgeons are experienced in endovascular and endoscopic surgeries, which emulates a similar experience.

The second reported advantages of the exoscope were its image quality, high contrast, high brightness, and high resolution when using a 4K-3D monitor. Regarding image resolution, the images obtained directly from the eye lens of the microscope might be difficult to compare with those obtained from the monitor and complementary metal oxide semiconductor (CMOS) image sensor of the exoscope [13]. Interestingly, the results of question 2 indicated that the image quality of the exoscope scored highly. The higher contrast and brightness of the exoscope may have contributed to this result. In the conventional microscope, almost half of the light source was lost in the optical path, especially in the peripheral visual field [4]. In contrast, the exoscope can transmit images obtained by the CMOS image sensor directly to the 4K-3D monitor without significant loss [2]. Additionally, anybody in the operating room, including the assistant surgeon, scrub nurse, students, and visitors, share the same monitor with the surgeon, which may play an important role in surgical learning and teaching.

In exoscopic bypass surgery, surgeons can increase magnification by up to 26 times with digital zoom in combination with optical zoom [8]. When using digital zoom, the resolution is still 2K (1920×1080), which is sufficient for cerebrovascular surgery. This feature was useful during anastomosis for the observation of the intimal wall and suturing as well as speeding up the anastomosis via instantaneous magnification switching on the foot switch. Of all types of exoscopes, ORBEYE has five focus modes, which adjust the diaphragm of the lens. We selected setting 1 because it has the strongest stereoscopic effect and shallow depth of field, similar to a conventional microscope. We believe the most important aspect of cerebrovascular surgery, including STA-MCA bypass, is the accurate three-dimensionality. In contrast, when settings 4 or 5 are used, surgeons achieve a greater depth of field than with a conventional microscope. This reduced need for frequent refocusing can speed up procedures in situations where fine manipulation is unnecessary.

Despite these advantages, the use of an exoscope also has several limitations. The first disadvantage of using an exoscope is the "red-color shift." The exoscope emphasizes red more than the conventional microscope does [7]. To resolve this problem, we changed the color mode of ORBEYE to setting 4, which suppressed the red color compared with the default setting.

The second disadvantage of the exoscope is the "90-degree problem," wherein the assistant's operating field and the display on the assistant monitor are misaligned by 90 degrees [12]. In conventional microscopes, surgeons can adjust the direction of the operating field in the assistant's lens as desired, whereas the exoscope allows only a 180-degree rotation in the assistant's monitor. If the assistant monitor itself is rotated 90 degrees and placed vertically to resolve this problem, the stereoscopic view is lost for the following reasons [3, 9]. The ORBEYE uses "circular polarization" to provide different visual information to each eye, which enables a stereoscopic view. However, the hue is known to differ depending on the angle shift. Thus, the angle between the 3D glasses and the monitor should be kept constant. To resolve this problem, the assistant could share the main monitor with the surgeon instead of using the assistant monitor. Use of the ceiling-mounted monitor may also help resolve this issue.

The third disadvantage of using the exoscope is the image vibration with a maximum magnification at the time of suturing. Although previous reports have not identified this problem, we confirmed it with reproducibility. Because the ORBEYE is more than twice as light as the conventional microscope, the stability of the optical unit may be inferior to that of the conventional microscope. Therefore, the ORBEYE may be affected by vibration from cooling fans or quake-absorbing structures. In the current condition, it is necessary to use a maximum magnification partially on the point and to reduce the load of the cooling fan. The author canceled the vibration of the operative videos using "stabilization" in the video editor software.

Finally, exoscopes require about 80 ms of latency for image processing and data transfer according to our measurements, whereas the manufacturer claimed "zero delay" [8]. We should pay attention to this latency during procedures, although no significant discomfort was observed.

Study Limitations

This study has several limitations. First, this study was limited to the data acquired retrospectively from a single center. This small number of patients is insufficient for the analysis of the outcomes. Second, no complete randomization of the therapeutic modalities was observed, which could result in selection bias. Third, the surgeons were not unified, and the results may be influenced by their respective learning curves. Despite these limitations, this study was able to report the advantages and disadvantages of exoscopic STA-MCA bypass as revealed through initial experiences.

Conclusion

The advantages of the exoscope were image quality, its compact body, and its comfortable resting position, which could reduce the fatigue of neurosurgeons. The instantaneous digital zoom was particularly useful during bypass surgery. Despite some specific disadvantages, the clinical outcomes of the exoscope were comparable to those of the conventional microscope. Thus, we speculate that exoscopes will be more commonly used in the neurosurgical field in the near future.

Data availability: Supporting data are available from the corresponding author upon reasonable request.

Declarations
Competing interests: No competing interests exist in the submission of the manuscript, and the manuscript was approved by all authors for publication. No special funding was received for this study.

Ethics approval: All aspects of this study were approved by the Ethics Committee of Saitama Medical University International Medical Center (2021-230). The need for written informed consent was waived due to the study's retrospective design.

References

1. Ahmad FI, Mericli AF, DeFazio MV, Chang EI, Hanasono MM, Pederson WC, Kaufman M, Selber JC. Application of the ORBEYE three-dimensional exoscope for microsurgical procedures. Microsurgery. 2020;40(4):468–72.
2. Fiani B, Jarrah R, Griepp DW, Adukuzhiyil J. The role of 3D exoscope Systems in Neurosurgery: an optical innovation. Cureus. 2021;13(6):e15878.
3. Hong J, Kim Y, Choi HJ, Hahn J, Park JH, Kim H, Min SW, Chen N, Lee B. Three-dimensional display technologies of recent interest: principles, status, and issues [invited]. Appl Opt. 2011;50(34):H87–H115.
4. Lang WH, Muchel FL. ZEISS microscopes for microsurgery. ZEISS Microscopes Microsurg. 1981; https://doi.org/10.1007/978-3-642-81644-4.
5. Maeda T, Oogigawa H, Onodera K, Sato H, Suzuki K, Kurita H. Pros and cons of Exoscopic intracranial aneurysm repair. Surg Cerebral Stroke. 2023;51(5):397–404.
6. Mamelak AN, Danielpour M, Black KL, Hagike M, Berci G. A high-definition exoscope system for neurosurgery and other microsurgical disciplines: preliminary report. Surg Innov. 2008;15(1):38–46.
7. Noro S, Seo Y, Honjo K, Okuma M, Asayama B, Amano Y, Kyono M, Hashimoto M, Hanai K, Nakamura H. Visualization and Maneuverability features of a robotic arm three-dimensional exoscope and operating microscope for clipping an Unruptured intracranial aneurysm: video comparison and technical evaluation. Oper Neurosurg (Hagerstown). 2022;22(1):101–5.
8. Olympus corporation ORBEYE. In: https://medical.olympusamerica.com/products/orbeye.
9. Richtberg S, Girwidz R. Use of linear and circular polarization: the secret LCD screen and 3D cinema. Phys Teach. 2017;55(7):406.
10. Shibano A, Kimura H, Tatehara S, et al. Efficacy of a high-definition three-dimensional exoscope in simultaneous transcranial and endoscopic Endonasal surgery: a case report. NMC Case Rep J. 2022;9:243–7.
11. Takahashi S, Toda M, Nishimoto M, Ishihara E, Miwa T, Akiyama T, Horiguchi T, Sasaki H, Yoshida K. Pros and cons of using ORBEYE™ for microneurosurgery. Clin Neurol Neurosurg. 2018;174:57–62.
12. Tamura R, Kuranari Y, Katayama M. A three-surgeon–six-hand operation using a 4K-3D exoscope for neurological surgery: a case report. Front Surg. 2022;9:866476.
13. Iwama T. Properties and characteristics of surgical microscopes for microneurosurgery. Jap J Neurosurg. 2010;19(7):504–9.
14. Yaşargil MG. A legacy of microneurosurgery: memoirs, lessons, and axioms. Neurosurgery. 1999;45(5):1025–91.
15. Yasargil M, Krayenbuhl H, Jacobson J. Microneurosurg arterial reconstruct. Surgery. 1970;67(1):221–33.

Open Access This chapter is licensed under the terms of the Creative Commons Attribution 4.0 International License (http://creativecommons.org/licenses/by/4.0/), which permits use, sharing, adaptation, distribution and reproduction in any medium or format, as long as you give appropriate credit to the original author(s) and the source, provide a link to the Creative Commons license and indicate if changes were made.

The images or other third party material in this chapter are included in the chapter's Creative Commons license, unless indicated otherwise in a credit line to the material. If material is not included in the chapter's Creative Commons license and your intended use is not permitted by statutory regulation or exceeds the permitted use, you will need to obtain permission directly from the copyright holder.

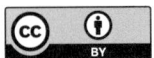

Flow-Augmentation Bypass Surgery: Indications and Decision-Making

Giuseppe Esposito, Martina Sebök, Jorn Fierstra, and Luca Regli

Summary

Flow-augmentation bypass aims to enhance blood flow to hypoperfused brain regions in patients with cerebrovascular steno-occlusive diseases. This surgical procedure is indicated for ischemic and hemorrhagic moyamoya vasculopathy and for selected patients with chronic steno-occlusive disease and acute ischemic stroke. Flow-augmentation bypass has been rigorously evaluated in randomized clinical trials, including the EC-IC Bypass Trial, the Carotid Occlusion Surgery Study (COSS), the Japanese Adult Moyamoya (JAM) trial, and the recent Carotid and Middle Cerebral Artery Occlusion Surgery Study (CMOSS). In this article, we examine the current indications and outline the diagnostic and therapeutic decision-making processes for patients with steno-occlusive disease who are candidates for flow-augmentation bypass surgery.

Introduction

Flow-augmentation bypass aims to restore the flow to hypoperfused brain territories in patients with cerebrovascular steno-occlusive diseases such as moyamoya vasculopathy, chronic steno-occlusive disease, and acute ischemic stroke

[1]. Flow-augmentation bypass methods are traditionally classified into direct, indirect, and combined procedures. A direct bypass creates an immediate anastomosis between a donor artery, typically the superficial temporal artery (STA), and an intracranial recipient artery, providing instant blood flow to the brain. Indirect techniques involve placing vascularized tissue, such as muscle, dura, or pericranium, onto the cerebral cortex to favor neoangiogenesis over time: this results in delayed revascularization. Combined procedures integrate both direct and indirect methods in a single surgical session, in this way offering the benefits of immediate and delayed revascularization [1, 2]. The effectiveness of a flow-augmentation extracranial-intracranial (EC-IC) bypass surgery has been critically studied in randomized clinical trials (RCTs): the EC-IC Bypass Trial [3], the Carotid Occlusion Surgery Study (COSS) [4], the Japanese Adult Moyamoya (JAM) trial [5], and recently the CMOSS (Carotid and Middle Cerebral Artery Occlusion Surgery Study) [6].

Overview of Current Indications

Moyamoya Vasculopathy

Flow-augmentation bypass is the only effective treatment for symptomatic Moyamoya patients with hemodynamic insufficiency. Bypass has been shown to reduce both ischemic and hemorrhagic stroke rates and to prevent neurocognitive decline [1, 7]. Its effectiveness in preventing ischemic strokes and cognitive deterioration in moyamoya patients has not been confirmed through RCTs, but observational studies clearly demonstrate the benefits of bypass surgery, and favorable outcomes from revascularization have been documented in both children and adults [8, 9]. Untreated patients have an unfavorable annual ischemic stroke rate of 13.3%; moreover, a high rate of disease progression and of subsequent symptoms in nonsurgically treated hemispheres

G. Esposito (✉) · L. Regli
Department of Neurosurgery, Clinical Neuroscience Center, University Hospital Zurich, University of Zurich, Zurich, Switzerland

Zurich Microsurgery Lab, Department of Neurosurgery, University Hospital Zurich, Zurich, Switzerland
e-mail: giuseppe.esposito@usz.ch; luca.regli@usz.ch

M. Sebök · J. Fierstra
Department of Neurosurgery, Clinical Neuroscience Center, University Hospital Zurich, University of Zurich, Zurich, Switzerland
e-mail: martina.seboek@usz.ch; jorn.fierstra@usz.ch

has been reported [10, 11]. Nowadays, surgery is recommended for both children and adults with ischemic symptoms and compromised hemodynamics. Careful observation is advised for asymptomatic patients with normal cerebral hemodynamics [1, 12].

The role of surgical treatment in patients with moyamoya disease presenting with intracerebral hemorrhage was highlighted by the JAM trial. This RCT demonstrated that direct bypass for adult patients with hemorrhagic moyamoya disease reduces the rebleeding rate and improves prognosis over 5 years. This indicates that improving the hemodynamic state of the revascularized hemisphere decreases the hemodynamic strain on the fragile moyamoya collateral vessels that are prone to rupture [1, 5].

Revascularization surgery for moyamoya disease involves both direct and indirect methods, tailored to the patient's age, the specific vascular areas needing revascularization, and the individual's unique angioanatomy. Unanimous agreement has not been reached on the optimal type of bypass surgery. The most common direct revascularization procedure remains the STA-MCA (superficial temporal artery to middle cerebral artery) bypass. Surgeons often use a combination of direct and indirect techniques. In general, adult patients are typically treated with direct bypass methods, such as the STA-MCA bypass, whereas children are more commonly treated with indirect or combined revascularization approaches [1].

Although most bypass techniques focus on the MCA territory, enhancing cerebral blood flow to the frontal areas is particularly important in moyamoya patients, especially in the pediatric population. Bifrontal hypoperfusion adversely affects intellectual development, cognitive function, and patients' motor control of the lower extremities and sphincters. Therefore, the timely revascularization of the frontal lobes is essential to prevent neurocognitive decline. In addition to direct STA to anterior cerebral artery (STA-ACA) bypass, indirect and combined bypass techniques have been proposed to optimize blood supply to the bifrontal region [1, 13, 14].

Atherosclerotic Occlusive Disease of the ICA and MCA

To date, randomized controlled trials (RCTs) such as the EC-IC Bypass Trial, the COSS, and the recent CMOSS have not demonstrated a clear benefit from bypass surgery over medical therapy for patients with atherosclerotic internal carotid artery (ICA) occlusion and hemodynamic impairment [3, 4, 6]. As a result, the use of flow-augmentation EC-IC bypass in ischemic cerebrovascular disease has been limited. However, despite advances in medical therapy, patients with severe steno-occlusive disease continue to experience significant event rates [15]. Notably, even in light of these RCT findings, neurologist and cerebrovascular boards continue to refer selected patients for flow-augmentation bypass. These patients may present with more-severe disease and differ from those included in the RCTs, as observed in our experience and reported by other institutions [16].

First and foremost, bypass surgery is now considered only when optimal medical management fails to prevent stroke and recurrent symptoms. In the COSS trial, the primary symptomatic inclusion criterion was a transitory ischemic attack (TIA) or stroke within the previous 120 days [4, 16]. However, the published COSS data do not specify how many patients experienced multiple versus single ischemic events. In a recent study by Wessels et al. [16] involving 179 patients who underwent bypass for atherosclerotic cerebrovascular disease, 80% experienced recurrent hemodynamic events, and approximately 76% suffered recurrent ischemic strokes.

Second, these patients referred for bypass often exhibit more-severe hemodynamic impairment, more-intense symptoms, and more-complex vascular occlusion patterns, such as inadequate collateral pathways. They frequently present with flow and hemodynamic profiles indicative of profoundly compromised cerebrovascular reserve capacity, symptomatic oligemia, and persistent severe ischemic symptoms despite intensive medical therapy [16, 17]. These patients often present with multiple occlusions of brain-feeding arteries [16, 18]. Additionally, many have multiple vessel occlusions, which can markedly diminish collateral circulation capacity [16]. In the COSS trial, only 18 out of 195 patients (9.2%) had significant ($\geq$70%) contralateral carotid stenosis [4, 16]. In contrast, in the recent series of Wessels et al. [16], 50% of the patients had significant ($\geq$70%) stenosis in multiple vascular segments in addition to unilateral ICA occlusion. This highlights that patients undergoing bypass today differ substantially from the COSS population.

Third, further analysis suggests that the failure of the COSS trial to demonstrate a reduction in ipsilateral 2-year stroke recurrence with cerebral bypass revascularization was likely due to the limitations of the semiquantitative, hemispheric oxygen extraction fraction (OEF) ratio method (OEF ratio >1.13 used in COSS) rather than flaws in patient selection based on hemodynamic compromise [19–21]. Currently, patients considered for bypass revascularization are those with symptomatic carotid occlusion with recurrent symptoms and with significant hemodynamic impairment—often more severe than the OEF ratio >1.13 used in COSS—placing them at high risk for subsequent stroke [18, 21]. Therefore, alternative and, in particular, quantitative imaging techniques are essential to accurately assess the hemodynamic status in patients with ischemic stroke due to ICA occlusion [19].

Certain subgroups of patients were not specifically addressed in the RCTs—for example, individuals with chronic retinal ischemia leading to progressive visual loss and those with ongoing hemodynamic symptoms despite optimal medical therapy [22, 23]. Some patients may experience ischemic episodes triggered by postural changes or blood pressure fluctuations, such as those with debilitating orthostatic hypoperfusion syndrome or limb-shaking TIAs [1, 22].

Finally, another subgroup that might benefit from bypass surgery includes patients with acute or subacute stroke, where brain tissue remains at risk due to persistent oligemia despite optimal medical and interventional management [18, 21, 24]. Surgical flow augmentation via STA-MCA bypass for penumbra salvation has yielded promising outcomes in selected case series [21, 24]. Recent data from a Zurich group suggest that symptomatic patients with persistent penumbra in the acute stroke phase or recurrent symptoms in the subacute stroke phase, particularly those with hemodynamic impairment (paradoxical cerebrovascular reactivity (CVR)) and inadequate collateral circulation, may represent a highly selected group who could benefit from early cerebral revascularization surgery [21]. These patients could derive significant benefits from bypass surgery, provided that it can be performed with sufficiently low morbidity, as demonstrated in certain case series [5, 16, 17].

Although RCTs did not demonstrate a clear benefit from bypass surgery over medical therapy [3, 4, 21], several studies have shown significant improvements in hemodynamic parameters following bypass surgery in carefully selected patients [25–28]. A reduction in stroke recurrence after bypass has been reported [21]. Nguyen et al. [29] recently conducted a systematic review of 50 articles and found that long-term stroke rates and favorable outcomes for surgical revascularization for steno-occlusive disease have improved over time and are much better than previously reported. This improvement in outcomes is likely due to more-refined patient selection since the COSS trial. At most institutions performing flow-augmentation bypass surgery, patients must have failed optimal medical management, experienced recurrent perfusion-dependent ischemia, and had anatomical characteristics favorable for revascularization surgery [29]. These procedures are carried out by highly skilled surgeons, and patients receive comprehensive perioperative care by specialized teams [29]. After the RCTs, lower-volume centers and less-experienced surgeons ceased performing the procedure, leading to a more homogeneous group of experienced surgeons reporting these improved results [29]. The clinical challenge, however, remains the accurate identification of patients at higher risk for future stroke (despite medical therapy), who are those most likely to benefit from bypass surgery [21].

Studying Brain Hemodynamic and Collaterals

At the University Hospital Zurich, two innovative magnetic resonance imaging (MRI) techniques have been implemented in recent years to assess cerebral hemodynamics and collateralization and assess patients with cerebrovascular steno-occlusive diseases: (I) blood oxygenation level-dependent (BOLD) functional MRI cerebrovascular reactivity (CVR), which uses a standardized CO_2 vasodilatory challenge to quantitatively evaluate CVR on a voxel-by-voxel basis, and (II) noninvasive optimal vessel analysis (NOVA; VasSol Inc.), a quantitative magnetic resonance angiography (qMRA) technique that measures the volume flow rate (VFR) in mL/min in cerebral vessels [18, 21].

BOLD-CVR is a valuable tool for examining cerebral hemodynamics and assessing stroke risk in patients with symptomatic cerebrovascular steno-occlusive diseases, such as atherosclerosis and moyamoya [19, 30]. NOVA-qMRA provides an accurate measurement of blood flow in mL/min in cerebral vessels and allows for a reliable assessment of flow status and cerebral collateral pathways in cases of large vessel occlusion [31]. In addition to evaluating hemodynamic status, analyzing collateral blood supply is of importance for determining the need for flow-augmentation bypass surgery because collateral flow significantly affects perfusion and hemodynamics [31, 32].

Candidates for bypass surgery, whether due to moyamoya disease or atherosclerotic vasculopathy, admitted or referred to the University Hospital of Zurich, are receiving a detailed hemodynamic and flow evaluation using BOLD-CVR and NOVA-qMRA [17, 21, 33, 34]. Surgical revascularization with an STA-MCA bypass is indicated for symptomatic patients who exhibit a paradoxical BOLD-CVR (steal phenomenon) in at least half of the occluded vascular territory [18]. For patients with atherosclerotic large vessel occlusion, we use an M1-VFR ratio <50% and a hemispheric VFR ratio <70% as thresholds, indicating insufficient collateralization via the Willis circle (Acom or Pcom) or insufficient extra-intracranial collateralization through the ophthalmic artery [18]. If these collateralization patterns are inadequate, a third pattern of collateralization activates, leading to increased leptomeningeal flow through the P2-segment [35]. We demonstrated a correlation between the hemodynamics and the collateral flow measured via BOLD-CVR and NOVA-qMRA. In patients with symptomatic carotid occlusion, impaired BOLD-CVR is partly linked to an increased PCA-P2 volume flow rate, potentially indicating the activation of leptomeningeal collaterals in severe hemodynamic conditions. Both imaging techniques could aid clinicians in creating personalized treatment strategies for patients with symptomatic ICA occlusion [33].

Intra- and Postoperative Measurements

At the University Hospital Zurich, bypass flow is monitored intraoperatively by using a flexible perivascular transit-time flow probe (Charbel MicroFlowprobe; Transonic Systems, Inc., Ithaca, NY, USA). Postoperatively, before discharge, patients undergo a qMRA-NOVA scan. This technique allows for the noninvasive measurement of bypass patency and flow and an analysis of collateral status and pathways [17, 36]. In post-bypass NOVA-qMRA assessments, the hemispheric VFR (hVFR) on the ipsilateral side includes the bypass flow values, calculated as the sum of VFR from the A2, M1, and P2 segments and from the bypass itself. Previous studies have demonstrated the reliability and utility of this noninvasive method for the serial monitoring of bypass function, suggesting that qMRA may serve as an alternative to standard angiography for follow-ups to bypass grafts [37].

After undergoing a transcranial Doppler 4–6 weeks after surgery, patients are monitored 3 months later by using BOLD-CVR to assess changes in hemodynamics [21]. Improved CVR, excellent bypass flow, and positive clinical outcomes (such as the absence of stroke recurrence) are key indicators that surgical candidates were appropriately selected. These results further highlight the effectiveness of advanced neuroimaging techniques like BOLD-CVR and NOVA in evaluating patients.

Flow-augmentation revascularization through an STA-MCA bypass is a relatively uncommon procedure that should be carried out at specialized, high-volume referral centers. These centers need to be equipped with advanced quantitative neuroimaging and possess highly specialized neurovascular units, including intensive care facilities for optimal postoperative management. Advanced neuroimaging enables precise candidate selection based on objective criteria. Continuous follow-up is important to monitor neurological outcomes and recurrent stroke incidents. At University Hospital Zurich, bypass candidates are studied via advanced neuroimaging, with treatment decisions made during interdisciplinary conferences involving neurologists, neurosurgeons, and neuroradiologists. The goal is to provide high-quality diagnostics, treatment, and follow-up to achieve the best possible patient care and clinical outcomes.

Conclusions

Flow-augmentation bypass improves blood flow to brain regions with reduced perfusion and remains the only effective treatment for symptomatic moyamoya patients with compromised brain hemodynamics. Additionally, this procedure is essential for managing selected patients with atherosclerotic steno-occlusive disease as a last-resort option for patients who experience recurrent symptoms despite optimal medical treatment, show severe brain hemodynamic impairment, and present inadequate collateral circulation. In this context, we have outlined the current indications, diagnostic approaches, and therapeutic decision-making for patients with steno-occlusive disease who are candidates for flow-augmentation bypass surgery. These patients should be concentrated at specialized, high-volume bypass centers where STA-MCA bypass surgery can be performed with an acceptable level of risk.

References

1. Esposito G, Amin-Hanjani S, Regli L. Role of and indications for bypass surgery after Carotid Occlusion Surgery Study (COSS)? Stroke. 2016;47(1):282–90.
2. Esposito G, Sebök M, Amin-Hanjani S, Regli L. Cerebral bypass surgery: level of evidence and grade of recommendation. Acta Neurochir Suppl. 2018;129:73–7.
3. EC/IC Bypass Study Group. Failure of extracranial-intracranial arterial bypass to reduce the risk of ischemic stroke. Results of an international randomized trial. N Engl J Med. 1985;313(19):1191–200.
4. Powers WJ, Clarke WR, Grubb RL Jr, Videen TO, Adams HP Jr, Derdeyn CP. Extracranial-intracranial bypass surgery for stroke prevention in hemodynamic cerebral ischemia: the Carotid Occlusion Surgery Study randomized trial. JAMA. 2011;306(18):1983–92.
5. Miyamoto S, Yoshimoto T, Hashimoto N, Okada Y, Tsuji I, Tominaga T, et al. Effects of extracranial-intracranial bypass for patients with hemorrhagic moyamoya disease: results of the Japan Adult Moyamoya trial. Stroke. 2014;45(5):1415–21.
6. Ma Y, Wang T, Wang H, Amin-Hanjani S, Tong X, Wang J, et al. Extracranial-intracranial bypass and risk of stroke and death in patients with symptomatic artery occlusion: the CMOSS randomized clinical trial. JAMA. 2023;330(8):704–14.
7. Kronenburg A, Esposito G, Fierstra J, Braun KP, Regli L. Combined bypass technique for contemporary revascularization of unilateral MCA and bilateral frontal territories in Moyamoya vasculopathy. Acta Neurochir Suppl. 2014;119:65–70.
8. Rosen C, McKetton L, Russell J, Sam K, Poublanc J, Crawley A, et al. Long-term changes in cerebrovascular reactivity following EC-IC bypass for intracranial steno-occlusive disease. J Clin Neurosci. 2018;54:77–82.
9. Han JS, Abou-Hamden A, Mandell DM, Poublanc J, Crawley AP, Fisher JA, et al. Impact of extracranial-intracranial bypass on cerebrovascular reactivity and clinical outcome in patients with symptomatic moyamoya vasculopathy. Stroke. 2011;42(11):3047–54.
10. Gross BA, Du R. The natural history of moyamoya in a North American adult cohort. J Clin Neurosci. 2013;20(1):44–8.
11. Kuroda S, Ishikawa T, Houkin K, Nanba R, Hokari M, Iwasaki Y. Incidence and clinical features of disease progression in adult moyamoya disease. Stroke. 2005;36(10):2148–53.
12. Kronenburg A, Braun KP, van der Zwan A, Klijn CJ. Recent advances in moyamoya disease: pathophysiology and treatment. Curr Neurol Neurosci Rep. 2014;14(1):423.
13. Weinberg DG, Rahme RJ, Aoun SG, Batjer HH, Bendok BR. Moyamoya disease: functional and neurocognitive outcomes in the pediatric and adult populations. Neurosurg Focus. 2011;30(6):E21.

14. Khan N, Schuknecht B, Boltshauser E, Capone A, Buck A, Imhof HG, et al. Moyamoya disease and Moyamoya syndrome: experience in Europe; choice of revascularisation procedures. Acta Neurochir. 2003;145(12):1061–71. discussion 71
15. Elder TA, White TG, Woo HH, Siddiqui AH, Nunna R, Siddiq F, et al. Future of endovascular and surgical treatments of atherosclerotic intracranial stenosis. Stroke. 2024;55(2):344–54.
16. Wessels L, Hecht N, Vajkoczy P. Patients receiving Extracranial to intracranial bypass for atherosclerotic vessel occlusion today differ significantly from the COSS population. Stroke. 2021;52(10):e599–604.
17. Sebök M, Höbner LM, Grob A, Fierstra J, Schubert T, Wegener S, et al. Flow capacity of a superficial temporal artery as a donor in a consecutive series of 100 patients with superficial temporal artery-middle cerebral artery bypass. J Neurosurg. 2024;142:1–8.
18. Sebök M, Esposito G, Niftrik C, Fierstra J, Schubert T, Wegener S, et al. Flow augmentation STA-MCA bypass evaluation for patients with acute stroke and unilateral large vessel occlusion: a proposal for an urgent bypass flowchart. J Neurosurg. 2022;137:1–9.
19. Sebök M, van der Wouden F, Mader C, Pangalu A, Treyer V, Fisher JA, et al. Hemodynamic failure staging with blood oxygenation level-dependent cerebrovascular reactivity and acetazolamide-challenged ((15)O-)H(2)O-Positron emission tomography across individual cerebrovascular territories. J Am Heart Assoc. 2023;12(24):e029491.
20. Carlson AP, Yonas H, Chang YF, Nemoto EM. Failure of cerebral hemodynamic selection in general or of specific positron emission tomography methodology?: Carotid Occlusion Surgery Study (COSS). Stroke. 2011;42(12):3637–9.
21. Sebök M, Höbner LM, Fierstra J, Schubert T, Wegener S, Kulcsár Z, et al. Flow-augmentation STA-MCA bypass for acute and subacute ischemic stroke due to internal carotid artery occlusion and the role of advanced neuroimaging with hemodynamic and flow-measurement in the decision-making: preliminary data. Quant Imaging Med Surg. 2024;14(1):777–88.
22. Reynolds MR, Derdeyn CP, Grubb RL Jr, Powers WJ, Zipfel GJ. Extracranial-intracranial bypass for ischemic cerebrovascular disease: what have we learned from the Carotid Occlusion Surgery Study? Neurosurg Focus. 2014;36(1):E9.
23. Powers WJ, Clarke WR, Adams HP Jr, Derdeyn CP, Grubb RL Jr. Commentary: Extracranial-intracranial bypass for stroke in 2012: response to the critique of the carotid occlusion surgery study "It was déjà vu all over again". Neurosurgery. 2012;71(3):E772–6.
24. Guida L, Sebök M, Wegener S, Fierstra J, van Niftrik B, Luft AR, et al. Flow-augmentation bypass in the treatment of acute ischemic stroke. J Neurosurg Sci. 2021;65(3):269–76.
25. Burkhardt JK, Winklhofer S, Fierstra J, Wegener S, Esposito G, Luft A, et al. Emergency Extracranial-intracranial bypass to Revascularize salvageable brain tissue in acute ischemic stroke patients. World Neurosurg. 2018;109:e476–e85.
26. Low SW, Teo K, Lwin S, Yeo LL, Paliwal PR, Ahmad A, et al. Improvement in cerebral hemodynamic parameters and outcomes after superficial temporal artery-middle cerebral artery bypass in patients with severe stenoocclusive disease of the intracranial internal carotid or middle cerebral arteries. J Neurosurg. 2015;123(3):662–9.
27. Ishikawa T, Houkin K, Abe H, Isobe M, Kamiyama H. Cerebral haemodynamics and long-term prognosis after extracranial-intracranial bypass surgery. J Neurol Neurosurg Psychiatry. 1995;59(6):625–8.
28. Klijn CJ, Kappelle LJ, van der Zwan A, van Gijn J, Tulleken CA. Excimer laser-assisted high-flow extracranial/intracranial bypass in patients with symptomatic carotid artery occlusion at high risk of recurrent cerebral ischemia: safety and long-term outcome. Stroke. 2002;33(10):2451–8.
29. Nguyen VN, Motiwala M, Parikh K, Miller LE, Barats M, Nickele CM, et al. Extracranial-intracranial cerebral revascularization for atherosclerotic vessel occlusion: an updated systematic review of the literature. World Neurosurg. 2023;173:199–207.e8.
30. van Niftrik CHB, Sebök M, Germans MR, Halter M, Pokorny T, Stumpo V, et al. Increased risk of recurrent stroke in symptomatic large vessel disease with impaired BOLD cerebrovascular reactivity. Stroke. 2024;55(3):613–21.
31. Bae YJ, Jung C, Kim JH, Choi BS, Kim E. Quantitative magnetic resonance angiography in internal carotid artery occlusion with primary collateral pathway. J Stroke. 2015;17(3):320–6.
32. Ruland S, Ahmed A, Thomas K, Zhao M, Amin-Hanjani S, Du X, et al. Leptomeningeal collateral volume flow assessed by quantitative magnetic resonance angiography in large-vessel cerebrovascular disease. J Neuroimaging. 2009;19(1):27–30.
33. Walser A, Fierstra J, Höbner LM, Bellomo J, Schubert T, Germans M, et al. Correlation between P2-PCA volume flow rate and BOLD cerebrovascular reactivity in patients with symptomatic carotid artery occlusion. AJNR Am J Neuroradiol. 2024;18:ajnr.A8626.
34. Garbani Nerini L, Bellomo J, Höbner LM, Stumpo V, Colombo E, van Niftrik CHB, et al. BOLD cerebrovascular reactivity and NOVA quantitative MR angiography in adult patients with Moyamoya vasculopathy undergoing cerebral bypass surgery. Brain Sci. 2024;14(8):762.
35. Sebök M, Niftrik C, Lohaus N, Esposito G, Amki ME, Winklhofer S, et al. Leptomeningeal collateral activation indicates severely impaired cerebrovascular reserve capacity in patients with symptomatic unilateral carotid artery occlusion. J Cereb Blood Flow Metab. 2021;41(11):3039–51.
36. Amin-Hanjani S, Meglio G, Gatto R, Bauer A, Charbel FT. The utility of intraoperative blood flow measurement during aneurysm surgery using an ultrasonic perivascular flow probe. Neurosurgery. 2006;58(4 Suppl 2):ONS-305-12; discussion ONS-12.
37. Amin-Hanjani S, Shin JH, Zhao M, Du X, Charbel FT. Evaluation of extracranial-intracranial bypass using quantitative magnetic resonance angiography. J Neurosurg. 2007;106(2):291–8.

Open Access This chapter is licensed under the terms of the Creative Commons Attribution 4.0 International License (http://creativecommons.org/licenses/by/4.0/), which permits use, sharing, adaptation, distribution and reproduction in any medium or format, as long as you give appropriate credit to the original author(s) and the source, provide a link to the Creative Commons license and indicate if changes were made.

The images or other third party material in this chapter are included in the chapter's Creative Commons license, unless indicated otherwise in a credit line to the material. If material is not included in the chapter's Creative Commons license and your intended use is not permitted by statutory regulation or exceeds the permitted use, you will need to obtain permission directly from the copyright holder.

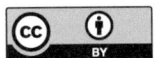

Part IV
Neuroimaging

New Classification of the Degree of Cerebrovascular Insufficiency in Patients with Moyamoya Disease Measured According to ASL-MRI Perfusion

Anna A. Shulgina, Vasily A. Lukshin, Anton A. Korshunov, Dmitry Yu Usachev, and Igor N. Pronin

Introduction

One of the main stages in the diagnostics of patients with steno-occlusive cerebrovascular pathology is the assessment of the degree of cerebrovascular insufficiency (CVI) based on the measurement of cerebral perfusion. The presence and severity of signs of CVI determine the severity of the disease and the prognosis of its natural course. The detection of CVI signs with modern neuroimaging methods is based on measuring cerebral blood flow (CBF) at the baseline and after stimulation. In particular, these parameters help to determine indications for the surgical revascularization of the brain given that cerebral perfusion impairment is a reliable prognostic risk factor for ischemic stroke [1]. After the inconclusive results of a large international trial, namely the Carotid Occlusion Surgery Study (COSS) [2], currently the main natural clinical model of chronic cerebral ischemia are patients with moyamoya angiopathy (MMA), a group of chronic cerebrovascular diseases characterized by the progressive stenosis of the circle of Willis arteries with the development of a basal collateral network ("moyamoya vessels").

Various diagnostic methods can evaluate cerebral blood flow [3], most of which, however, require the administration of radioactive or contrast agents and are associated with radiation exposure and the risk of side effects. This creates significant technical difficulties and limits the use of these methods in general practice as a routine diagnostic standard for perfusion studies [4].

Recently, the technique of noncontrast ASL perfusion has been actively developed. This method is not associated either with radiation exposure or with the administration of contrast agents, and therefore, it can be performed during all stages of treatment and in almost all categories of patients. The results of the first applications of arterial spin labeling were published in 1998 [5], but the actual spread of the technique in wide clinical practice is beginning to occur only now. Although comparative studies have shown a high correlation of CBF values in ASL-perfusion studies with PET, SPECT, and DSC [6–8], the application of this technique is limited in some cases by the technical complexity of the quantitative assessment of the results and the appearance of different artifacts. Among them, the most difficult for interpretation are arterial transit artifacts (ATAs), which are described among patients with moyamoya angiopathy [9]. Arterial transit artifacts are hyperintensive signals along of the circle of Willis arteries on the side of stenosis or occlusion or along the leptomeningeal vessels on the convexital surface of the hemispheres [10]. The long delay of labeled arterial spins in the cortical arteries is considered as the main cause of ATAs that leads to the appearance of very-high-intensity signals that exceed the true CBF values by several folds. This leads to difficulties in the quantitative assessment of cerebral blood flow. Therefore, the development of a classification system and methods for measuring cerebral blood flow according to ASL-perfusion studies is highly relevant and requires further investigation.

Aim

This chapter aims to develop a methodology to assess the degree of cerebrovascular insufficiency in patients with moyamoya angiopathy (MMA) that is based on an MR-perfusion study of cerebral blood flow (CBF) and the presence of arterial transit artifacts (ATAs) by using arterial spin labeling (ASL). The proposed ASL classification of CVI can be verified by comparing the distinguished degrees of perfusion deficiency with individual characteristics of patients' angio-architectonics and clinical symptoms.

A. A. Shulgina (✉) · V. A. Lukshin · A. A. Korshunov
D. Y. Usachev · I. N. Pronin
Burdenko Neurosurgical Center, Moscow, Russia
e-mail: AShulgina@nsi.ru

Materials and Methods

This study included 47 patients with different types of moyamoya angiopathy. The clinical data of patients are presented in Table 1. Among these patients, 86% were children and 14% adults. The mean age was 10.7 years. Most of the patients were female (W: M = 6: 1). The predominant type of moyamoya angiopathy was moyamoya disease (66%). Moyamoya syndrome was observed in 34% of cases. The ischemic type of the disease was observed in 92% of cases, where the most common clinical presentation featured completed stroke consequences (54%). Clinical symptoms were evaluated by using, National Institutes of Health Stroke Scale (NIHSS) scores [11], with a mean score of 3.4 ± 1.8 points.

In total, 148 perfusion studies were analyzed: 47 before surgical treatment and 101 control studies at different times after surgery. To compare changes in cerebral blood flow with angiography data more correctly, a separate analysis was carried out for each hemisphere. In total, the ASL-perfusion patterns of 296 hemispheres were studied, among them 94 studies before surgery.

The study was carried out on a GE Signa HDxt 3.0 Tesla MR scanner using three-dimensional pseudo-continuous ASL perfusion (3D pCASL) with the following parameters: 3D fast spin echo (FSE), 8-helical scanning that captures the entire brain volume and that subsequently reforms with a section thickness of 4 mm; field of view (FOV) = 240 × 240 mm; 128 × 128 matrix, zero filling (ZIP) 512; repetition time (TR) = 4717 ms; echo time (TE) = 9.8 ms; number of excitations (NEX) = 3; postlabeling delay (PLD) = 1525 ms; pixel bandwidth = 976.6 Hz/pixel. The duration of scanning was 4 minutes and 30 seconds. The arterial blood was marked in a layer 4 mm thick in the axial plane of the neck, perpendicular to the course of the internal carotid artery. The data were processed on an AW Server 3.2 Ext 2.0 workstation using the ReadyView program. As a result, perfusion maps of regional cerebral blood flow (CBF) were constructed (Fig. 1a). Regions of interest (ROIs) were selected in each hemisphere in axial view in seven zones (five in the cortical regions at the level of the centrum semiovale, one in the white matter, and one in the region of the basal ganglia):

1. The territory of the anterior cerebral artery (ACA)
2. The territory of the middle cerebral artery (MCA)
3. The territory of the posterior cerebral artery (PCA)
4. The watershed territory of ACA-MCA
5. The watershed territory of MCA-PCA
6. The area of white matter at the level of the centrum semiovale
7. The area of the basal ganglia at the level of the ventricles of the brain

To more accurately distinguish between the gray and white matter areas of the brain and more reliably manually drawn these areas, the obtained cerebral blood flow maps (Fig. 1a) were fused with the T2-FLAIR sequence using the NeuroRegistration program (AW Server 3.2 Ext. 2.0, General Electric). T2-FLAIR, unlike CBF maps, allows the border of white and gray matter to be visualized more clearly (Fig. 1b). After that, in the fused images (Fig. 1c), the necessary ROIs were manually drawn in the interested zones (Fig. 1d, e) while taking into account the presence of arterial transit artifacts (ATAs). To obtain more-reliable CBF values, ROIs were drawn in way to exclude ATAs in the area of study (Fig. 1f).

An ATA was defined as an area with a very bright signal whose value exceeded the value of blood flow in areas adjacent to the ATA and did not correspond to physiological norms [12]. The correctness of the choice of ATA was confirmed by the conclusions of two experienced neuroradiologists, who were blinded from the clinical data of the patients,

Table 1 Characteristics of the distinguished degrees of perfusion deficit

Degree	N	Characteristics	ATA	ASL pattern
0	66	"Compensation" The values of cerebral blood flow correspond to the values of healthy people **CBF = 64.5 ± 16.2 mL/min/100 g** [CI 61.2–69.2]	No	Fig. 2a
1	116	"Subcompensation" Moderate reduction in cerebral blood flow **CBF = 61.5 ± 16.6 mL/min/100 g** [CI 57.3–63.4]	Yes	Fig. 2b
2	82	"Initial decompensation" Significant decrease in cerebral blood flow **CBF = 26.5 ± 7.2 mL/min/100 g** [CI 25.0–28.2]	Yes	Fig. 2c
3	32	"Decompensation" Extremely low cerebral blood flow **CBF = 16.0 ± 4.7 mL/min/100 g** [CI 15.6–18.8]	No	Fig. 2d

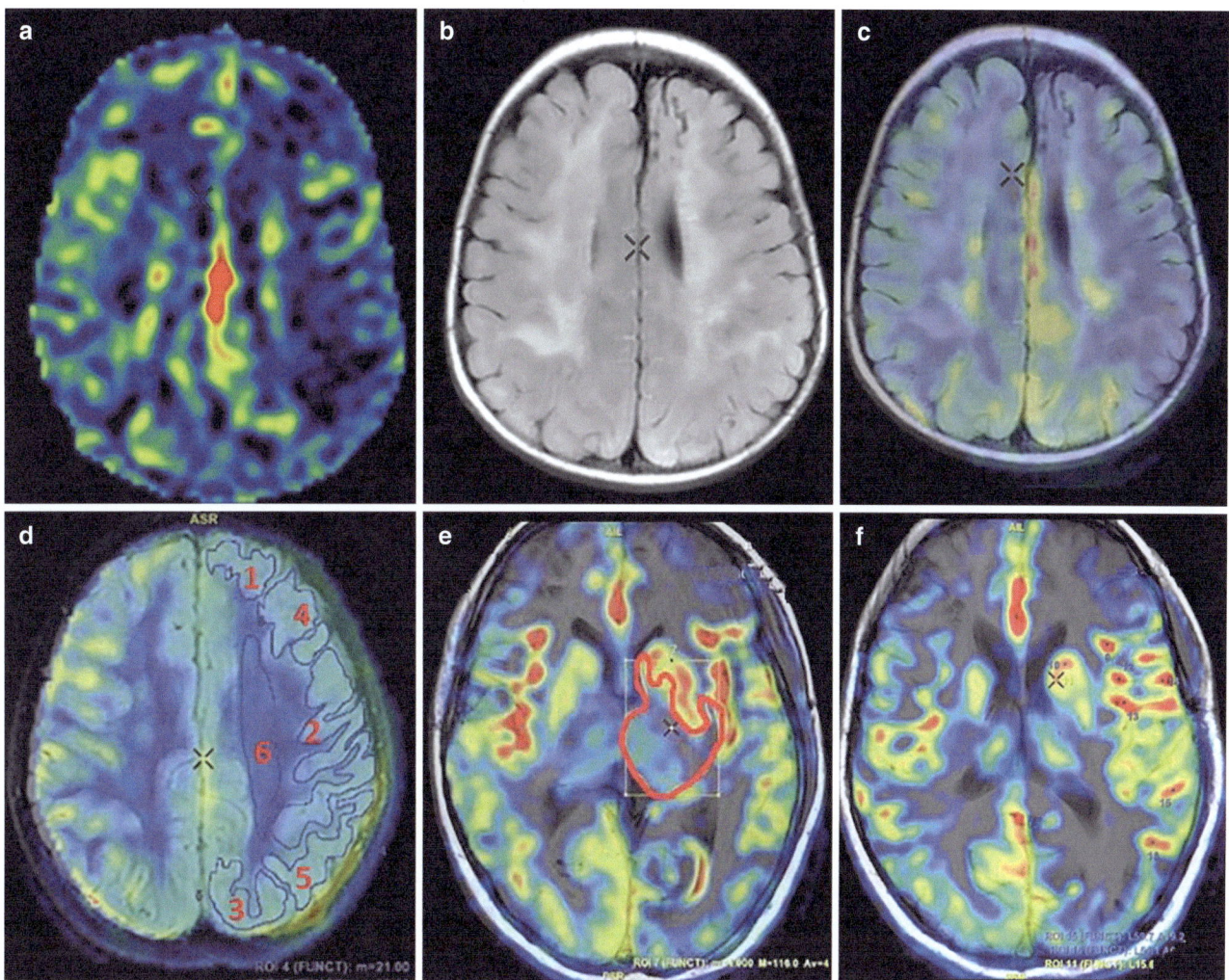

Fig. 1 The technique for measuring CBF using ASL. (**a**) cerebral blood flow (CBF) map. (**b**) T2-FLAIR weighted image that allows the borders of the gray and white matter of the brain to be visualized. (**c**) fused CBF map with T2-FLAIR. (**d**) manually drawn regions of interest: 1—the territory of ACA, 2—the territory of MCA, 3—the territory of PCA, 4—the watershed territory of ACA-MCA, 5—the watershed territory of MCA-PCA, 6—the area of white matter at the level of the centrum semiovale. (**e**) the ROI in the area of basal ganglia, where the region of interest is drawn to exclude ATA. (**f**) registration of values, severity, and localization of ATA

on the basis of well-known criteria widely described in the literature [9, 13, 14]. The quantitative values of the ATA (CBF value in the central point of the artifact), the degree of their severity (no/single/extensive), and their localization (similar to the ROIs described above) were estimated (Fig. 1f). For each study, the maximum and minimum CBF values in the zone of artifacts were recorded.

Direct angiography and 3D time of flight (TOF) magnetic resonance angiography were performed on all 47 patients before the surgical treatment to assess the stage of moyamoya angiopathy and the presence and severity of collateral blood flow. By means of selective direct angiography, the stage of the disease according to Suzuki classification (for patients with moyamoya disease) (94 hemispheres) [15] and the presence of leptomeningeal and transdural collaterals (79 hemispheres) were assessed. Leptomeningeal collaterals from the PCA were evaluated by the number of lobes of hemispheres that were supplied from them—from one to three lobes—according to the classification proposed by Togao et al. [16]. Transdural collaterals from the system of the external carotid artery were evaluated according to their degree and graded as single/blood supplying one lobe of hemisphere/blood, supplying two lobes/blood, or supplying three lobes according to the modification of generally accepted classifications [16, 17]. Based on the MR angiography, the stage of the disease according to Houkin classification [18] and the level of ICA stenosis depending on the site of the ostium of the posterior communicating artery were determined. One-way analysis of variance (ANOVA) and Pearson's chi-square test were used to identify statistical differences between the groups. The statistical process-

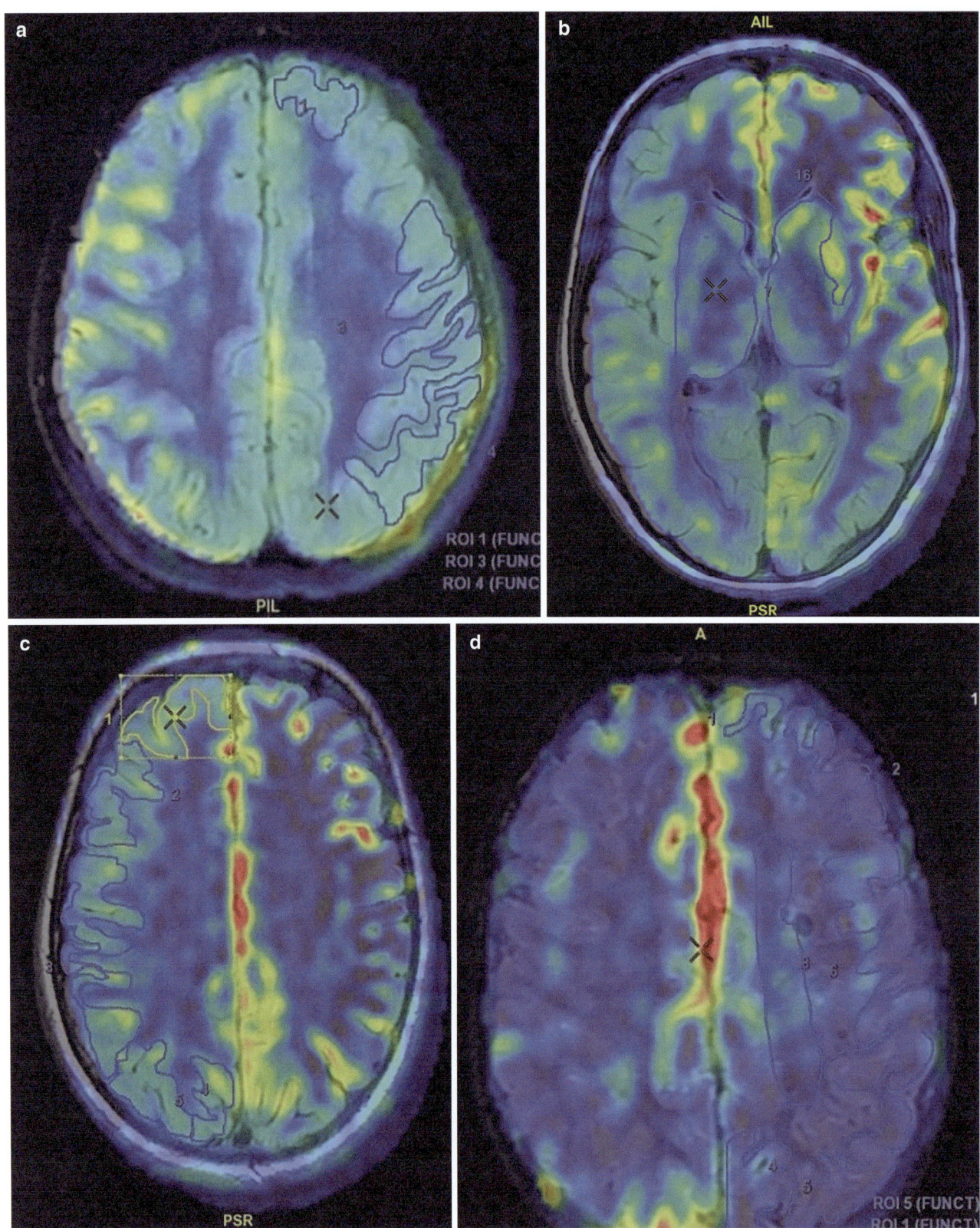

Fig. 2 (**a**) Degree 0. No perfusion deficit. No signs of ATA. Compensation of blood flow. (**b**) Degree 1. Moderate reduction in cerebral blood flow. Signs of ATA. Subcompensation of blood flow. (**c**) Degree 2. Significant decrease in cerebral blood flow. Signs of ATA. Initial decompensation of blood flow. (**d**) Degree 3. Extremely low cerebral blood flow. Disappearance of ATA. Decompensation of blood flow

ing of the material was performed in the IBM SPSS Statistics 23 program.

Results

To determine the criteria for assessing perfusion patterns, the values of cerebral blood flow in the territory of MCA were analyzed in all studies (296 hemispheres). According to the results of the analysis, bimodal distribution, divided by an average CBF value of 47.43 ± 23.2 mL/min/100 g, was noted. In light of the aim of the study, which is to identify signs of CVI, we decided to consider this average value of cerebral blood flow as a threshold between various forms of CBF compensation (>47 mL/min/100 g) and decompensation (<47 mL/min/100 g). A quantitative analysis of the distributions of CBF values for the selected degrees showed a wide dispersion of the obtained values, which indicates the possible heterogeneity of these groups. This required that these stages be refined by using additional criteria.

We selected the presence of arterial transit artifacts as such a criterion. In total, ATA was detected in 77% of studies (69% of the hemispheres). The minimum CBF values in ATA ranged from 51 to 205 mL/min/100 g (mean 120.2 ± 21.1 mL/min/100 g). The lower limit of the confidence interval ($p < 0.05$) was 117.43 mL/min/100 g. The maximum CBF values in ATA varied greatly, from 65 to 995 mL/min/100 g (mean 234.9 ± 105 mL/min/100 g). The effects of ATA can be explained by a slowdown in the blood flow in the collateral network of the brain and reflect the mechanisms of the "subcompensation" of cerebral circulation [13]. Therefore, appearance of ATA in the "compensation" group can be considered as manifestations of the "initial subcompensation" and considered as manifestations of the "initial decompensation" in the group with a gross perfusion deficit.

Thus, depending on the value of CBF and the presence of ATA, we distinguished 4 degrees of perfusion deficit, which are presented in Table 1.

An analysis of the CBF values in all studied areas revealed that values of degree 0 of perfusion deficit correspond to the values of the cerebral blood flow in healthy people (CBF in the territory of MCA = 64.5 ± 16.2 mL/min/100 g [CI 61.2–69.2]). This allowed us to consider this degree as a stage of "compensation." The third degree was characterized by the lowest values of cerebral blood flow (CBF = 16.0 ± 4.7 mL/min/100 g [CI 15.6–18.8]) without the presence of ATA, which indicates the absence of leptomeningeal collateral blood flow, so it was considered as severe "decompensation." The first and second degrees were distinguished by the presence of ATA. The first degree of perfusion deficit had slightly lower values of CBF than did the stage of compensation (degree 0) (CBF = 61.5 ± 16.6 mL/min/100 g [CI 57.3–63.4]), which is why it was classified as "subcompensation." The second degree was characterized by low CBF values (CBF = 26.5 ± 7.2 mL/min/100 g [CI 25.0–28.2]), but the signs of collateral blood flow (ATA) can be seen on MRI, which is why it was classified as "initial decompensation". Univariate analysis of variance (ANOVA) showed the presence of statistically significant differences in CBF values for the proposed degrees of cerebrovascular insufficiency in all analyzed ROIs.

To verify the proposed method for the assessment of the patterns of ASL-perfusion studies and to estimate its ability to reflect the stages of the MMA course, the distinguished degrees of perfusion deficit were compared with the angiographic and clinical characteristics of the patients. This comparative analysis revealed a statistically significant relationship between the Suzuki and Houkin stage of the disease and the degree of perfusion deficit ($p < 0.0001$); a more pronounced perfusion deficit was observed in the advanced stages of MMA ($p < 0.0001$). Also, a more severe degree of perfusion deficit corresponded to a hemodynamically more unfavorable type of MMA with the ICA stenosis proximal to the ostium of the PComA ($\chi^2 = 62.813, p < 0.0001$).

The study of the causes of ATA formation revealed a statistically significant pattern of their detection in patients with a well-developed system of leptomeningeal collaterals in the studied hemisphere—they were seen in 86% of cases ($\chi2 = 20.394, p < 0.001$). Transdural collaterals were detected in 69% of patients with ATA, but no reliable relationship between them was found ($\chi2 = 1.198, p = 0.274$). Also, a statistically significant relationship between the severity of neurological deficit in NIHSS scores and the distinguished degrees of cerebrovascular insufficiency was revealed (ANOVA, $F_{2,44} = 6.914, p = 0.02$).

A more severe neurological deficit was more often observed in the groups of "initial decompensation" and "decompensation." Thus, when the proposed method is used to assess ASL-perfusion patterns in patients with MMA, it has a good agreement with the clinical and angiographic characteristics of the disease and does not contradict the well-known and widespread classifications.

Discussion

Recently, the development of diagnostic methods has been moving toward reducing invasiveness, and therefore, MR-perfusion methods are increasingly being used in the diagnosis of cerebrovascular insufficiency. Currently, one of the most promising technologies in the diagnosis of patients with steno-occlusive cerebrovascular pathology, in particular with moyamoya angiopathy, is ASL perfusion. Although this technique allows the values of cerebral blood flow in all areas of the brain to be reliably quantified, interpretation and comparing the data obtained from different studies are often difficult. This is because of the lack of general methods for determining regions of interest (ROIs) and the appearance of special artifacts in the studies. ROIs are often drawn by covering large areas, including both the cortex and white matter [19–21], even though the values of cerebral blood flow in these areas differ in a healthy person [12]. Usually, this leads to an underestimation of received results, which is why conducting separate assessments of cortex CBF and white matter CBF is crucial. To exclude this error, some studies have performed an approximate comparison of the selected regions with the anatomical modes of MRI, but this is not reliable technique [7]. In our study, to quantify cerebral blood flow more accurately, we used the fusion of CBF maps with the T2-FLAIR sequence. The simultaneous visualization of both the perfusion map and the brain anatomy allowed ROIs to be drawn separately for gray matter and for white matter. In addition, CBF should be separately measured in the blood supply territories of different intracranial vessels, and only one vast region of interest covering the surface of the entire hemisphere of the brain should not be used, as is often suggested in published studies [7, 21].

Another reason for obtaining the incorrect quantitative data on CBF values is the presence of artifacts specific to the steno-occlusive cerebrovascular pathology. They include arterial transit artifacts that appear due to the long delay of labeled blood in the cortical arteries. CBF values in ATAs can exceed the true values of cerebral blood flow by several times, which hampers quantifying CBF in the presence of artifacts. Different specialists take different approaches to ATAs. In studies where artifacts were included in ROIs [20, 21], a very high dispersion of CBF values in the cortical regions of the brain was observed—from 12 to 149 mL/min/100 g before the operation and from 17 to 118 mL/min/100 g after the operation. Such results are more likely associated with the inclusion of ATAs in the studied areas. Zaharchuk et al. in 2011 proposed four groups of perfusion deficit on the basis of a qualitative analysis of ASL-perfusion images: degree 0 denotes the minimal ASL signal without ATAs, degree 1 denotes a moderate reduction in ASL signal with ATA, degree 2 denotes a high ASL signal with ATAs, degree 3 denotes normal values of ASL perfusion [22]. Lee et al. [23], on the basis of the same groups, compared the changes of ASL perfusion after surgical treatment and showed that the presence and the severity of ATA changes after surgery, in particular, decrease after successful revascularization. However, these studies were limited to qualitative and semiquantitative analyses of images without measuring the exact values of cerebral blood flow. The technique for setting ROI outside artifact zones, which was used in our study, allowed us to obtain quantitative values of cerebral blood flow in all the studied areas.

Previous studies have confirmed that the appearance of ATAs on ASL images corresponds to the presence of collateral vessels with slow blood flow according to direct angiography [22] and is associated with a better prognosis of ischemic stroke [24]. These facts allowed us to consider ATAs as elements of the subcompensation of cerebral blood flow. Therefore, in our study, the presence of ATAs was the criterion for distinguishing intermediate groups ("subcompensation" and "initial decompensation").

Previous studies have revealed a significant relationship between the angiographic and clinical characteristics of moyamoya disease and the degree of decrease in CBF according to the ASL perfusion [22, 25]. Noguchi et al. in 2013 revealed a statistically significant correlation between the severity of the decrease in cerebral blood flow according to ASL and the degree of progression of moyamoya disease according to MR angiography ($p < 0.01$) as well as the severity of clinical symptoms ($p < 0.01$) [25]. Zaharchuk et al. in 2011 showed the relation between ATAs and the presence of collateral blood flow according to direct angiography [22]. Our study also revealed a significant relationship between the proposed degrees of cerebrovascular insufficiency and the angiographic and clinical data of the patients. Thus, our results provide a pathogenetic rationale for the distinguished degrees of perfusion deficit and do not contradict the data from the world literature.

Continuous improvement in diagnostic perfusion techniques aims to reduce the effect of artifacts on the results of measuring cerebral blood flow. For this reason, a modified ASL technique was recently proposed with a long delay after labeling, a delay of at least 4 seconds (long label long delay ASL, or LLLD ASL), which allows for reducing the number of artifacts [26]. However, by using the image interpretation methods proposed in this study, the disadvantages of ASL perfusion with standard post-labeling delay in the form of ATA can be turned into advantages if the meaning of all study patterns is taken into account.

Conclusions

ASL perfusion is an effective quantitative method for measuring cerebral blood flow and revealing cerebrovascular insufficiency in patients with moyamoya angiopathy. The presence of arterial transit artifacts reflects the presence of leptomeningeal collaterals and can be considered as a sign of the subcompensation of cerebral circulation. In patients with MMA, artifacts were detected in 69% of the studied hemispheres. The minimal CBF for ATAs is greater than 117 mL/min/100 g. On the basis of the values of cerebral blood flow and the presence of ATA, the following four degrees of cerebrovascular insufficiency can be distinguished: degree 0 denotes "compensation," degree 1 denotes "subcompensation," degree 2 denotes "initial decompensation," and degree 3 denotes "decompensation." The proposed degrees of cerebrovascular insufficiency reliably reflect the severity of neurological deficit, the stage of the disease, and the presence of leptomeningeal and transdural collaterals.

Declarations

Conflict of interest The authors have no conflict of interests to declare.

Informed consent For this type of study, formal consent is not required.

Human and animal rights This chapter does not contain any studies with animals performed by any of the authors.

References

1. Lee M, et al. Quantitative hemodynamic studies in moyamoya disease: a review. Neurosurg Focus. 2009;26(4):E5.
2. Grubb RL Jr, et al. Surgical results of the carotid occlusion surgery study. J Neurosurg. 2013;118(1):25–33.
3. Wintermark M, et al. Comparative overview of brain perfusion imaging techniques. Stroke. 2005;36(9):11.
4. Latchaw RE, et al. Adverse reactions to xenon-enhanced CT cerebral blood flow determination. Radiology. 1987;163(1):251–4.
5. Detre JA, et al. Noninvasive MRI evaluation of cerebral blood flow in cerebrovascular disease. Neurology. 1998;50(3):633–41.
6. Goetti R, et al. Quantitative cerebral perfusion imaging in children and young adults with Moyamoya disease: comparison of arterial spin-labeling-MRI and H(2)[(15)O]-PET. AJNR Am J Neuroradiol. 2014;35(5):1022–8.
7. Goetti R, et al. Arterial spin labelling MRI for assessment of cerebral perfusion in children with moyamoya disease: comparison with dynamic susceptibility contrast MRI. Neuroradiology. 2013;55(5):639–47.
8. Noguchi T, et al. Arterial spin-labeling MR imaging in moyamoya disease compared with SPECT imaging. Eur J Radiol. 2011;80(3):18.
9. Petcharunpaisan S, Ramalho J, Castillo M. Arterial spin labeling in neuroimaging. World J Radiol. 2010;2(10):384–98.
10. Amukotuwa SA, Yu C, Zaharchuk G. 3D Pseudocontinuous arterial spin labeling in routine clinical practice: a review of clinically significant artifacts. J Magn Reson Imaging. 2016;43(1):11–27.
11. Kwah LK, Diong J. National Institutes of Health Stroke Scale (NIHSS). J Physiother. 2014;60(1):61.
12. Biagi L, et al. Age dependence of cerebral perfusion assessed by magnetic resonance continuous arterial spin labeling. J Magn Reson Imaging. 2007;25(4):696–702.
13. Kohno N, et al. The clinical significance of arterial transit artifact on arterial spin labeling in patients with acute ischemic stroke. AME Med J. 2017;2(9):140.
14. Mutke MA, et al. Clinical evaluation of an arterial-spin-labeling product sequence in steno-occlusive disease of the brain. PLoS One. 2014;9(2):e87143.
15. Suzuki J, Takaku A. Cerebrovascular "moyamoya" disease. Disease showing abnormal net-like vessels in base of brain. Arch Neurol. 1969;20(3):288–99.
16. Togao O, et al. Cerebral hemodynamics in Moyamoya disease: correlation between perfusion-weighted MR imaging and cerebral angiography. AJNR Am J Neuroradiol. 2006;27(2):391–7.
17. Baltsavias G, Khan N, Valavanis A. The collateral circulation in pediatric moyamoya disease. Childs Nerv Syst. 2015;31(3):389–98.
18. Houkin K, et al. Novel magnetic resonance angiography stage grading for moyamoya disease. Cerebrovasc Dis. 2005;20(5):347–54.
19. Sugino T, et al. Arterial spin-labeling magnetic resonance imaging after revascularization of moyamoya disease. J Stroke Cerebrovasc Dis. 2013;22(6):811–6.
20. Quon JL, et al. Arterial spin-labeling cerebral perfusion changes after revascularization surgery in pediatric moyamoya disease and syndrome. J Neurosurg Pediatr. 2019;23(4):486–92.
21. Ha JY, et al. Arterial spin Labeling MRI for quantitative assessment of cerebral perfusion before and after cerebral revascularization in children with Moyamoya disease. Korean J Radiol. 2019;20(6):985–96.
22. Zaharchuk G, et al. Arterial spin-labeling MRI can identify the presence and intensity of collateral perfusion in patients with moyamoya disease. Stroke. 2011;42(9):2485–91.
23. Lee S, et al. Monitoring cerebral perfusion changes after revascularization in patients with Moyamoya disease by using arterial spin-labeling MR imaging. Radiology. 2018;288(2):565–72.
24. Chalela JA, et al. Magnetic resonance perfusion imaging in acute ischemic stroke using continuous arterial spin labeling. Stroke. 2000;31(3):680–7.
25. Noguchi T, et al. Arterial spin-labeling MR imaging in Moyamoya disease compared with clinical assessments and other MR imaging findings. Eur J Radiol. 2013;82(12):1.
26. Fan AP, et al. Long-delay arterial spin labeling provides more accurate cerebral blood flow measurements in Moyamoya patients: a simultaneous positron emission tomography/MRI study. Stroke. 2017;48(9):2441–9.

Open Access This chapter is licensed under the terms of the Creative Commons Attribution 4.0 International License (http://creativecommons.org/licenses/by/4.0/), which permits use, sharing, adaptation, distribution and reproduction in any medium or format, as long as you give appropriate credit to the original author(s) and the source, provide a link to the Creative Commons license and indicate if changes were made.

The images or other third party material in this chapter are included in the chapter's Creative Commons license, unless indicated otherwise in a credit line to the material. If material is not included in the chapter's Creative Commons license and your intended use is not permitted by statutory regulation or exceeds the permitted use, you will need to obtain permission directly from the copyright holder.

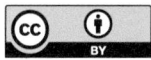

ADC Threshold Indicating the Ischemic Region for Predicting Efficacy in Thrombectomy

Hideyuki Ishihara, Fumiaki Oka, Takuma Nishimoto, Masatoshi Yamane, Kazutaka Sugimoto, and Hirokazu Sadahiro

Introduction

Three randomized trials have shown the efficacy of endovascular thrombectomy (EVT) over medical care alone in patients with a large ischemic region (Alberta Stroke Program Early Computed Tomography Score (ASPECTS) 3 to 5) [6, 10, 14]. However, compared with EVT in patients without a large ischemic region (ASPECTS ≥ 6), the number of cases with improvement is limited. Being able to select patients for whom EVT is likely to be effective would be useful given the burden of this treatment on the patient, the risk, and its medical efficiency. An imaging evaluation of ischemic penumbra is ideal for this purpose because the goal of treatment for hyperacute ischemic stroke is to save ischemic penumbra.

Areas with an apparent diffusion coefficient (ADC) $<620 \times 10^{-6}$ mm^2/s (ADC_{620}) on diffusion-weighted imaging (DWI) are generally diagnosed as ischemic regions; however, there might be differences in brain tissue damage depending on the magnitude of the decrease in ADC. Thus, we hypothesized that areas with a mild decrease in ADC contain salvageable brain tissue. In the present study, to identify the optimal ADC value for assessing an ischemic region, we examined whether ADCs before EVT affected outcomes in patients with acute ischemic stroke with ASPECTS < 6 and causative occlusion of the internal carotid artery (ICA) or proximal middle cerebral artery (MCA) (M1) in the early time window.

Methods

After institutional review board approval from Yamaguchi University, a retrospective chart review was performed on patients with acute occlusion of the intracranial ICA or proximal MCA (M1) and large ischemic regions defined as DWI ASPECTS < 6 who were admitted to Yamaguchi University Hospital between January 2014 and December 2021. Only patients who had DWI ASPECTS < 6, had an ischemic core volume <150 mL, and achieved more than thrombolysis in cerebral infarction (TICI) 2b recanalization were included in the study. Associations of clinical characteristics and ischemic region volumes defined by various ADC thresholds with a favorable outcome (modified Rankin Scale (mRS) 0–2 and 0–3 at 90 days) after EVT were examined. The optimal ADC threshold for a favorable outcome was determined on the basis of this analysis. Estimates of ischemic regions from DWI were obtained by using Vitrea software (Canon Medical Systems). Ischemic region volume was analyzed in 10×10^{-6} mm^2/s steps for ADC between ADC $< 480 \times 10^{-6}$ mm^2/s (ADC_{480}) and ADC_{620}.

Statistical Analysis

Categorical variables are shown as numbers and percentages, and they were analyzed via the χ^2 test and the Fisher exact test, as appropriate. Continuous variables are expressed as medians and interquartile range. Some continuous variables were not normally distributed and were analyzed via the Wilcoxon rank-sum test. A univariate logistic regression model was used to compare clinical features and ischemic region volumes defined by different ADC thresholds for patients with mRS 0–3 vs. 4–6 at 90 days. The optimal ADC threshold for identifying patients who are likely to respond to EVT was determined via ROC curve analysis by using thresholds of ADC_{480} to ADC_{620}. The area under the ROC curve

H. Ishihara (✉) · F. Oka · T. Nishimoto · K. Sugimoto
H. Sadahiro
Department of Neurosurgery, Yamaguchi University School of Medicine, Ube, Yamaguchi, Japan
e-mail: hishi@yamaguchi-u.ac.jp

M. Yamane
Department of Radiology, Yamaguchi University Hospital, Ube, Yamaguchi, Japan

(AUC) for the optimal ADC threshold was determined. The closer the AUC is to 1, the better the association with a favorable outcome. A multivariate logistic regression model was used to identify independent predictors of mRS 0–3 at 90 days in patients with a large ischemic region who underwent EVT. On the basis of previous studies, age, gender, initial NIHSS score, and the use of intravenous recombinant tissue plasminogen activator (IV rt-PA) were included as adjusting covariates. All statistical analyses were conducted by using JMP 15.0 (SAS Institute Inc, Cary, NC). All reported p-values are two tailed, and $p < 0.05$ was considered to be significant.

Results

This analysis included 48 patients with a median age of 78 years and a median NIHSS score of 23 at admission. The occlusion sites were the ICA (46%) and the M1 segment (46%) and M2 segment (8%) of the MCA. Of the 48 patients, 18 (38%) had mRS 0–3 and 30 (62%) mRS 4–6 at 90 days. A comparison of baseline characteristics for cases with mRS 0–3 vs. 4–6 at 90 days is shown in Table 1. Patients with mRS 0–3 at 90 days were significantly younger (mean [IQR] 72.0 [66.8–73.0] vs. 81.0 [73.0–86.3] years, $p < 0.01$) and had a shorter onset to door time (median [IQR] 118 [49–180] vs. 243 [100–450] min, $p < 0.01$) and onset to reperfusion time (mean [IQR] 247 [150–320] vs. 351 [250–599] min, $p = 0.02$) compared to those with mRS 4–6 at 90 days. Sex, medical history, baseline NIHSS, baseline ASPECTS, the occlusion site, IV rt-PA, and any intracranial hemorrhage (ICH) or symptomatic ICH within 48 hours did not differ significantly between the groups.

In ROC analysis, an ischemic region defined by ADC_{540} had the highest AUC (AUC = 0.85) (Table 2). In multivariate analysis, there were independent associations between onset to reperfusion time (OR 0.991, 95% CI 0.981–1.000, $p = 0.013$) and ADC_{540} (OR 0.887, 95% CI 0.807–0.976, $p = 0.001$) with mRS 0–3 at 90 days (Table 3).

Table 1 Baseline characteristics for patients with 90-day mRS 0–3 vs. 4–6

Item	mRS 0–3 ($n = 18$)	mRS 4–6 ($n = 30$)	p-Value
Age (y)	72.0 (66.8–73.0)	81.0 (73.0–86.3)	0.0006*
Male sex	11 (61.1)	12 (40.0)	0.1564
Medical history			
Hypertension	13 (72.2)	18 (60.0)	0.3914
Diabetes mellitus	1 (5.6)	5 (16.7)	0.3883
Etiology			0.6148
Cardioembolic	13 (72.2)	25 (83.3)	
Atherosclerotic	4 (22.2)	4 (13.3)	
Undetermined	1 (5.6)	1 (3.3)	
Baseline NIHSS (points)	19 (17–25)	24 (18–27)	0.0814
Baseline ASPECTS (points)	5 (3–5)	4 (2–5)	0.1662
Occlusion side (left)	11 (61.1)	17 (56.7)	0.7624
Occlusion site			0.3690
IC	8 (44.4)	14 (46.7)	
M1	7 (38.9)	15 (50.0)	
M2	3 (16.7)	1 (3.3)	
IV rt-PA	15 (83.3)	16 (53.3)	0.0603
TICI 3	4 (22.2)	7 (23.3)	1.0000
1st pass	9 (50.0)	18 (60.0)	0.4990
Onset to door (min)	118 (49–180)	243 (100–450)	0.0075*
Onset to reperfusion (min)	247 (150–320)	351 (250–599)	0.0021*
Any ICH within 48 hr	7 (38.9)	21 (70.0)	0.0681
sICH within 48 hr	1 (5.6)	3 (10.0)	1.0000

Note: *mRS* modified Rankin Scale, *NIHSS* National Institutes of Health Stroke Scale, *ASPECTS* Alberta Stroke Program Early Computed Tomography Score, *ICA* internal carotid artery, *M1* middle cerebral artery sphenoidal segment, *M2* middle cerebral artery insular segment, *IV rt-PA* intravenous recombinant tissue plasminogen activator, *TICI* thrombolysis in cerebral infarction, *ICH* intracranial hemorrhage, and *sICH* symptomatic intracranial hemorrhage. *P < 0.05

Table 2 ROC curve analysis of the relationship between ischemic region volume (as defined by each ADC threshold) and a favorable outcome (90-day mRS 0–3)

ADC Threshold (ischemic region volume, mL)	AUC Curve	Cutoff Value (mL)	Sensitivity	Specificity
<620	0.77407	70.0	53.3	100.0
<610	0.78333	65.2	56.7	100.0
<600	0.79630	58.5	60.0	94.4
<590	0.80833	56.2	60.0	100.0
<580	0.81574	53.8	60.0	100.0
<570	0.81389	46.5	63.3	94.4
<560	0.82315	43.8	66.7	94.4
<550	0.83241	41.6	66.7	94.4
<540	0.84815	40.4	63.3	100.0
<530	0.83796	38.3	60.0	100.0
<520	0.83519	36.0	60.0	100.0
<510	0.83426	33.9	60.0	100.0
<500	0.83333	31.4	60.0	100.0
<490	0.81852	28.6	60.0	100.0
<480	0.82593	25.5	60.0	100.0

Note: *ROC* receiver operating characteristic, *mRS* modified Rankin Scale, *ADC* apparent diffusion coefficient, and *AUC* area under the curve.

Table 3 Multivariate analysis of predictors for a favorable outcome (90-day mRS 0–3)

Variables	Odds Ratio (95% CI)	p-Value
Age (/y)	0.882 (0.755–1.031)	0.0861
Sex (male)	1.744 (0.246–12.361)	0.5762
Baseline NIHSS (/point)	0.896 (0.736–1.091)	0.2569
Use of IV rt-PA	0.977 (0.092–10.303)	0.985
Onset to reperfusion (/min)	0.991 (0.981–1.001)	0.0134*
ADC < 540 (/mL)	0.887 (0.806–0.975)	0.0014*

Note: *mRS* modified Rankin Scale, *NIHSS* National Institutes of Health Stroke Scale, *IV rt-PA* intravenous recombinant tissue plasminogen activator, and *ADC* apparent diffusion coefficient. *P < 0.05

Representative cases are shown in Fig. 1. Case 1 was a 79-year-old female patient with left M1 cardioembolic occlusion. Her NIHSS score on admission was 32, and the onset to MR examination time was 65 min. On DWI, ADC_{620} was 70 mL and ADC_{540} was 28 mL. Case 2 was a 73-year-old male patient with left M1 cardioembolic occlusion. His NIHSS score on admission was 22 and the onset to MR examination time was 230 min. ADC_{620} was 54 mL, and ADC_{540} was 42 mL. Both cases underwent EVT, and their TICI was 3. The neurological symptoms of Case 1 improved, and the patient was discharged home 18 days after onset with an mRS of 1. In Case 2, neurological symptoms were not significantly improved, and the patient was transferred to a rehabilitation hospital with an mRS of 4.

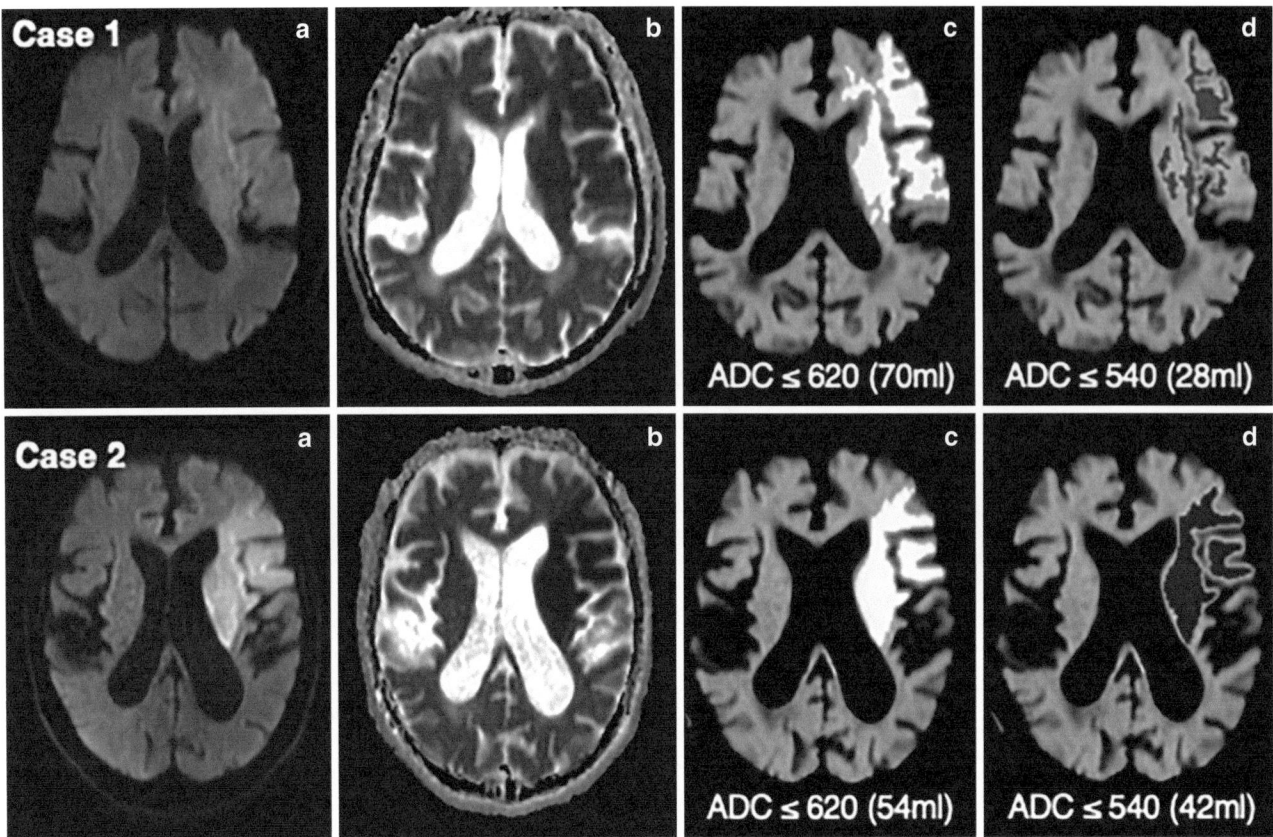

Fig. 1 Representative cases of ischemic region volume estimation based on ADC values, where Case 1 had a mild ADC reduction and Case 2 a severe ADC reduction: (**a**) DWI, (**b**) ADC map, (**c**) ADC_{620} lesion, and (**d**) ADC_{540} lesion

Discussion

In this study, the ischemic region volume was used as a basis to investigate the characteristics of patients who benefited from thrombectomy among those with a large ischemic region. The results showed that the ischemic region volume assessed on DWI significantly affected functional outcomes and that ADC_{540} was a stronger predictor of these outcomes than the more generally used ADC_{620} threshold.

In acute ischemic stroke, DWI-positive lesions are generally considered to be markers of an irreversible ischemic region. Animal studies have shown that ADCs decrease in the central area where ischemia is most intense and gradually spread to the periphery [9]. Clinically, early recanalization with EVT has been shown to increase ADCs and to improve functional outcomes [5, 7]. The grounds for the use of ADC_{620} as the threshold for an irreversible ischemic region are based on an analysis of MR images in DWI before IV rt-PA and fluid-attenuated inversion recovery (FLAIR) images in the chronic phase [8]. The ADC reflects the amount and velocity of water molecules in tissues, and because an ADC lesion indirectly reflects an ischemic region, the magnitude of change in ADC values is considered to reflect the degree of tissue damage [12]. Mild ADC reduction can be reversed to avoid cerebral infarction with early reperfusion [3, 11], and lesions with a mean ADC ≥ 520 have been suggested to be salvageable via early reperfusion [13]. These findings are consistent with our results.

Regions with mild ADC reduction are thought to include the penumbra, which suggests that this change might also be a useful index for determining treatment indications. An imaging evaluation of ischemic penumbra is ideal because the goal of treatment for hyperacute ischemic stroke is to save ischemic penumbra. The DEFUSE 3 study showed that the PWI-DWI mismatch was useful for penumbra evaluation in the late time window [1]. A meta-analysis of Highly Effective Reperfusion evaluated in Multiple Endovascular Stroke Trials (HERMES) showed a significant association between ischemic core volume and functional outcome, but mismatch volume was not proven to be useful for the selection of cases in which EVT is effective in the early time window [2, 4]. The present study suggests that the PWI-DWI mismatch may underestimate the penumbra. This might be the reason why the usefulness of PWI-DWI mismatch in the early time window has not been established.

This study has several limitations, including the retrospective single center design and small sample size. However, this approach allowed detailed analysis using MR images obtained under the same conditions. The study targeted patients with DWI ASPECTS < 6, so the results may not be applicable to patients with DWI ASPECTS > 5. However, our findings indicate that the severity of ischemic brain tissue damage correlates with a decrease in ADC, and a similar tendency may exist in patients with DWI ASPECTS > 5.

Conclusion

Earlier reperfusion and a smaller ischemic region were related to a favorable outcome in patients with acute vessel occlusion with a large ischemic region. An ischemic region defined by ADC_{540} correlated more strongly with functional outcome than that defined by ADC_{620}. An area with a slight change from ADC_{540} to ADC_{620} might contain ischemic penumbra.

Author Contributions Hideyuki Ishihara contributed to the study conception and design. Material preparation, data collection, and data analysis were performed by Fumiaki Oka, Takuma Nishimoto, Masatoshi Yamane, Kazutaka Sugimoto, and Hirokazu Sadahiro. The first draft of the manuscript was written by [Hideyuki Ishihara], and all authors commented on previous versions of the manuscript. All authors read and approved the final manuscript.

Funding Information Institutional sources only.

Declarations

Conflicts of interest The authors declare no competing interests or funding.

Ethical approval This retrospective study was approved by the Institutional Review Board of Yamaguchi University Hospital (approval number: H2020-095-3).

References

1. Albers GW, Marks MP, Lansberg MG. Thrombectomy for stroke with selection by perfusion imaging. N Engl J Med. 2018;378:1849–50. https://doi.org/10.1056/NEJMc1803856.
2. Campbell BCV, Majoie CBLM, Albers GW, Menon BK, Yassi N, Sharma G, van Zwam WH, van Oostenbrugge RJ, Demchuk AM, Guillemin F, White P, Dávalos A, van der Lugt A, Butcher KS, Cherifi A, Marquering HA, Cloud G, Macho Fernández JM, Madigan J, Oppenheim C, Donnan GA, Roos YBWE, Shankar J, Lingsma H, Bonafé A, Raoult H, Hernández-Pérez M, Bharatha A, Jahan R, Jansen O, Richard S, Levy EI, Berkhemer OA, Soudant M, Aja L, Davis SM, Krings T, Tisserand M, San Román L, Tomasello A, Beumer D, Brown S, Liebeskind DS, Bracard S, Muir KW, Dippel DWJ, Goyal M, Saver JL, Jovin TG, Hill MD, Mitchell PJ, collaborators H. Penumbral imaging and functional outcome in patients with anterior circulation ischaemic stroke treated with endovascular thrombectomy versus medical therapy: a meta-analysis of individual patient-level data. Lancet Neurol. 2019;18:46–55. https://doi.org/10.1016/S1474-4422(18)30314-4.
3. Fiehler J, Knudsen K, Kucinski T, Kidwell CS, Alger JR, Thomalla G, Eckert B, Wittkugel O, Weiller C, Zeumer H, Röther J. Predictors of apparent diffusion coefficient normalization in stroke patients. Stroke. 2004;35:514–9. https://doi.org/10.1161/01.STR.0000114873.28023.C2.
4. Goyal M, Menon BK, van Zwam WH, Dippel DW, Mitchell PJ, Demchuk AM, Dávalos A, Majoie CB, van der Lugt A, de Miquel MA, Donnan GA, Roos YB, Bonafe A, Jahan R, Diener HC, van den Berg LA, Levy EI, Berkhemer OA, Pereira VM, Rempel J, Millán M, Davis SM, Roy D, Thornton J, Román LS, Ribó M, Beumer D, Stouch B, Brown S, Campbell BC, van Oostenbrugge RJ, Saver JL, Hill MD, Jovin TG, collaborators H. Endovascular thrombectomy after large-vessel ischaemic stroke: a meta-analysis of individual patient data from five randomised trials. Lancet. 2016;387:1723–31. https://doi.org/10.1016/S0140-6736(16)00163-X.
5. Hsia AW, Luby M, Cullison K, Burton S, Armonda R, Liu AH, Leigh R, Nadareishvili Z, Benson RT, Lynch JK, Latour LL. Rapid apparent diffusion coefficient evolution after early revascularization. Stroke. 2019;50:2086–92. https://doi.org/10.1161/STROKEAHA.119.025784.
6. Huo X, Ma G, Tong X, Zhang X, Pan Y, Nguyen TN, Yuan G, Han H, Chen W, Wei M, Zhang J, Zhou Z, Yao X, Wang G, Song W, Cai X, Nan G, Li D, Wang AY, Ling W, Cai C, Wen C, Wang E, Zhang L, Jiang C, Liu Y, Liao G, Chen X, Li T, Liu S, Li J, Gao F, Ma N, Mo D, Song L, Sun X, Li X, Deng Y, Luo G, Lv M, He H, Liu A, Mu S, Liu L, Jing J, Nie X, Ding Z, Du W, Zhao X, Yang P, Wang Y, Liebeskind DS, Pereira VM, Ren Z, Miao Z, Investigators A-A. Trial of endovascular therapy for acute ischemic stroke with large infarct. N Engl J Med. 2023; https://doi.org/10.1056/NEJMoa2213379.
7. Panni P, Lapergue B, Maïer B, Finitsis S, Clarençon F, Richard S, Marnat G, Bourcier R, Sibon I, Dargazanli C, Blanc R, Consoli A, Eugène F, Vannier S, Spelle L, Denier C, Boulanger M, Gauberti M, Saleme S, Macian F, Rosso C, Naggara O, Turc G, Ozkul-Wermester O, Papagiannaki C, Albucher JF, Darcourt J, Le Bras A, Evain S, Wolff V, Pop R, Timsit S, Gentric JC, Bourdain F, Veunac L, Arquizan C, Gory B, Investigators EETiIS. Clinical impact and predictors of diffusion weighted imaging (DWI) reversal in stroke patients with diffusion weighted imaging Alberta Stroke Program Early CT Score 0-5 treated by thrombectomy: diffusion weighted imaging reversal in large volume stroke. Clin Neuroradiol. 2022;32:939–50. https://doi.org/10.1007/s00062-022-01156-z.
8. Purushotham A, Campbell BC, Straka M, Mlynash M, Olivot JM, Bammer R, Kemp SM, Albers GW, Lansberg MG. Apparent diffusion coefficient threshold for delineation of ischemic core. Int J Stroke. 2015;10:348–53. https://doi.org/10.1111/ijs.12068.
9. Reith W, Hasegawa Y, Latour LL, Dardzinski BJ, Sotak CH, Fisher M. Multislice diffusion mapping for 3-D evolution of cerebral ischemia in a rat stroke model. Neurology. 1995;45:172–7. https://doi.org/10.1212/wnl.45.1.172.
10. Sarraj A, Hassan AE, Abraham MG, Ortega-Gutierrez S, Kasner SE, Hussain MS, Chen M, Blackburn S, Sitton CW, Churilov L, Sundararajan S, Hu YC, Herial NA, Jabbour P, Gibson D, Wallace AN, Arenillas JF, Tsai JP, Budzik RF, Hicks WJ, Kozak O, Yan B, Cordato DJ, Manning NW, Parsons MW, Hanel RA, Aghaebrahim AN, Wu TY, Cardona-Portela P, Pérez de la Ossa N, Schaafsma JD, Blasco J, Sangha N, Warach S, Gandhi CD, Kleinig TJ, Sahlein D, Elijovich L, Tekle W, Samaniego EA, Maali L, Abdulrazzak MA, Psychogios MN, Shuaib A, Pujara DK, Shaker F, Johns H, Sharma A, Yogendrakumar V, Ng FC, Rahbar MH, Cai C, Lavori P, Hamilton S, Nguyen T, Fifi JT, Davis S, Wechsler L, Pereira VM, Lansberg MG, Hill MD, Grotta JC, Ribo M, Campbell BC, Albers GW, Investigators S. Trial of endovascular thrombectomy for large ischemic strokes. N Engl J Med. 2023; https://doi.org/10.1056/NEJMoa2214403.

11. Shinoda N, Hori S, Mikami K, Bando T, Shimo D, Kuroyama T, Kuramoto Y, Matsumoto M, Hirai O, Ueno Y. Utility of relative ADC ratio in patient selection for endovascular revascularization of large vessel occlusion. J Neuroradiol. 2017;44:185–91. https://doi.org/10.1016/j.neurad.2016.12.015.
12. Tong DC, Adami A, Moseley ME, Marks MP. Relationship between apparent diffusion coefficient and subsequent hemorrhagic transformation following acute ischemic stroke. Stroke. 2000;31:2378–84. https://doi.org/10.1161/01.str.31.10.2378.
13. Umemura T, Hatano T, Ogura T, Miyata T, Agawa Y, Nakajima H, Tomoyose R, Sakamoto H, Tsujimoto Y, Nakazawa Y, Wakabayashi T, Hashimoto T, Fujiki R, Shiraishi W, Nagata I. ADC level is related to DWI reversal in patients undergoing mechanical thrombectomy: a retrospective cohort study. AJNR Am J Neuroradiol. 2022;43:893–8. https://doi.org/10.3174/ajnr.A7510.
14. Yoshimura S, Sakai N, Yamagami H, Uchida K, Beppu M, Toyoda K, Matsumaru Y, Matsumoto Y, Kimura K, Takeuchi M, Yazawa Y, Kimura N, Shigeta K, Imamura H, Suzuki I, Enomoto Y, Tokunaga S, Morita K, Sakakibara F, Kinjo N, Saito T, Ishikura R, Inoue M, Morimoto T. Endovascular therapy for acute stroke with a large ischemic region. N Engl J Med. 2022;386:1303–13. https://doi.org/10.1056/NEJMoa2118191.

Open Access This chapter is licensed under the terms of the Creative Commons Attribution 4.0 International License (http://creativecommons.org/licenses/by/4.0/), which permits use, sharing, adaptation, distribution and reproduction in any medium or format, as long as you give appropriate credit to the original author(s) and the source, provide a link to the Creative Commons license and indicate if changes were made.

The images or other third party material in this chapter are included in the chapter's Creative Commons license, unless indicated otherwise in a credit line to the material. If material is not included in the chapter's Creative Commons license and your intended use is not permitted by statutory regulation or exceeds the permitted use, you will need to obtain permission directly from the copyright holder.

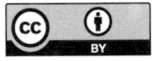

Novel Hemodynamic Parameters for Cerebral Ischemia in Patients with Occlusive Cerebrovascular Disease Using Dual ASL Perfusion Imaging

Jyoji Nakagawara

Background and Aims

Moyamoya disease (MMD) requires long-term follow-up regardless of whether the patient is treated surgically or conservatively. In outpatient care, magnetic resonance imaging/magnetic resonance angiography (MRI/MRA) is performed regularly to evaluate the progression and worsening of the disease stage, focusing on the appearance of new brain tissue lesions such as cerebral infarction, white matter lesions, and microbleeds on MRI and on the development of cerebrovascular lesions such as progressive stenosis of intracranial arteries and any increase in moyamoya vessels on MRA [8]. However, the appearance of brain tissue lesions or the development of cerebrovascular lesions without the onset of symptoms requires screening imaging to easily determine the presence or absence of hemodynamic cerebral impairment.

Perfusion MRI via arterial spin labeling (ASL) by using arterial blood spins as endogenous tracers can be easily performed in the outpatient setting, but it could not precisely estimate cerebral ischemia severity in patients with occlusive cerebrovascular disease (CVD), because the delayed arrival of arterial spins in the affected vascular territories could not be corrected via single post-labeling delay (PLD) setting [10]. In this study, new hemodynamic parameters for screening cerebral ischemia severity using dual ASL perfusion imaging under double PLD setting will be proposed.

Methods

In this study, 67 patients (10~83 years) with MMD and 22 patients (35~72 years) with large artery atherosclerosis (LAA) were included, and hemodynamic parameters were investigated by using dual ASL perfusion imaging via 3.0 T MRI. In ASL perfusion imaging, blood vessels in the neck were irradiated with radiofrequency (RF) for a certain period of time to invert arterial blood spins (labeling time: 1800 ms), and the distribution of arterial blood spins that reached the brain tissue after a certain time (post-labeling delay: PLD) was reconstructed as a perfusion image. Pulsed continuous ASL (pCASL) was selected as the arterial labeling method, and double PLDs were set to 1525 ms for early images and 2525 ms for late images. The data collection time was counted at 2.19 min for early images and 3.55 min for late images to obtain 36 axial slices with a 4 mm slice thickness.

In general, in the ASL perfusion images of cases without occlusive CVD, arterial blood spins are uniformly supplied from the arteries in the neck through cerebral vessels to the brain tissue and are distributed to the brain tissue according to the distribution of cerebral blood flow at PLD 1525 ms, and its sufficiency to the brain tissue is maintained at PLD 2525 ms, so no significant dissociation between the two images occurs [1]. On the other hand, occlusive CVD such as MMD and LAA could cause an uneven supply of arterial blood spins into cortical arteries and delayed arrival and filling up in cerebral tissue, resulting in dissociation in the distribution of arterial blood spins in cortical arteries and cerebral tissue at PLD 1525 ms and PLD 2525 ms.

Therefore, for each ASL perfusion image, new hemodynamic parameters were established on the basis of the distribution of arterial blood spins in cerebral tissue and in cortical arteries. New hemodynamic parameters for dual ASL perfusion imaging are defined as follows: In early images, "early slow-in" is defined as the delayed arrival of arterial blood spins in cerebral tissue, and "early stagnation" is defined as stagnated arterial blood spins in cortical arteries. In late images, "late filling up" is defined as the complete or incomplete fulfillment of arterial blood spins in cerebral tissue, and this reflects the severity of cerebral ischemia (the degree of the development of collateral blood circulation). "Late

---

J. Nakagawara (✉)
Department of Neurosurgery, Umeda Brain-Spine-Neurology Clinic, Osaka, Japan

stagnation or overstagnation" is defined as stagnated arterial blood spins in cortical arteries, and overstagnation reflects compensatory cerebral vasodilation. Changes in the arterial blood spins in cerebral tissue should be estimated separately from changes in the arterial blood spins in cortical arteries.

Results

The incidence of new hemodynamic parameters assumed from the distribution of arterial blood spins in the brain tissue and cortical arteries was investigated in 67 MMD patients and 22 LAA patients (Table 1). On one hand, in the MMD patients' group, early images showed "early slow-in" in 65/67 (97%) and "early stagnation" in 48/67 (72%). Late images demonstrated "late incomplete filling up" (suspected moderate ischemia) in 22/67 (33%), "late complete filling up" in 45/67 (67%), "late stagnation" in 48/67 (72%), and "overstagnation" in 8/67 (12%). On the other hand, in the LAA patients' group, early images showed "early slow-in" in 22/22 (100%) and "early stagnation" in 7/22(32%). Late images demonstrated "late incomplete filling up" (suspected moderate ischemia) in 3/22 (14%), "late complete filling up" in 19/22 (86%), "late stagnation" in 10/22 (45%), and "overstagnation" in 2/22 (9%).

Among 67 MMD patients, four cases with symptomatic ischemia showed incomplete filling up with mild stagnation in late images. These findings were suspected as moderate cerebral ischemia, and they could be foremost candidates for cerebral blood flow-single photon emission computed tomography (CBF-SPECT) or positron emission tomography (PET) examination.

A comparison of the two groups yielded that late incomplete filling up and early and late stagnation were observed more frequently in the MMD group. A comparison of late filling up to cerebral tissue between the two groups showed a higher rate of late incomplete filling up (moderate ischemia: 33% vs. 17%) on late images in the MMD group. A comparison of arterial blood spin stagnation within cortical arteries between the two groups showed early stagnation on early images (72% vs. 32%) and late stagnation (72% vs. 45%) and overstagnation (12% vs. 9%) on late images; both images showed a higher rate of the stagnation of arterial blood spins within cortical arteries in the MMD group.

Case Presentations

Dual ASL Perfusion Imaging of Mild Ischemia

Figure 1 presents the dual ASL perfusion imaging findings of a case of moyamoya disease with mild cerebral ischemia. The patient was a 10-year-old girl. She presented with mild left-hand weakness (transient ischemic attack). Early images showed the delayed arrival of arterial blood spins (early slow-in) in the bilateral anterior cerebral artery and middle cerebral artery territories and showed the stagnation of arterial blood spins (early stagnation) within bilateral Sylvian fissure to the frontal cortical arteries. Late images showed the late incomplete filling up of arterial blood spins in the bilateral anterior cerebral artery territories, late complete filling up in the bilateral middle cerebral artery territories, and the excessive stagnation of arterial blood spins (late overstagnation) within the bilateral Sylvian fissure to the frontal cortical arteries. Hemodynamic cerebral ischemia was judged to be relatively mild and amenable to follow-up. Overstagnation suggests that compensatory vasodilation and prolonged circulation time could easily occur in MMD patients.

Dual ASL Perfusion Imaging of Moderate Ischemia

Figure 2 presents the dual ASL perfusion imaging findings of a case of moyamoya disease with moderate cerebral ischemia. The patient was a 23-year-old woman. She presented with repeated left-hand weakness (transient ischemic attack). Early images showed a marked slow-in of arterial blood spins in the bilateral anterior cerebral artery and the middle cerebral artery territories and the early stagnation of arterial blood spin in the vicinity of the bilateral Sylvian fissures. Late images showed the late incomplete filling up of arterial blood spins in the bilateral anterior cerebral arteries and the left middle cerebral artery territories, moderate incomplete

Table 1 The incidence of new hemodynamic parameters in 67 MMD patients and 22 LAA patients

Early images:

    Early slow-in (delayed arrival of arterial blood spins in cerebral tissue)

    Early stagnation (stagnated arterial blood spins in cortical arteries)

Late images:

    Late complete filling up (complete fulfillment of arterial blood spins in cerebral tissue)

    Late incomplete filling up (incomplete fulfillment of arterial blood spins in cerebral tissue)

    Late stagnation (stagnated arterial blood spins in cortical arteries)

    Overstagnation (overstagnated arterial blood spins in cortical arteries)

Note: *MMD* moyamoya disease and *LAA* large artery atherosclerosis

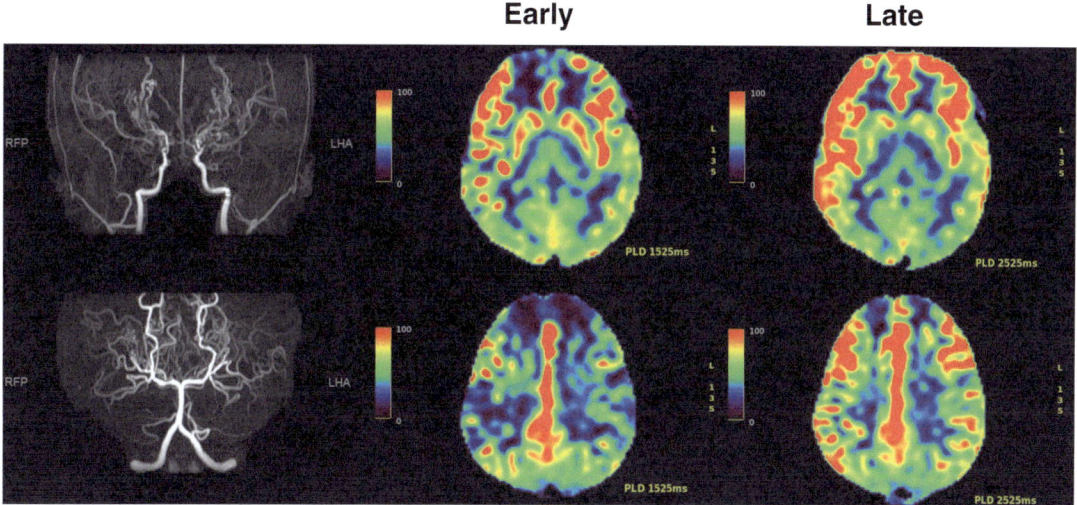

Fig. 1 Dual ASL perfusion imaging in MMD patient with mild cerebral ischemia

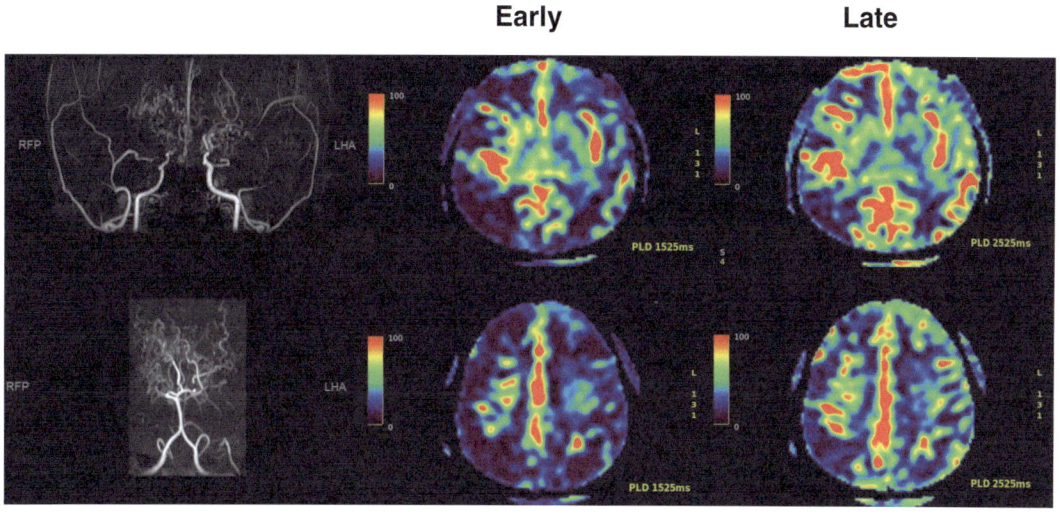

Fig. 2 Dual ASL perfusion imaging in MMD patient with moderate cerebral ischemia

filling up in the right middle cerebral artery territories, and the limited stagnation of arterial blood spins near the bilateral Sylvian fissures. Hemodynamic cerebral ischemia was determined to be moderate, and the patient was considered eligible for cerebral perfusion SPECT and PET scan for severity evaluation. Overstagnation was not associated with incomplete filling up in late images.

Discussions

ASL perfusion images that indicate the early brain distribution of arterial blood spins as an endogenous tracer could be reconstructed noninvasively and briefly [2]. Its clinical application ranges widely, and its usefulness as a surrogate for fluorodeoxyglucose positron emission tomography (FDG-PET) in dementia, perfusion changes in acute and chronic stroke, small fistulas in cerebral arteriovenous malformations and dural arteriovenous fistulas, epileptic focus, and brain tumor grading has been reported [3]. In addition, its usefulness in the evaluation of hyperperfusion after revascularization procedures has been reported in relation to MMD patients [7].

In dual ASL perfusion imaging for normal control, early and late images can show almost the same distribution of arterial blood spin input. This finding suggests that arterial blood spin input could be distributed identically from early PLD to late PLD. However, arterial blood spin input via collateral vessels in patients with occlusive CVD have not yet been investigated. In general, arterial blood spin input via collateral vessels could demonstrate "slow wash-in and slow wash-out" in the affected vascular territories. Hence, dual ASL perfusion imaging could capture the stagnation of arterial blood spins within cortical arteries and the fulfillment of arterial blood spins to cerebral tissue in the vascular territories at the periphery of the occlusive lesion on a time axis from two images by setting two PLDs, enabling the screening of cerebral ischemia severity in the same territories.

Figure 3 schematically shows the relationship between the delay arrival (slow-in) and its fulfillment (filling up) of arterial blood spins in cerebral tissue on a time axis, assuming healthy subjects, MMD with mild cerebral ischemia, and MMD with moderate cerebral ischemia. In healthy subjects, there is no delay in the arrival of arterial blood spins, and the full filling up of arterial blood spins in cerebral tissue is achieved at PLD 1525 ms and maintained at PLD 2525 ms. In contrast, in MMD with mild cerebral ischemia, there is a delay in the arrival of arterial blood spins (early slow-in) at PLD 1525 ms, but the complete filling up of arterial blood spins in cerebral tissue is achieved at PLD 2525 ms (late complete filling up). Furthermore, MMD with moderate cerebral ischemia features an exacerbation of the delayed arrival of arterial blood spins (remarkable early slow-in) at PLD 1525 ms, and an incomplete filling up of arterial blood spins in cerebral tissue is achieved at PLD 2525 ms (late incomplete filling up).

Thus, as the severity of hemodynamic cerebral ischemia increases, the delayed arrival and incomplete filling up of arterial blood spins to cerebral tissue becomes more obvious, and the degree of the filling up of arterial blood spins in late images (late filling up) can be used clinically as an indicator to assess the severity of cerebral ischemia or the degree of the development of collateral blood channels. In the present study, the incidence of late incomplete filling up in the MMD group was higher than that in the LAA group (33% vs. 17%), and the incidence of late complete filling up was lower than that in the LAA group (64% vs. 86%), indicating that more severe cases of hemodynamic cerebral ischemia appear in the MMD group.

On the other hand, in ASL perfusion imaging, when the distribution of arterial blood spins to cerebral tissue is delayed due to occlusion of the main cerebral artery, arterial blood spins could stagnate in cortical arteries, and the presence of arterial blood spins in cortical arteries has been considered a problem when assessing cerebral tissue perfusion [9]. The higher rate of the stagnation of arterial blood spins

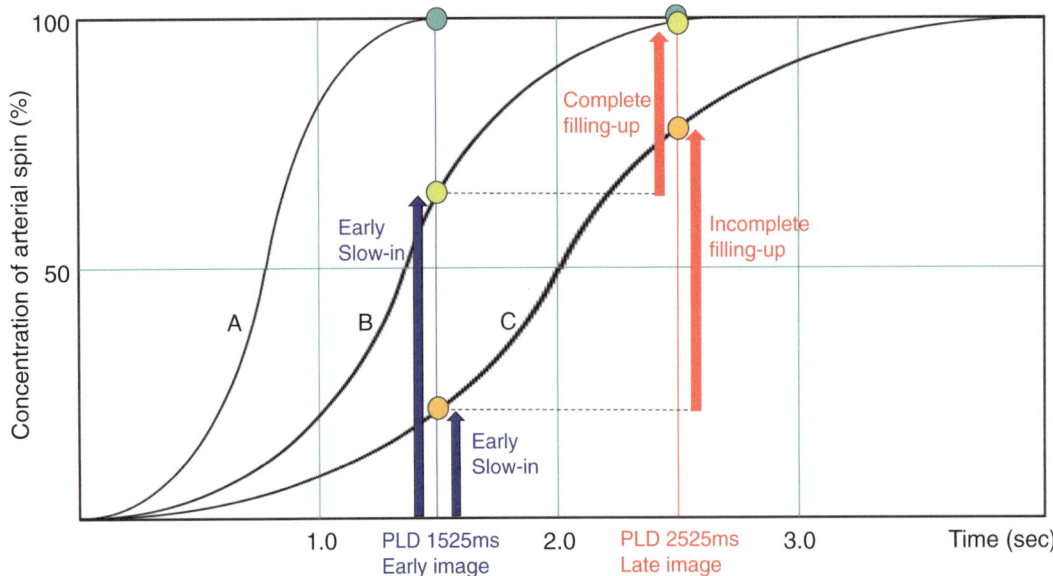

Fig. 3 The relationship between delayed arrival and the fulfillment of arterial blood spins in cerebral tissue. Curve A: In a healthy case, complete filling up is achieved at PLD 1525 ms and maintained at PLD 2525 ms. Curve B: In patients with mild ischemia, early slow-in is observed at PLD 1525 ms, and complete filling up is achieved at PLD 2525 ms. Curve C: In patients with moderate ischemia, remarkable early slow-in is observed at PLD 1525 ms, and incomplete filling up is achieved at PLD 2525 ms

in cortical arteries in the MMD group than in the LAA group (72% vs. 32% and 72% vs. 45%, respectively) on both early and late images may be due to the significant delay in circulation time and compensatory vasodilation in the MMD group. As shown by recent PET studies, the characteristic features of hemodynamic cerebral ischemia in MMD patients include delayed circulation time and significant vasodilatory compensatory capacity compared to those in LAA patients [6]. The higher rate of overstagnation in cortical arteries on late imaging (12% vs. 9%) in the MMD group may also be due to marked compensatory vasodilatation.

To reconstruct regional cerebral blood flow (CBF) images similar to PET-CBF or CBF-SPECT from ASL perfusion images using arterial blood spins as endogenous tracers, time series data on arterial blood spins need to be obtained at each pixel of cerebral tissue (multi-PLD ASL) and arterial blood spin components within cortical arteries need to be removed [5]. From this perspective, cerebral tissue perfusion in a single PLD setting in cases with occlusive CVD cannot be evaluated, because the distribution of arterial blood spins in cortical arteries could overlap with the distribution of arterial blood spins in cerebral tissue in the ASL perfusion image [4]. On the other hand, dual ASL perfusion imaging enables us to distinguish between the fulfillment of arterial blood spins in cerebral tissue and the stagnation of arterial blood spins in cortical arteries by setting up two PLDs; however, when evaluating the dual ASL perfusion images of patients with hemodynamic cerebral ischemia, the mechanism of the stagnation of arterial blood spins through collateral vessels needs to be better understood.

From the above, it was concluded that dual ASL perfusion imaging can screen and evaluate the severity of hemodynamic cerebral ischemia and the degree of the development of collateral blood flow in patients with occlusive CVD by setting the delayed arrival and fulfillment of arterial blood spins reaching cerebral tissue and the stagnation of arterial blood spins within cortical arteries as cerebral hemodynamic parameters and evaluating each separately.

Conclusion

Using dual ASL perfusion imaging, the early slow-in and late filling up of arterial blood spins into cerebral tissue and the early and late stagnation of arterial blood spins within cortical arteries could be identified separately as novel hemodynamic parameters. The severity of hemodynamic cerebral ischemia and the development of collateral circulation could be assessed only from the early slow-in and late filling up (complete or incomplete) of arterial blood spins. The early and late stagnation of arterial blood spins could not reflect cerebral ischemia, and a higher rate of these parameters in the MMD group could reflect compensatory vasodilation and prolonged circulation time.

Declarations

Conflicts of interest The author declares no conflicts of interest associated with this manuscript. The manuscript has not been published previously and is not under consideration for publication elsewhere.

Informed consent Informed consent was obtained from the patients included in this study.

References

1. Alsop DC, Detre JA, Golay X, Günther M, Hendrikse J, Hernandez-Garcia L, Lu H, MacIntosh BJ, Parkes LM, Smits M, van Osch MJP, Wang DJJ, Wong EC, Zaharchuk G. Recommended implementation of arterial spin-labeled perfusion MRI for clinical applications: a consensus of the ISMRM perfusion study group and the European consortium for ASL in dementia. Magn Reson Med. 2015;73(1):102–16.
2. Fujiwara Y, Ishida S, Kimura H. Perfusion Imaging using Arterial Spin Labeling (ASL). Japanese J Magnet Resonan Med. 2020;40(4):149–68.
3. Haller S, Zaharchuk G, Thomas DL, Lovblad K-O, Barkhof F, Golay X. Arterial spin labeling perfusion of the brain: emerging clinical applications. Radiology. 2016;281(2):337–56.
4. Hara S, Tanaka Y, Ueda Y, Hayashi S, Inaji M, Ishiwata K, Ishii K, Maehara T, Nariai T. Noninvasive evaluation of CBF and perfusion delay of moyamoya disease using arterial spin-labeling MRI with multiple postlabeling delays: comparison with 15 O-gas PET and DSC-MRI. Am J Neuroradiol. 2017;38(4):696–702.
5. Johnston ME, Lu K, Maldjian JA, Jung Y. Multi-TI arterial spin labeling MRI with variable TR and bolus duration for cerebral blood flow and arterial transit time mapping. IEEE Trans Med Imaging. 2015;34:1392–402.
6. Nakagawara J. Progress of pathophysiological diagnosis using 15O gas PET for cerebrovascular disease. No Shinkei Geka. 2017;45(9):831–46.
7. Sugino T, Mikami T, Miyata K, Suzuki K, Houkin K, Mikuni N. Arterial spin-labeling magnetic resonance imaging after revascularization of moyamoya disease. J Stroke Cerebrovasc Dis. 2013;22(6):811–6.
8. Tominaga T, Suzuki N, Miyamoto S, Koizumi A, Kuroda S, Takahashi J, Fujimura M, Houkin K. Recommendations for the Management of Moyamoya Disease: a statement from research committee on spontaneous occlusion of the circle of Willis (Moyamoya disease) [2nd edition]. Surg Cerebral Stroke (JPN). 2018;46:1–24.
9. Zaharchuk G, Do HM, Marks MP, Rosenberg J, Moseley ME, Steinberg GK. Arterial spin-labeling MRI can identify the presence and intensity of collateral perfusion in patients with moyamoya disease. Stroke. 2011;42(9):2485–91.
10. Zaharchuk G. Arterial spin labeling for acute stroke: practical considerations. Transl Stroke Res. 2012;3(2):228–35.

Open Access This chapter is licensed under the terms of the Creative Commons Attribution 4.0 International License (http://creativecommons.org/licenses/by/4.0/), which permits use, sharing, adaptation, distribution and reproduction in any medium or format, as long as you give appropriate credit to the original author(s) and the source, provide a link to the Creative Commons license and indicate if changes were made.

The images or other third party material in this chapter are included in the chapter's Creative Commons license, unless indicated otherwise in a credit line to the material. If material is not included in the chapter's Creative Commons license and your intended use is not permitted by statutory regulation or exceeds the permitted use, you will need to obtain permission directly from the copyright holder.

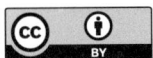

Part V

Cavernoma and Others

Epidemiology and Aetiology of Cerebral Cavernous Malformations

Hiroki Hongo, Satoru Miyawaki, and Nobuhito Saito

Introduction

Cerebral cavernous malformations (CCMs) are vascular malformations of the central nervous system that comprise a cluster of sinusoidal vascular channels prone to rupture. They can have various clinical presentations, ranging from asymptomatic to fatal haemorrhagic stroke. The underlying aetiology of these lesions remains to be understood. However, several observational and molecular genetic studies have elucidated the epidemiology, clinical course, and mechanisms of CCMs. This knowledge can facilitate appropriate therapeutic decisions and opportunities to develop novel treatment options. Here, we discuss the epidemiological and genetic aspects of CCMs.

Epidemiology and Natural History of Cerebral Cavernous Malformations (CCMs)

CCMs constitute the second-most-common type of vascular malformation of the central nervous system, following developmental venous anomalies (DVAs) [13]. The prevalence of CCMs ranges from 0.16% to 0.5% in the general population, although the estimated value of CCMs varies depending on what population the studies are based on, such as autopsy, clinically based, and population-based magnetic resonance imaging (MRI) [9]. CCMs are increasingly discovered incidentally owing to the widespread use of brain MRI. Both men and women are equally affected with CCMs. Approximately 20% of patients with CCMs have multiple lesions [23]. Patients with CCMs are most frequently diagnosed between the third and fourth decades of life, although CCMs can present at any age, including children [27]. Although CCMs can occur anywhere in the central nervous system, most lesions occur in the supratentorial region, followed by the brainstem and cerebellum.

Patients with CCMs usually have a benign clinical course and remain asymptomatic throughout their lifetime. However, CCMs can present with a wide range of symptoms, including headaches, seizures, and focal neurological deficits. Moreover, the vascular channels of patients with CCMs consist of thinner vessel walls that are prone to rupture and sometimes cause intracerebral/spinal haemorrhage, which is potentially fatal. Several studies have investigated the risk of haemorrhage during the natural course of CCMs. Although the estimated haemorrhage risks vary—largely because of differences in the study designs, including the definition of haemorrhage—in 2008, the Angioma Alliance Scientific Advisory Board developed a definition of *haemorrhage* that requires acute or subacute onset symptoms referable to the anatomical location of the lesion accompanied by a haemorrhage testified mainly by a radiograph [2]. A recent meta-analysis of individual patient data reported an average 5-year bleeding rate of 15.8% based on this definition [11]. In this study, the brainstem location and presentation of haemorrhage were identified as risk factors that were independently associated with haemorrhage. The risk of intracerebral haemorrhage is also known to decline over time; one prospective study demonstrated that the annual risk of haemorrhage was 19.8% in the first year, which decreased to 5.0% in the fifth year [23]. In contrast, the bleeding rate of lesions found incidentally is considered as low as 0.08%, as reported in a previous study [20].

H. Hongo (✉) · S. Miyawaki · N. Saito
Department of Neurosurgery, Faculty of Medicine, The University of Tokyo, Tokyo, Japan
e-mail: hongoh-nsu@h.u-tokyo.ac.jp

Genetic Mutations

In patients with CCMs, sporadic and hereditary (familial) forms have been recognised. The former is typically solitary, whereas the latter is characterised by multifocal lesions (Fig. 1). The hereditary CCMs are inherited in an autosomal dominant manner. This observation has led researchers to use genetic approaches to explore the pathogenesis of CCMs. Specifically, linkage analysis was used to search for loci propagating with the phenotype among pedigree patients, including those with CCMs. This approach maps genes that cause CCMs to three loci: 7q, 3q, and 7p [4]. Further specification identifies *CCM1* (*KRIT1*), *CCM2*, and *CCM3* (*PDCD10*) as causative genes of familial CCMs [3, 14, 15]

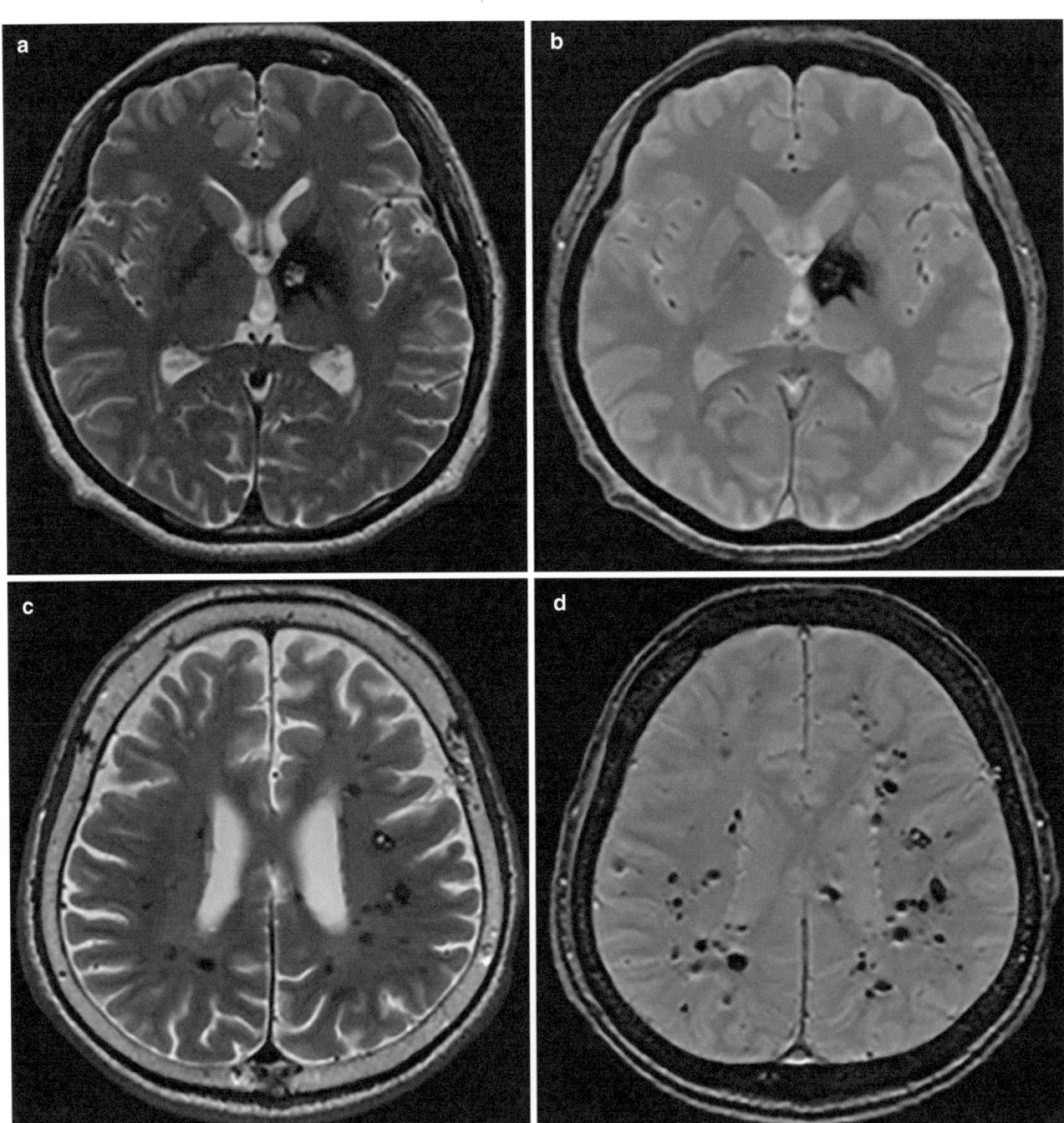

Fig. 1 Magnetic resonance imaging of patients with sporadic and familial cerebral cavernous malformations (CCMs): T2-weighted (**a**) and T2*-weighted (**b**) images of a patient with sporadic CCMs with a solitary lesion and T2-weighted (**c**) and T2*-weighted (**d**) images of a patient with familial CCMs with multiple CCM lesions, where the latter shows characteristically numerous lesions identified as hypointense on the T2*-weighted image

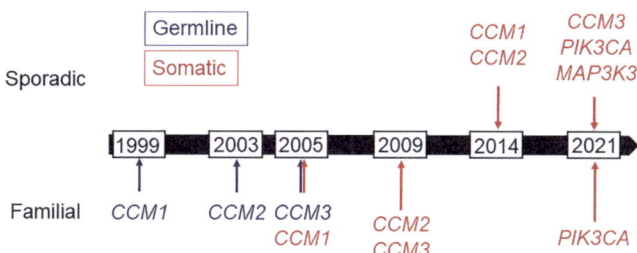

Fig. 2 Timeline of the identification of genes mutated in sporadic and familial cerebral cavernous malformations

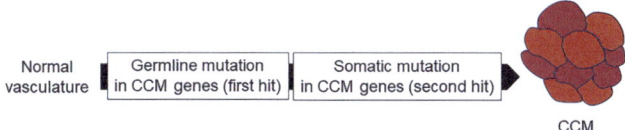

Fig. 3 Schema of the widely accepted pathogenesis of familial cerebral cavernous malformations

(Fig. 2). At present, at least one of the *CCM1*, *CCM2*, or *CCM3* mutations is a germline mutation in almost all familial CCMs cases [26]. Most genetic abnormalities are either truncating mutations, such as nonsense and frameshift mutations, or large deletions, which result in the loss of gene function. Familial CCMs are characterised by multiple lesions, whereas sporadic CCMs are generally solitary, suggesting a two-hit mechanism in which the loss of both copies of the gene results in loss of function and leads to lesion formation. Accordingly, in addition to germline mutations that are harboured in all cells in the body, somatic mutations, which are harboured only in CCM lesions, have begun to be sought, and biallelic mutations have been identified in patients with all three forms (*CCM1*, *CCM2*, and *CCM3*) of inherited CCMs [1] (Fig. 3). In these patients, somatic mutations are harboured in the vascular endothelial cells of the lesions. Next-generation sequencing has enabled us to more easily detect somatic mutations harboured only in a fraction of heterogeneous lesions. This technique, in addition to familial CCMs, is be used to identify somatic mutations in patients with sporadic CCMs, including a patient with two somatic *CCM1* pathogenic mutations, confirming that both familial and sporadic CCMs can be caused by a two-hit mechanism [19].

However, in sporadic CCMs, the detection rate of pathogenic mutations in these three CCM genes is low. This suggests that sporadic CCMs arise from somatic mutations in genes other than these genes and prompts researchers to explore somatic mutations in genes other than these three genes. Recently, somatic *PIK3CA* and *MAP3K3* mutations have been identified in CCMs, in addition to germline and somatic mutations in CCM genes [8, 30]. Mutations in *PIK3CA* and *MAP3K3* occur in endothelial cells, similar to mutations in CCM genes. Somatic *PIK3CA* mutations have been identified in familial and sporadic CCMs. These mutations co-occur with mutations in the three CCM genes and *MAP3K3*. In lesions with somatic mutations in both *PIK3CA* and one of the CCM genes, mutations in the *PIK3CA* and CCM genes are identified in the same cells, suggesting that the mutations act synergistically in the pathogenesis of CCMs [22]. In contrast, *MAP3K3* mutations are predominantly identified in patients with sporadic CCMs and are mutually exclusive of CCM gene mutations [30]. Thus, the identification of novel mutations associated with CCM is ongoing.

Genotype–Phenotype Correlations

Some genotype–phenotype correlations have been reported. Regarding familial CCMs, patients having *CCM2* mutations have a lower number of lesions than those having *CCM1* or *CCM3* mutations [5]. The clinical phenotype of patients with *CCM3* mutations is more aggressive than that of patients with *CCM1* or *CCM2* mutations, with an earlier age at disease onset, greater lesion burden, and more-frequent haemorrhages [24]. Patients with familial CCMs sometimes present with cutaneous vascular lesions, which are more frequently found in patients with *CCM1* mutations than in those with *CCM2* or *CCM3* mutations [6].

In sporadic CCMs, patients with *PIK3CA* mutations have a higher risk of haemorrhage than those with *MAP3K3* mutations [8]. Lesions with *PIK3CA* mutations are found predominantly in the brain and are larger [8]. Regarding MRI appearance, lesions with acute or subacute bleeding are more likely to have *PIK3CA* mutations; however, popcorn-like lesions indicating chronic haemorrhage more frequently have *MAP3K3* mutations [30].

Molecular Pathogenesis

The discovery of mutations in *CCM1*, *CCM2*, and *CCM3* promotes the development of in vivo CCM models. Among several animal species, such as mice and zebrafish, murine models have provided significant insights into the pathogenesis of CCMs. Globally, murine models losing one of the CCM genes are developed and found to be embryonically lethal owing to vascular defects, suggesting that *CCM1*, *CCM2*, and *CCM3* are essential for proper angiogenesis [31, 32]. To explore the cell types that originate from CCM formation, conditional CCM models were created, which can modulate the expression of certain proteins in a specific subset of cell types, demonstrating that the endothelial cell-specific loss of one of the CCM genes can also cause abnormal cardiovascular development, suggesting the necessity of the expression of CCM proteins in vascular endothelial cells. More-recent studies have created mice with postnatal loss-of-CCM genes in vascular endothelial cells—or, more specifically, brain endothelial cells—which develop vascular lesions similar to human CCM lesions and are used as faithful CCM models to study CCM pathogenesis [22, 33]. In addition to these mice, to examine the function of mutations in *PIK3CA* and *MAP3K3*, adeno-associated virus-mediated transduction, which can induce the overexpression of mutant proteins in a subset of cells depending on the type of virus, has also been used in some recent studies [12, 22]. Although some conflicting studies have demonstrated that pericyte- or neuron-specific loss-of-CCM genes can result in the formation of vascular lesions resembling CCMs [17, 29], suggesting a highly complicated mechanism of CCM development, vascular endothelial cells are widely accepted as the primary sites where driver gene mutations cause the disease.

The underlying molecular mechanisms of CCM development have been elucidated by using these mouse models. *CCM1*, *CCM2*, and *CCM3* form a complex and play a role in pathogenesis [7]. The primary role of this complex is to regulate mitogen-activated protein kinase 3 (MEKK3)-Krüppel-like factor 2/4 (KLF2/4) signalling [33]. Loss-of-function mutations in the three genes result in the activation of MEKK3 and transcription factors KLF2 and KLF4 downstream of the protein. Moreover, the loss of function of the complex results in the activation of the RHO/Rho-associated protein kinase, which is also considered a major mechanism [31]. Other mechanisms have also been reported, such as endothelial-to-mesenchymal transition and the locally elevated expression of anticoagulant endothelial receptors, thrombomodulin, and the endothelial protein C receptor [16, 18].

PIK3CA encodes the catalytic p110a subunit of PI3K. In endothelial cells, p110a is activated and upregulates PI3K and its downstream pathways, which are required for vascular development. *PIK3CA* mutations frequently identified in CCMs, c.1624G > A (p.Glu542Lys), c.1633G > A (p.Glu545Lys), and c.3140 A > G (p.His1047Arg), are also known mutation hotspots in several cancers, including breast, colon, and endometrial cancers. These mutations activate downstream pathways and are thus considered probable drivers of CCM formation.

MAP3K3 encodes MEKK3. As mentioned above, the activation of the MEKK3-KLF2/4 pathway is one of the primary mechanisms of CCMs, and the hotspot mutation *MAP3K3* c.1323 C > G (p.Ile441Met) activates the downstream pathway. Thus, the mutation can potentially be a driver of the disease by exhibiting similar functional consequences to the loss of function of CCM genes, which activate the pathway.

Association Between CCMs and Developmental Venous Anomalies

The coexistence of CCMs and DVAs is well known. DVAs are the most common vascular anomalies of the brain and are present in 6–14% of the adult population [25]. Approximately 20–30% of patients with sporadic CCMs have DVAs when assessed by using MRI [21]. De novo CCM formation around DVAs has also been reported [28]. These data suggest a causative association between CCMs and DVAs. A probable pathogenesis of CCM formation around the DVAs is that increased haemodynamic pressure within DVAs induces repeated microhaemorrhages and activates angiogenic factors, such as vascular endothelial growth factor, which results in the initiation of CCM formation. In contrast, familial CCMs are rarely accompanied by DVAs. This suggests that the developmental mechanisms differ between sporadic CCMs and familial CCMs. A recent study screened for *PIK3CA* and *MAP3K3* mutations in sporadic CCMs and accompanying DVA samples [25]. Consequently, in lesions harbouring both *PIK3CA* and *MAP3K3* mutations, the accompanying DVA samples harboured only *PIK3CA* mutations. This finding suggests that DVAs develop first in normal vasculature by acquiring *PIK3CA* mutation and that the associated CCMs are derived from cells in the DVAs that gain *MAP3K3* mutation in addition to *PIK3CA* mutation (Fig. 4). Further genetic studies are required to elucidate the detailed association between CCMs and DVAs.

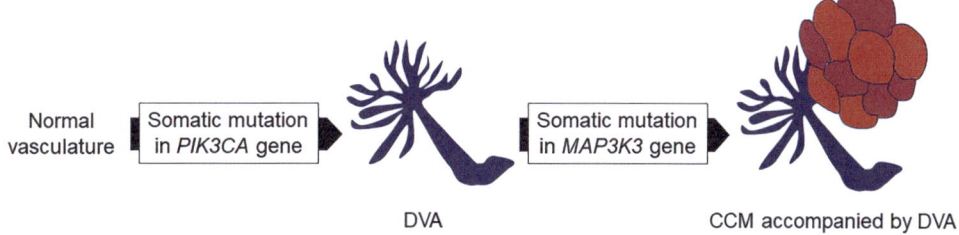

Fig. 4 Schema of the possible pathogenesis of sporadic cerebral cavernous malformations accompanied by developmental venous anomalies

GJA4: A Novel Cavernous Malformation–Associated Gene

Knowledge about the mutations and molecular mechanisms underlying the aetiology of CCMs has increased. However, other mechanisms may remain that can be anticipated from the recent identification of novel gene mutations, such as *PIK3CA* and *MAP3K3*, which are involved in pathogenesis. We recently identified *GJA4* mutation in orbital cavernous venous malformations (OCVMs) [10]. OCVMs are low-flow vascular malformations similar to CCMs, and their causative mutations have not yet been identified. By sequencing several vascular malformations, including OCVMs and CCMs, *GJA4* mutation is frequently present in OCVMs. *GJA4* is a transmembrane protein that forms hemichannels, which connect the cytoplasm to the extracellular space, and gap junctions, which connect the cytoplasm of adjacent cells in the endothelium and smooth muscles of blood vessels. This mutation is identified predominantly in lesions of endothelial cells. A functional analysis revealed the mutation to be a gain-of-function mutation that induces a hyperactive hemichannel, which subsequently induces the loss of the normal function of endothelial cells. Therefore, abnormal *GJA4* hemichannel activity may play a role in the pathogenesis of vascular malformations. In addition, an identical *GJA4* mutation was recently identified in intracranial angioleiomyomas and haematic and cutaneous venous malformations, suggesting that this mutation may be the driver of a broad range of vascular malformations. The abnormality of hemichannel and gap junctions is involved in the pathogenesis of vascular malformations. Therefore, this discovery provides novel insights into the molecular pathogenesis of cavernous malformations and contributes to our understanding of their underlying mechanisms.

Conclusions

This review describes the epidemiology, natural course, and aetiology of CCMs, with a focus on their genetic aspects. Several observational studies have provided information about their clinical behaviours, which will contribute to improving surgical intervention decisions. Moreover, the currently evolving molecular genetic approach has revealed their pathophysiology, providing insights into the development of novel therapeutic strategies.

Funding Information This work was supported by a grant-in-aid for scientific research (B) (No. 21H03041) from the Japan Society for the Promotion of Science to Dr Saito, a grant-in-aid for early-career scientists (No. 22K16677) from the Japan Society for the Promotion of Science to Dr Hongo, and a grant from the Uehara Memorial Foundation to Dr Hongo.

Declarations

Conflict of Interest The authors declare that they have no conflict of interest.

References

1. Akers AL, Johnson E, Steinberg GK, Zabramski JM, Marchuk DA. Biallelic somatic and germline mutations in cerebral cavernous malformations (CCMs): evidence for a two-hit mechanism of CCM pathogenesis. Hum Mol Genet. 2009;18:919–30. https://doi.org/10.1093/hmg/ddn430.
2. Al-Shahi Salman R, Berg MJ, Morrison L, Awad IA, Angioma Alliance Scientific Advisory B. Hemorrhage from cavernous malformations of the brain: definition and reporting standards. Angioma Alliance Scientific Advisory Board. Stroke. 2008;39:3222–30. https://doi.org/10.1161/STROKEAHA.108.515544.
3. Bergametti F, Denier C, Labauge P, Arnoult M, Boetto S, Clanet M, Coubes P, Echenne B, Ibrahim R, Irthum B, Jacquet G, Lonjon M, Moreau JJ, Neau JP, Parker F, Tremoulet M, Tournier-Lasserve E, Societe Francaise de N. Mutations within the programmed cell death 10 gene cause cerebral cavernous malformations. Am J Hum Genet. 2005;76:42–51. https://doi.org/10.1086/426952.
4. Craig HD, Günel M, Cepeda O, Johnson EW, Ptacek L, Steinberg GK, Ogilvy CS, Berg MJ, Crawford SC, Scott RM, Steichen-Gersdorf E, Sabroe R, Kennedy CT, Mettler G, Beis MJ, Fryer A, Awad IA, Lifton RP. Multilocus linkage identifies two new loci for a mendelian form of stroke, cerebral cavernous malformation, at 7p15-13 and 3q25.2-27. Hum Mol Genet. 1998;7:1851–8. https://doi.org/10.1093/hmg/7.12.1851.
5. Denier C, Labauge P, Bergametti F, Marchelli F, Riant F, Arnoult M, Maciazek J, Vicaut E, Brunereau L, Tournier-Lasserve E. Genotype-phenotype correlations in cerebral cavernous malformations patients. Ann Neurol. 2006;60:550–6. https://doi.org/10.1002/ana.20947.

6. Grippaudo FR, Piane M, Amoroso M, Longo B, Penco S, Chessa L, Giubettini M, Santanelli F. Cutaneous venous malformations related to KRIT1 mutation: case report and literature review. J Mol Neurosci. 2013;51:442–5. https://doi.org/10.1007/s12031-013-0053-1.
7. Hilder TL, Malone MH, Bencharit S, Colicelli J, Haystead TA, Johnson GL, Wu CC. Proteomic identification of the cerebral cavernous malformation signaling complex. J Proteome Res. 2007;6:4343–55. https://doi.org/10.1021/pr0704276.
8. Hong T, Xiao X, Ren J, Cui B, Zong Y, Zou J, Kou Z, Jiang N, Meng G, Zeng G, Shan Y, Wu H, Chen Z, Liang J, Xiao X, Tang J, Wei Y, Ye M, Sun L, Li G, Hu P, Hui R, Zhang H, Wang Y. Somatic MAP3K3 and PIK3CA mutations in sporadic cerebral and spinal cord cavernous malformations. Brain. 2021;144:2648–58. https://doi.org/10.1093/brain/awab117.
9. Hongo H, Miyawaki S, Teranishi Y, Ishigami D, Ohara K, Sakai Y, Shimada D, Umekawa M, Koizumi S, Ono H, Nakatomi H, Saito N. Genetics of brain arteriovenous malformations and cerebral cavernous malformations. J Hum Genet. 2023;68:157–67. https://doi.org/10.1038/s10038-022-01063-8.
10. Hongo H, Miyawaki S, Teranishi Y, Mitsui J, Katoh H, Komura D, Tsubota K, Matsukawa T, Watanabe M, Kurita M, Yoshimura J, Dofuku S, Ohara K, Ishigami D, Okano A, Kato M, Hakuno F, Takahashi A, Kunita A, Ishiura H, Shin M, Nakatomi H, Nagao T, Goto H, Takahashi SI, Ushiku T, Ishikawa S, Okazaki M, Morishita S, Tsuji S, Saito N. Somatic GJA4 gain-of-function mutation in orbital cavernous venous malformations. Angiogenesis. 2023;26:37–52. https://doi.org/10.1007/s10456-022-09846-5.
11. Horne MA, Flemming KD, Su IC, Stapf C, Jeon JP, Li D, Maxwell SS, White P, Christianson TJ, Agid R, Cho W-S, Oh CW, Wu Z, Zhang J-T, Kim JE, ter Brugge K, Willinsky R, Brown RD, Murray GD, Salman RA-S. Clinical course of untreated cerebral cavernous malformations: a meta-analysis of individual patient data. Lancet Neurol. 2016;15:166–73. https://doi.org/10.1016/s1474-4422(15)00303-8.
12. Huo R, Yang Y, Sun Y, Zhou Q, Zhao S, Mo Z, Xu H, Wang J, Weng J, Jiao Y, Zhang J, He Q, Wang S, Zhao J, Wang J, Cao Y. Endothelial hyperactivation of mutant MAP3K3 induces cerebral cavernous malformation enhanced by PIK3CA GOF mutation. Angiogenesis. 2023; https://doi.org/10.1007/s10456-023-09866-9.
13. Idiculla PS, Gurala D, Philipose J, Rajdev K, Patibandla P. Cerebral cavernous malformations, developmental venous anomaly, and its coexistence: a review. Eur Neurol. 2020;83:360–8. https://doi.org/10.1159/000508748.
14. Laberge-le Couteulx S, Jung HH, Labauge P, Houtteville JP, Lescoat C, Cecillon M, Marechal E, Joutel A, Bach JF, Tournier-Lasserve E. Truncating mutations in CCM1, encoding KRIT1, cause hereditary cavernous angiomas. Nat Genet. 1999;23:189–93. https://doi.org/10.1038/13815.
15. Liquori CL, Berg MJ, Siegel AM, Huang E, Zawistowski JS, Stoffer T, Verlaan D, Balogun F, Hughes L, Leedom TP, Plummer NW, Cannella M, Maglione V, Squitieri F, Johnson EW, Rouleau GA, Ptacek L, Marchuk DA. Mutations in a gene encoding a novel protein containing a phosphotyrosine-binding domain cause type 2 cerebral cavernous malformations. Am J Hum Genet. 2003;73:1459–64. https://doi.org/10.1086/380314.
16. Lopez-Ramirez MA, Pham A, Girard R, Wyseure T, Hale P, Yamashita A, Koskimäki J, Polster S, Saadat L, Romero IA, Esmon CT, Lagarrigue F, Awad IA, Mosnier LO, Ginsberg MH. Cerebral cavernous malformations form an anticoagulant vascular domain in humans and mice. Blood. 2019;133:193–204. https://doi.org/10.1182/blood-2018-06-856062.
17. Louvi A, Chen L, Two AM, Zhang H, Min W, Gunel M. Loss of cerebral cavernous malformation 3 (Ccm3) in neuroglia leads to CCM and vascular pathology. Proc Natl Acad Sci USA. 2011;108:3737–42. https://doi.org/10.1073/pnas.1012617108.
18. Maddaluno L, Rudini N, Cuttano R, Bravi L, Giampietro C, Corada M, Ferrarini L, Orsenigo F, Papa E, Boulday G, Tournier-Lasserve E, Chapon F, Richichi C, Retta SF, Lampugnani MG, Dejana E. EndMT contributes to the onset and progression of cerebral cavernous malformations. Nature. 2013;498:492–6. https://doi.org/10.1038/nature12207.
19. McDonald DA, Shi C, Shenkar R, Gallione CJ, Akers AL, Li S, De Castro N, Berg MJ, Corcoran DL, Awad IA, Marchuk DA. Lesions from patients with sporadic cerebral cavernous malformations harbor somatic mutations in the CCM genes: evidence for a common biochemical pathway for CCM pathogenesis. Hum Mol Genet. 2014;23:4357–70. https://doi.org/10.1093/hmg/ddu153.
20. Moore SA, Brown RD Jr, Christianson TJ, Flemming KD. Long-term natural history of incidentally discovered cavernous malformations in a single-center cohort. J Neurosurg. 2014;120:1188–92. https://doi.org/10.3171/2014.1.JNS131619.
21. Petersen TA, Morrison LA, Schrader RM, Hart BL. Familial versus sporadic cavernous malformations: differences in developmental venous anomaly association and lesion phenotype. AJNR Am J Neuroradiol. 2010;31:377–82. https://doi.org/10.3174/ajnr.A1822.
22. Ren AA, Snellings DA, Su YS, Hong CC, Castro M, Tang AT, Detter MR, Hobson N, Girard R, Romanos S, Lightle R, Moore T, Shenkar R, Benavides C, Beaman MM, Muller-Fielitz H, Chen M, Mericko P, Yang J, Sung DC, Lawton MT, Ruppert JM, Schwaninger M, Korbelin J, Potente M, Awad IA, Marchuk DA, Kahn ML. PIK3CA and CCM mutations fuel cavernomas through a cancer-like mechanism. Nature. 2021;594:271–6. https://doi.org/10.1038/s41586-021-03562-8.
23. Salman RA-S, Hall JM, Horne MA, Moultrie F, Josephson CB, Bhattacharya JJ, Counsell CE, Murray GD, Papanastassiou V, Ritchie V, Roberts RC, Sellar RJ, Warlow CP. Untreated clinical course of cerebral cavernous malformations: a prospective, population-based cohort study. Lancet Neurol. 2012;11:217–24. https://doi.org/10.1016/s1474-4422(12)70004-2.
24. Shenkar R, Shi C, Rebeiz T, Stockton RA, McDonald DA, Mikati AG, Zhang L, Austin C, Akers AL, Gallione CJ, Rorrer A, Gunel M, Min W, De Souza JM, Lee C, Marchuk DA, Awad IA. Exceptional aggressiveness of cerebral cavernous malformation disease associated with PDCD10 mutations. Genet Med. 2015;17:188–96. https://doi.org/10.1038/gim.2014.97.
25. Snellings DA, Girard R, Lightle R, Srinath A, Romanos S, Li Y, Chen C, Ren AA, Kahn ML, Awad IA, Marchuk DA. Developmental venous anomalies are a genetic primer for cerebral cavernous malformations. Nat Cardiovasc Res. 2022;1:246–52. https://doi.org/10.1038/s44161-022-00035-7.
26. Spiegler S, Rath M, Paperlein C, Felbor U. Cerebral cavernous malformations: an update on prevalence, molecular genetic analyses, and genetic counselling. Mol Syndromol. 2018;9:60–9. https://doi.org/10.1159/000486292.
27. Stapleton CJ, Barker FG 2nd. Cranial cavernous malformations: natural history and treatment. Stroke. 2018;49:1029–35. https://doi.org/10.1161/STROKEAHA.117.017074.
28. Su IC, Krishnan P, Rawal S, Krings T. Magnetic resonance evolution of de novo formation of a cavernoma in a thrombosed developmental venous anomaly: a case report. Neurosurgery. 2013;73:E739–744; discussion E745. https://doi.org/10.1227/NEU.0000000000000002.
29. Wang K, Zhang H, He Y, Jiang Q, Tanaka Y, Park IH, Pober JS, Min W, Zhou HJ. Mural cell-specific deletion of cerebral cavernous malformation 3 in the brain induces cerebral cavernous malformations. Arterioscler Thromb Vasc Biol. 2020;40:2171–86. https://doi.org/10.1161/ATVBAHA.120.314586.
30. Weng J, Yang Y, Song D, Huo R, Li H, Chen Y, Nam Y, Zhou Q, Jiao Y, Fu W, Yan Z, Wang J, Xu H, Di L, Li J, Wang S, Zhao J, Wang J, Cao Y. Somatic MAP3K3 mutation defines a subclass of cere-

bral cavernous malformation. Am J Hum Genet. 2021;108:942–50. https://doi.org/10.1016/j.ajhg.2021.04.005.
31. Whitehead KJ, Chan AC, Navankasattusas S, Koh W, London NR, Ling J, Mayo AH, Drakos SG, Jones CA, Zhu W, Marchuk DA, Davis GE, Li DY. The cerebral cavernous malformation signaling pathway promotes vascular integrity via Rho GTPases. Nat Med. 2009;15:177–84. https://doi.org/10.1038/nm.1911.
32. Whitehead KJ, Plummer NW, Adams JA, Marchuk DA, Li DY. Ccm1 is required for arterial morphogenesis: implications for the etiology of human cavernous malformations. Development. 2004;131:1437–48. https://doi.org/10.1242/dev.01036.
33. Zhou Z, Tang AT, Wong WY, Bamezai S, Goddard LM, Shenkar R, Zhou S, Yang J, Wright AC, Foley M, Arthur JS, Whitehead KJ, Awad IA, Li DY, Zheng X, Kahn ML. Cerebral cavernous malformations arise from endothelial gain of MEKK3-KLF2/4 signalling. Nature. 2016;532:122–6. https://doi.org/10.1038/nature17178.

Open Access This chapter is licensed under the terms of the Creative Commons Attribution 4.0 International License (http://creativecommons.org/licenses/by/4.0/), which permits use, sharing, adaptation, distribution and reproduction in any medium or format, as long as you give appropriate credit to the original author(s) and the source, provide a link to the Creative Commons license and indicate if changes were made.

The images or other third party material in this chapter are included in the chapter's Creative Commons license, unless indicated otherwise in a credit line to the material. If material is not included in the chapter's Creative Commons license and your intended use is not permitted by statutory regulation or exceeds the permitted use, you will need to obtain permission directly from the copyright holder.

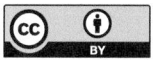

Part VI
Innovations

Experiences with and Practical Implications of Using a Hybrid Operating Room

Matthias Gmeiner, Vanessa Mazanec, Michael Sonnberger, and Andreas Gruber

Introduction

The idea of a hybrid operating room (OR) is not new and was originally proposed by Barstad et al. (1997), who used it for minimally invasive direct coronary artery bypass grafting and integrated hybrid procedures [1]. The increasing complexity of both interventional and surgical procedures has required new approaches, so the best of both worlds was combined, which resulted in the hybrid operating room [10]. The original technical implementation has little to do with today's OR, but due to rapid technological progress, significant advances have been possible. Today, systems that allow the user to perform intraoperative 3D rotational angiography have been established, which according to some studies provides a significant advantage in patient outcome in the treatment of cerebrovascular pathologies [6]. Furthermore, it enables the performing of a special type of computed tomography (CT), a so-called DynaCT, which allows an accurate anatomical understanding of a target vessel in relation to surrounding anatomical structures and metallic devices such as stents or clips, and in addition, perfusion measurement can be performed [17].

The popularity of the hybrid OR in neurosurgery, especially in cerebrovascular neurosurgery, may be related to the extremely low tolerable ischemia time, the high complexity of the surgical procedures, and the low error tolerance [7]. Because of this, success and quality control are essential to achieve optimal patient outcomes. However, the greatest advantage of this technology is its enabling surgeons to perform endovascular and surgical procedures simultaneously [6].

To make the best use of the aforementioned advantages, a high degree of interdisciplinarity, as well as expertise, is required [7]. One procedure that is frequently mentioned in connection with the hybrid operating room is the performance of a bypass followed by the endovascular treatment of a complex aneurysm [2, 11, 15]. Benefits frequently cited in previously published work include the shortening of procedure time, an improvement in treatment quality, and a reduction in procedure-associated complications [4, 6–8, 14, 15]. The aim of this chapter is to present the results of the use of a hybrid OR in the treatment of cerebrovascular pathologies at a neurovascular center and to highlight factors discovered that are relevant for the practice.

Methods and Materials

In this retrospective data analysis, all patients who had been treated because of cerebral vascular disease (cerebral aneurysm, arteriovenous malformation (AVM), arteriovenous (AV) fistulas, carotid pathologies) in the hybrid OR at the Department of Neurosurgery at Kepler University Hospital Linz between April 2020 and October 2022 were included. In all cases, intraoperative imaging and/or hybrid surgery was performed. In patients with cerebral aneurysms, indocyanide green videoangiography (ICG) and Doppler ultrasound were additionally performed before intraoperative angiography. Furthermore, the following parameters were collected: the type and localization of vascular disease, modality of surgical or endovascular treatment, outcome of intraoperative imaging, and influence on further surgical strategy.

M. Gmeiner (✉) · A. Gruber
Kepler University Hospital Linz, Department of Neurosurgery, Linz, Austria

Kepler University Hospital Linz, Medical Faculty, Linz, Austria
e-mail: matthias.gmeiner@kepleruniversitätsklinikum.at

V. Mazanec · M. Sonnberger
Kepler University Hospital Linz, Medical Faculty, Linz, Austria

Kepler University Hospital Linz, Institute for Neuroradiology, Linz, Austria

Results

A total of 152 patients met the inclusion criteria (Table 1).

Aneurysms

In total, 106 aneurysms were treated via clipping. Rupture was present in 4.8% (*n* = 22) of cases. The most frequent location was the middle cerebral artery (MCA; *n* = 61). Four patients were treated by using proximal or endovascular surgical vessel occlusion under bypass protection.

Carotid Stenosis/Occlusion

Also, 49 patients were treated because of carotid stenosis or occlusion, of whom 32 underwent carotid endarterectomy (CEA) and 17 were treated with bypass.

AVM/Dural AV-Fistula

Finally, 12 patients were treated because of an AVM or fistula.

Table 1 Pathologies and treatment

Vascular Pathology	n
Aneurysms	106
Patients	91
Middle cerebral artery	61
Anterior communicating artery	18
Anterior cerebral artery	15
Internal carotid artery	6
Posterior circulation	6
Ruptured	22
Clipping/bypass	102/4
Carotid stenosis/occlusion	49
Carotid endarterectomy	32
Bypass	17
Arteriovenous malformation/fistula	12
Overall patients	152

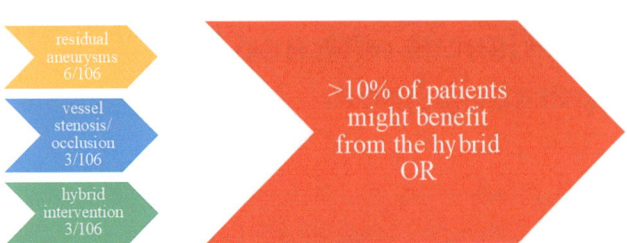

Fig. 1 Results after intraoperative angiography or hybrid intervention

Surgical Strategy, Intraoperative Angiography, and Hybrid Interventions

The surgical strategy is summarized in Fig. 1. In six of 106 patients (5.6%) treated via microsurgical clipping, a residual aneurysm was detected during intraoperative angiography, which led to the optimization of clip placement. Further, in three cases, vessel occlusion or stenosis occurred after clipping, and the surgical strategy had to be adapted: In two patients, the clip was repositioned, and in one case, a hybrid intervention was necessary. This hybrid procedure had to be performed due to persistent vessel occlusion despite several clip repositioning attempts (anterior communicating artery aneurysm). The pericallosal artery, which was occluded by a calcified plaque dislodged during clipping, was endovascularly dilated (percutaneous transluminal angioplasty, or PTA) and successfully recanalized. Another two planned hybrid interventions were performed by using endovascular parent artery occlusion (complex posterior cerebral artery or MCA aneurysm) under bypass protection.

In CEA or bypass surgery (carotid stenosis or occlusion), a residual critical stenosis persisted and was immediately treated only in one case. No ischemic complication occurred. Three of 12 patients (25%) with an AVM or AV fistulas had a remnant and could finally be treated completely.

Discussion

Recently, the hybrid OR has been introduced in various surgical disciplines [6]. However, advantages such as lower invasiveness, operation duration, mortality, and overall complication rates have been reported [6, 11]. In neurosurgery, a relevant increase in the quality of treatment might be achieved, especially in patients with complex vascular pathologies that are not amenable to endovascular or surgical therapy alone [3].

In previously published studies, aneurysm remnants were detected in 3.8–14% during postoperative angiography, and the percentage of vessel stenosis or occlusion was 3–8% [5, 14, 18]. Nowadays, standard intraoperative quality control is established by means of ICG video angiography and Doppler examination [9]. A further quality improvement through treatment in the hybrid operating room could be verified [4, 8, 14, 15]. During intraoperative angiography, a significantly higher detection rate of residual aneurysms could be determined via 3D compared to 2D angiography [5, 14]. In the field of other vascular pathologies, such as AVMs or fistulas, no superiority of 3D angiography could be demonstrated [8, 10].

In addition to intraoperative angiography, combined interdisciplinary interventions in the hybrid OR can contribute to both primary *one-stage* treatment and successful complication management [12, 13]. In one of our patients, despite clip repositioning, a vessel occlusion (plaque dislocated by a clip with resulting vessel occlusion) could not be resolved, and therefore, an unplanned acute hybrid intervention was performed. The vessel was successfully recanalized via endovascular PTA. Konakondla et al. published one case of intraoperative occlusion of the ipsilateral MCA during the clipping of a posterior communicating artery aneurysm. This complication was successfully treated via mechanical thrombectomy [13].

Mechanical thrombectomy with possible rescue stenting due to thromboembolic complications during CEA would also be possible at our center but was not necessary in any of our cases [20]. However, this strategy might contribute to avoiding severe complications.

Therapeutic vessel occlusion under bypass protection represents a classic example of hybrid interventions [2, 12, 16]. Thus, a complex aneurysm can be treated endovascularly under bypass protection, or a ruptured aneurysm can be partially embolized and then clipped to achieve an optimal surgical result [2, 16]. A similar approach in terms of partial embolization and subsequent surgical therapy can also be used in the treatment of AVMs [19]. In this context, the importance of the detection of AVM remnants during intraoperative angiography should be emphasized again.

Conclusion

No procedural complications occurred in this study. Intraoperative angiography is a safe and accurate method to optimize the surgical strategy and contributes to an improved patient outcome. Hybrid interventions with endovascular and surgical therapy become possible but require excellent interdisciplinary collaboration and expertise. Intraoperative complications can be reduced and, if they occur, can be treated quickly and optimally at a neurovascular center. Overall, the implementation of a hybrid OR can contribute to a significant increase in patient safety and treatment quality.

Declarations

Conflicts of interest The authors declare that they have no conflict of interest.

References

1. Barstad RM, Fosse E, Vatne K, Andersen K, Tønnessen T-I, Svennevig JL, Geiran OR. Intraoperative angiography in minimally invasive direct coronary artery bypass grafting. Ann Thorac Surg. 1997;64(6):1835–9.
2. Choi E, Lee JY, Jeon HJ, Cho B-M, Yoon DY. A hybrid operating room for combined surgical and endovascular procedures for cerebrovascular diseases: a clinical experience at a single Centre. Br J Neurosurg. 2019;33(5):490–4.
3. Choudhri O, Mukerji N, Steinberg GK. Combined endovascular and microsurgical management of complex cerebral aneurysms. Front Neurol. 2013;4:108.
4. Dammann P, Jägersberg M, Kulcsar Z, Radovanovic I, Schaller K, Bijlenga P. Clipping of ruptured intracranial aneurysms in a hybrid room environment-a case-control study. Acta Neurochir. 2017;159(7):1291–8.
5. Fong Y-W, Hsu S-K, Huang C-T, Hsieh C-T, Chen M-H, Huang J-S, Chang C-J, Su I-C. Impact of intraoperative 3-dimensional volume-rendering rotational angiography on clip repositioning rates in aneurysmal surgery. World Neurosurg. 2018;114:e573–80.
6. Gharios M, El-Hajj VG, Frisk H, Ohlsson M, Omar A, Edström E, Elmi-Terander A. The use of hybrid operating rooms in neurosurgery, advantages, disadvantages, and future perspectives: a systematic review. Acta Neurochir. 2023;165(9):2343–58.
7. Gmeiner M, Sonnberger M, Gollwitzer M, Sardi G, Hauser A, Aichholzer M, Stefanits H, Rauch P, Gruber A. Neurochirurgischer Hybrid-Operationssaal: Erste Erfahrungen an der Universitätsklinik für Neurochirurgie Linz // neurosurgical hybrid operating room: first experiences at the Kepler University Hospital Linz. J Für Neurol Neurochir Psychiatr. 2022;23(2):56–60.
8. Goren O, Bourdages G, Schirmer CM, Weiner G, Dalal SS, Griessenauer CJ. Intraoperative 3-dimensional rotational angiography in cerebrovascular surgery: a case series. World Neurosurg. 2020;141:e736–42.
9. Gruber A, Dorfer C, Standhardt H, Bavinzski G, Knosp E. Prospective comparison of intraoperative vascular monitoring technologies during cerebral aneurysm surgery. Neurosurgery. 2011;68(3):657–673; discussion 673.
10. Grüter BE, Strange F, Burn F, Remonda L, Diepers M, Fandino J, Marbacher S. Hybrid operating room settings for treatment of complex Dural Arteriovenous Fistulas. World Neurosurg. 2018;120:e932–9.
11. Jin H, Lu L, Liu J, Cui M. A systematic review on the application of the hybrid operating room in surgery: experiences and challenges. Updat Surg. 2022;74(2):403–15.
12. Kawamura Y, Sayama T, Maehara N, Nishimura A, Iihara K. Ruptured aneurysm of an aberrant internal carotid artery successfully treated with simultaneous intervention and surgery in a hybrid operating room. World Neurosurg. 2017;102:695.e1–5.
13. Konakondla S, Griessenauer CJ, Fong RP, Goren O, Schirmer CM. Zero-delay mechanical Thrombectomy for distal large vessel occlusion detected on intraoperative angiogram after microsurgical clipping of a posterior communicating artery aneurysm: value of hybrid operating room. World Neurosurg. 2018;119:278–81.
14. Marbacher S, Halter M, Vogt DR, Kienzler JC, Magyar CTJ, Wanderer S, Anon J, Diepers M, Remonda L, Fandino J. Value of

3-dimensional digital subtraction angiography for detection and classification of intracranial aneurysm remnants after clipping. Oper Neurosurg Hagerstown Md. 2021;21(2):63–72.
15. Marbacher S, Kienzler JC, Mendelowitsch I, D'Alonzo D, Andereggen L, Diepers M, Remonda L, Fandino J. Comparison of intra- and postoperative 3-dimensional digital subtraction angiography in evaluation of the surgical result after intracranial aneurysm treatment. Neurosurgery. 2020;87(4):689–96.
16. Murayama Y, Arakawa H, Ishibashi T, et al. Combined surgical and endovascular treatment of complex cerebrovascular diseases in the hybrid operating room. J NeuroInterventional Surg. 2013;5(5):489–93.
17. Namba K, Niimi Y, Song JK, Berenstein A. Use of dyna-CT angiography in neuroendovascular decision-making. Interv Neuroradiol. 2009;15(1):67–72.
18. Park J-H, Lee JY, Jeon HJ, Lim BC, Park SW, Cho BM. Safety and completeness of using indocyanine green videoangiography combined with digital subtraction angiography for aneurysm surgery in a hybrid operating theater. Neurosurg Rev. 2020;43(4):1163–71.
19. Song J, Li P, Tian Y, et al. One-stage treatment in a hybrid operation room to cure brain arteriovenous malformation: a single-center experience. World Neurosurg. 2021;147:e85–97.
20. Spiotta AM, Vargas J, Zuckerman S, Mokin M, Ahmed A, Mocco J, Turner RD, Turk AS, Chaudry MI, Myers P. Acute stroke after carotid endarterectomy: time for a paradigm shift? Multicenter experience with emergent carotid artery stenting with or without intracranial tandem occlusion thrombectomy. Neurosurgery. 2015;76(4):403–10.

Open Access This chapter is licensed under the terms of the Creative Commons Attribution 4.0 International License (http://creativecommons.org/licenses/by/4.0/), which permits use, sharing, adaptation, distribution and reproduction in any medium or format, as long as you give appropriate credit to the original author(s) and the source, provide a link to the Creative Commons license and indicate if changes were made.

The images or other third party material in this chapter are included in the chapter's Creative Commons license, unless indicated otherwise in a credit line to the material. If material is not included in the chapter's Creative Commons license and your intended use is not permitted by statutory regulation or exceeds the permitted use, you will need to obtain permission directly from the copyright holder.

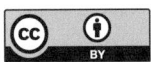

Artificial Intelligence and Augmented Reality in Vascular Neurosurgery

Tristan van Doormaal, Elisa Colombo, Tim Fick, Jesse A. M. van Doormaal, Tessa M. Kos, Mathijs de Boer, Pierre Robe, Eelco Hoving, Lambertus W. Bartels, and Luca Regli

Introduction

Over recent years, groundbreaking innovative technologies and devices have emerged in vascular neurosurgery as driving forces in the quest for outcome improvement. The increasing adoption of artificial intelligence (AI) and augmented reality (AR) within this field has become a prominent trend [1–5].

AI encompasses the development of intelligent systems capable of emulating human-like cognitive functions, including learning and problem-solving. Machine learning, a subfield of AI, is particularly relevant here because it focuses on the creation of algorithms and statistical models, enabling computer systems to learn from and make predictions or decisions on the basis of data and without being explicitly programmed. AI finds applications across various phases of patient care, encompassing prevention, preoperative assessment, perioperative management, and postoperative care. One impactful application of machine learning in the field of perioperative care in vascular neurosurgery is the training of algorithms for the conversion of two-dimensional (2D) medical images into 3D models [6]. This facilitates the creation of precise three-dimensional representations of complex vascular anatomy and pathology, offering invaluable insights into diagnosis and enabling informed surgical decision-making.

Augmented reality (AR) plays a pivotal role in 3D medical visualization. AR overlays virtual elements onto the real-world environment, affording a comprehensive view of anatomy [1, 7]. Furthermore, the concept of mixed reality (MxR) takes AR to a new level in that the virtual elements can interact with real-world elements (e.g., collide with it and appear behind it) presented through a head-mounted display (HMD) equipped with cameras that continuously scan the environment, which gives an even more realistic experience. Incorporating AR into vascular neurosurgery has the potential to enhance 3D insights into complex lesions and thereby significantly influence surgical planning, navigation, and intraoperative guidance, promising safer and more-effective procedures.

The primary challenge before us is seamlessly integrating these advanced concepts and developing them further to improve patient outcomes. To provide a basis for this future direction of our research group and potentially other groups, we present a review of all publications in our centers on the topic within the last 5 years. We combine this information with ongoing research projects to better understand the drawbacks, challenges, and the developmental steps to be followed.

T. van Doormaal (✉)
Department of Neurosurgery, University Medical Center Utrecht, Utrecht, Netherlands

Department of Neurosurgery, University Hospital Zurich, Zurich, Switzerland
e-mail: T.p.c.vandoormaal@umcutrecht.nl

E. Colombo · P. Robe · L. Regli
Department of Neurosurgery, University Hospital Zurich, Zurich, Switzerland

T. Fick · T. M. Kos
Department of Neurosurgery, University Medical Center Utrecht, Utrecht, Netherlands

Department of Neuro-oncology, Princess Máxima Center for Pediatric Oncology, Utrecht, Netherlands

J. A. M. van Doormaal · M. de Boer
Department of Neurosurgery, University Medical Center Utrecht, Utrecht, Netherlands

E. Hoving
Department of Neuro-oncology, Princess Máxima Center for Pediatric Oncology, Utrecht, Netherlands

L. W. Bartels
Image Sciences Institute, University Medical Center Utrecht, Utrecht, Netherlands

Methods

We selected articles featuring at minimum two of the members of our research group who have published within the past 5 years on topic combinations such as artificial intelligence and augmented reality; artificial intelligence and vascular neurosurgery; or augmented reality and vascular neurosurgery. We combined the information from these articles with information from ongoing research projects within our group. We used these resources to form the basis of a narrative discussion to more deeply explore the drawbacks and challenges of incorporating AI and AR into vascular neurosurgery and to find logical developmental phases in our research to shape the future.

All AR examples in the figures were made with Lumi software (Augmedit bv, Naarden, Netherlands).

Informed consent was obtained from all individual participants included in the described studies and participants anonymously depicted in the figures. All procedures performed in the described studies involving human participants were in accordance with the ethical standards of the institutional and/or national research committee and with the 1964 Helsinki Declaration and its later amendments or comparable ethical standards.

Results

We selected 14 peer-reviewed publications that fulfilled the criteria (Table 1). The selected research, along with ongoing research projects, resulted in the identification of four phases of development; (1) the integration of AI and AR to create adequate three-dimensional (3D) segmentations; (2) adding flow and pulsatility data to create 5D segmentations; (3) treatment planning in these models; and (4) treatment guidance using these models (Fig. 1). The main drawback described was the limited added value in the microscopic phase of neurovascular surgery due to view obstruction and a lack of accuracy. The main challenge described was the cur-

Table 1 Publications on topics combining artificial intelligence and augmented reality; artificial intelligence and vascular neurosurgery; or augmented reality and vascular neurosurgery featuring at minimum two publications by authors of our group published within the past 10 years

Year	Study	Journal
2018	AR glasses in the operating room [8]	*NTvG*
2019	Clinical Accuracy of Holographic Navigation Using Point-Based Registration on Augmented-Reality Glasses [9]	*Operative Neurosurgery*
2020	Current Accuracy of Augmented Reality Neuronavigation Systems: Systematic Review and Meta-Analysis [2]	*World Neurosurgery*
2021	Holographic patient tracking after bed movement for augmented reality neuronavigation using a head-mounted display [10]	*Acta Neurochirurgica*
2021	Fully Automatic Adaptive Meshing Based Segmentation of the Ventricular System for Augmented Reality Visualization and Navigation [11]	*World Neurosurgery*
2021	Fully automatic brain tumor segmentation for 3D evaluation in augmented reality [12]	*Neurosurgical Focus*
2022	Segmentation techniques of cerebral arteriovenous malformations for 3D visualisation: a systematic review [7]	*Brain and Spine*
2023	Comparing the influence of mixed reality, a 3D viewer, and MRI on the spatial understanding of brain tumours [13]	*Frontiers in Virtual Reality*
2023	Case report: Impact of mixed reality on anatomical understanding and surgical planning in a complex fourth ventricular tumor extending to the lamina quadrigemina [14]	*Frontiers in Surgery*
2023	Clinical potential of automated convolutional neural network-based hematoma volumetry after aneurysmal subarachnoid hemorrhage [5]	*J Stroke Cerebrovasc Dis*
2023	Effect of intraoperative mixed reality use on non-surgical team members in the neurosurgical operating room [3]	*World Neurosurgery*
2023	Application of Virtual and Mixed Reality for 3D Visualisation in Intracranial Aneurysm Surgery Planning: a systematic review [1]	*Frontiers in Surgery*
2023	Mixed Reality for Cranial Neurosurgical Planning: a single center applicability study with the first 107 subsequent holograms [15]	*Operative Neurosurgery*
2023	Evaluation Metrics for Augmented Reality in Neurosurgical Preoperative Planning, Surgical Navigation, and Surgical Treatment Guidance—A Systematic Review [16]	*Operative Neurosurgery*

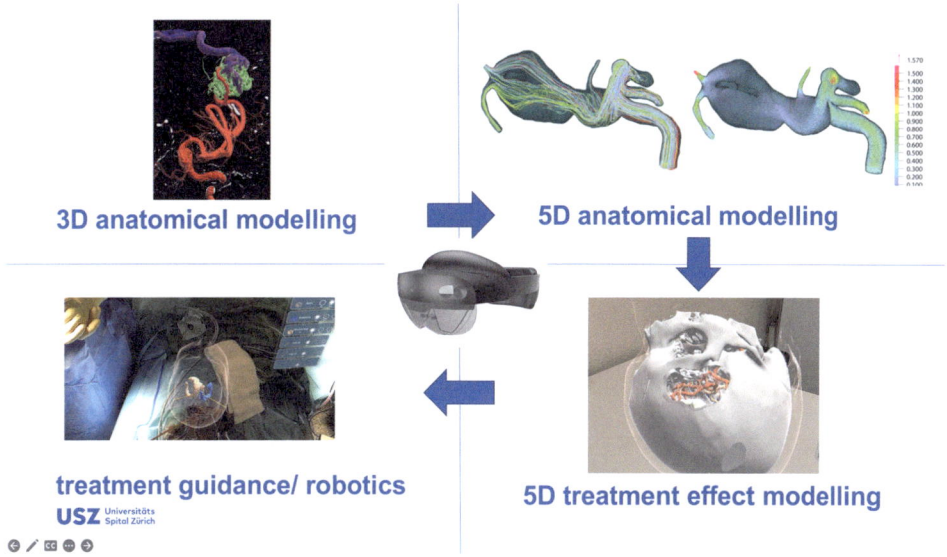

Fig. 1 The identified four phases in the development of mixed reality and artificial intelligence research according to our group

rent limitation in computational and graphical processing capabilities.

Discussion

Using the four developmental phases found in our research, we engage in a narrative discussion below.

Integration of AI and AR

The accurate segmentation of cerebral vessels is a challenging task due to the intricate geometry of these structures, limited spatial resolution, and sometimes suboptimal image contrast. To address this challenge, machine learning techniques, particularly artificial neural networks, have emerged as promising tools. Although the concept of using neural networks for image segmentation has been explored for several decades, not until recent advancements in computing power and cost-effective access to it did neural networks become a viable avenue for research in this field. A significant breakthrough came with the introduction of deep-learning models, such as the U-Net architecture and its variations, which have formed the foundational structure for many image segmentation tasks [17]. Notably, the nnU-Net framework introduced a set of rules that were based on dataset properties for selecting appropriate model settings, including parameters such as kernel size, the number of channels, and layer depth, commonly referred to as hyperparameters. These defined rules enabled nnU-Net to be applied to a wide range of segmentation tasks without the need for manual hyperparameter tun-

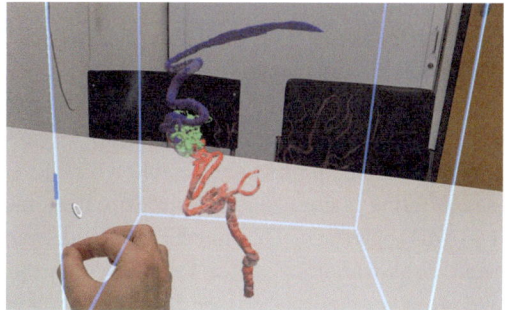

Fig. 2 First-person view in the outpatient clinic setting of a 3D segmentation of an intracranial AVM visualized through a MxR heads-up display

ing, streamlining the segmentation pipeline [18]. It potentially offers a fast and precise method not only for the automatic segmentation of intracranial and cerebropetal arteries but also for the detection and localization of intracranial aneurysms (IAs) using magnetic resonance (MR) [19–21] or computed tomography (CT) [6] and include them in a normal hologram containing skin, a skull, ventricles, and even subarachnoid blood [1, 5, 11]. The automatic segmentation of an arteriovenous malformation (AVM) is more complex [7]. In this case, magnetic resonance imaging (MRI) is the input of preference (Time of Flight (TOF) sequence with and without contrast), Computed Tomography Angiography (CTA) and Digital subtraction angiography (DSA) can show specific parts of the lesion as embolism materials and calcifications.

The successful adoption of AR has been observed in various domains within the field of neurosurgery [2, 10–12]. Notably, the utilization of 3D interactive holograms that can be seamlessly integrated with the real-world environment enhances anatomical perception and aids in surgical orientation [14] (Fig. 2). This also has been shown specifically for intracranial aneurysm surgery [1]. Moreover, these 3D holograms serve as valuable tools not only for experienced neurosurgeons but also, notably, for residents and nonoperative team members, enhancing their 3D insights [3, 13]. Despite these advancements, the widespread integration of AR into routine neurosurgical practices has not reached anticipated levels. One of the primary impediments to the broader adoption of AR was rooted in limitations related to computational and graphical processing capabilities [1, 16]. An important asset of integrating AI and AR is the automatization of as many steps as possible. Because a plethora of hardware and software is used in modern neurosurgical practice, each with its own user interface, the introduction of new technology as integrated AI and AR should be as intuitive as possible. A coherent pipeline for a seamless transition from 2D imaging to 3D imaging and ultimately to holographic representation necessitates an automated process that accommodates diverse file formats. This is particularly crucial when dealing with DICOM data, which exhibits wide variability. The standardization of these imaging files is imperative, leading to their conversion into volume files compatible with machine-learning-trained algorithms, such as NIFTI, for segmentation. Subsequently, the segmentation output should be converted into surface models compatible with AR, such as STL files, offering a single-click export to a head-mounted display (HMD) interface. This interface should enable the concurrent visualization of source images within the hologram and provide a control step over the delineation of automatic segmentations within these source images. Ensuring the pipeline's safety, security, and adaptability, given the rapid emergence of new algorithms, is best achieved through cloud technology [1, 7, 11, 14].

5D by Adding Flow and Pulsatility

In the case of cerebral aneurysms or arteriovenous malformations, complex flow patterns contribute to the genesis and progression of the pathology. Therefore, incorporating more-dynamic parameters into 3D cerebrovascular models seems useful. For certain cases, simplistic approaches were shown to provide adequate patient-specific flow models [22, 23]. Dedicated MRI techniques facilitate direct individual measurements in the cerebral vascular tree that can be used for modeling [24] (NOVA, Vassol, River Forest, IL, USA). However, advances in MR flow imaging have made time-resolved volumetric measurements of blood velocity vector fields in the entire brain possible, allowing the study of flow patterns, flow rates, collateral flow activation, arterial and venous pulsatility, pulse propagation velocities, pressure gradients, and wall shear stresses, among other parameters. These parameters promise to provide a detailed description and visualization of hemodynamic conditions in real time, including adaptations for pulsations and breathing With time as fourth dimension (flow) and pulsatility as fifth dimension this technological goal is defined by our group as 5D [25]. In our ongoing collaboration with this research group, our objective has been to collaboratively advance 5D MR flow imaging methods for individuals with intracranial aneurysms and arteriovenous malformations. Our overarching goal is to integrate these techniques into diverse 3D environments, including mixed reality (MxR), to enhance our comprehensive understanding of patient-specific hemodynamic characteristics among multidisciplinary teams.

Treatment Planning

The practical utility of models created with AI and AR integration extends to treatment planning. The objective of simulating diverse interventions is to quantitatively assess their implications for perfusion, changes in pressure in the treated pathology, and the overarching intracerebral hemodynamic consequences. Such modeling need not invariably involve intricate machine learning or complex mathematical approaches. For instance, through the utilization of a comparatively straightforward fluid-structure analysis model, our prior work demonstrated the ability to adequately predict the impact on cerebral hemodynamics resulting from the combination of bypass creation and selective parent vessel occlusion [26]. Simulating aneurysm clipping is a more intricate process, particularly in light of the growing demand for preoperatively determining clip sizes and simulating precise clipping angles, driven by the increasing diversity of clip sizes and shapes and the rising popularity of minimally invasive approaches with limited bone openings. Various preoperative preparation systems for aneurysm clipping exist. The advantage of utilizing augmented reality (AR) lies in its speed and cost-efficiency, as it eliminates the need for 3D printing or other fabrication methods while maintaining a true 3D simulation [1] (Fig. 3a, b). An even more significant advancement would involve the integration of flow prediction modeling to investigate the impact of microsurgical clipping, potentially mitigating unsuccessful clipping outcomes that adversely affect cerebral perfusion. Treatment planning for the microsurgical resection of an intracerebral AVM has been scarcely reported in the literature [7]. This is likely due to the complex nature of brain AVMs and the difficulty of rendering their detailed properties and treatment effects, where different imaging modalities, such as DSA, MRI and CT, have to be merged. Our group aims to take steps in this field in the following years.

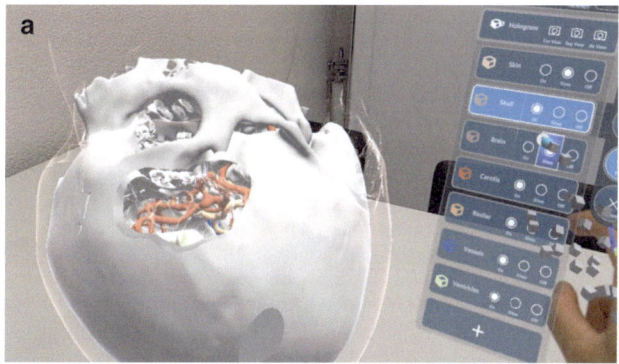

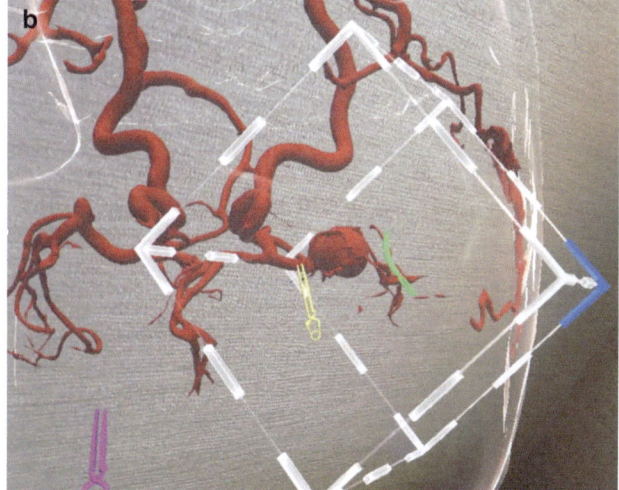

Fig. 3 (a) First-person view of trepanation planning in mixed reality of a carotid artery aneurysm (Lumi, Augmedit, Naarden, Netherlands): (b) first-person view of clip sizing in mixed reality of an middle cerebral artery (MCA) aneurysm

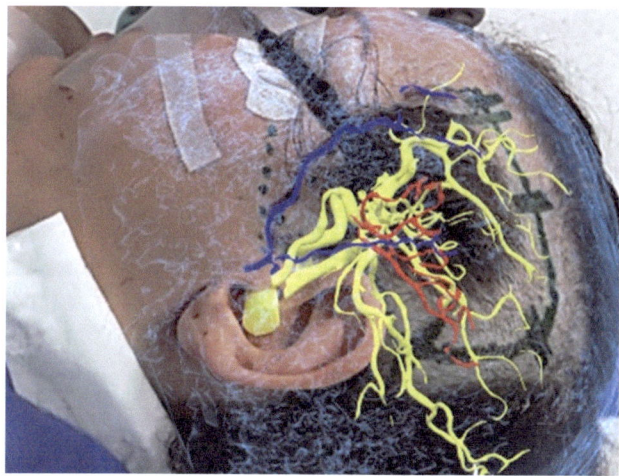

Fig. 4 First-person view of a hologram indicating the left STA (blue) and recipient MCA (red) branch to prepare for STA-MCA bypass surgery, where the more proximal vasculature is indicated in yellow

Treatment Guidance

To guide surgical treatment, first an accurate registration of the 3D object is needed for the patient. This can be performed with several techniques, although a uniform way to describe the accuracy of the registration is lacking [2, 16]. We suggested using target registration error (TRE) for this purpose [16]. In two other studies, we found that point-based registration with AR using quick-response (QR) codes attached to the patients to keep the hologram in place on the patient independent of the movement of the operation table seems accurate enough for the macroscopic phase of neurosurgical procedures [9, 10]. We subsequently performed this technique in different indications in vascular neurosurgery (aneurysms, AVM, and superficial temporal artery (STA) to middle cerebral artery (MCA) bypass surgery) [15] (Fig. 4). Although registering a hologram on a patient head in the operative position is visually very appealing, its true clinical benefit is the subject of debate. This should be studied in more depth using standardized evaluation metrics [16]. We will focus on this topic more in the near future. Once in the microscopic phase of the surgery, the use of a hologram is even more questionable; the hologram can be insufficiently accurate because often sub-millimeter precision is needed in vascular lesions and because it could also block the view of the surgeon in essential parts of the surgery. Most likely, a more significant contribution of AR in vascular surgery would be the guided introduction of an external ventricular shunt in the case of a subarachnoid bleeding. This procedure has properties that make it very suitable for AR guidance: its short duration, its purely macroscopic nature, and the fact that the current clinical standard (freehand placement) has an insufficient success rate (Kakarla 1 in first pass), of approximately 60% [27, 28]. We expect to publish the results of our own research in this field in the near future.

The efforts conducted in treatment guidance lay the groundwork for enabling fully automated guidance or even the robotic management of neurovascular pathology. A key element involves the automatic recognition of the pathology, including its surrounding functionally critical and vulnerable anatomical structures, thanks to using AI. In AR solutions, the resulting segmentation is then accurately registered in a coordinate system on the patient, which also potentially offers a foundational framework for a robotic system to approach the pathology and position a device within or around it. Continuous updates are essential to account for brain shifts and patient movements. The integration of ultrasound and intraoperative DSA, CT, or MRI holds potential solutions for addressing these challenges. Robot-assisted neurovascular interventions have already been successfully performed [29]. Our research group is actively collaborating with other research teams that are focused on achieving the complete automation of such treatments as the next progressive step.

Conclusion

Artificial intelligence and augmented reality are rapidly developing topics within vascular neurosurgery. In the research of our own group, we identified four phases of development: (1) the integration of AI and AR to create adequate three-dimensional (3D) segmentations; (2) adding flow and pulsatility data to create 5D segmentations; (3) treatment planning in these models; and (4) treatment guidance using these models. The main drawback described was the limited added value in the microscopic phase of neurovascular surgery due to view obstructions and a lack of accuracy. The main challenge described was the current limitation in computational and graphical processing capabilities. The research in this field could lay the groundwork for fully automatized treatment strategies in the future.

Declarations

Conflict of interest T. van Doormaal is the leader of the research group and also the cofounder and CMO of Augmedit bv (Naarden, the Netherlands), a company that provides AI-based AR for neurosurgeons. The figures shown in this publication are generated with the LumiNE light software of Augmedit.

References

1. Colombo E, Lutters B, Kos T, van Doormaal T. Application of virtual and mixed reality for 3D visualization in intracranial aneurysm surgery planning: a systematic review. Front Surg. 2023;10:1227510.
2. Fick T, van Doormaal JAM, Hoving EW, Willems PWA, van Doormaal TPC. Current accuracy of augmented reality neuronavigation systems: systematic review and meta-analysis. World Neurosurg. 2021;146:179–88.
3. Kos TM, Haaksman S, van Doormaal TPC, Colombo E. Effect of intraoperative mixed-reality use on nonsurgical team members in the neurosurgical operating room: an explorative study. World Neurosurg. 2023;180:e219–25.
4. Tangsrivimol JA, Schonfeld E, Zhang M, et al. Artificial intelligence in neurosurgery: a state-of-the-art review from past to future. Diagnostics. 2023;13(14):2429.
5. Thomson BR, Gürlek F, Buzzi RM, Schwendinger N, Keller E, Regli L, van Doormaal TP, Schaer DJ, Hugelshofer M, Akeret K. Clinical potential of automated convolutional neural network-based hematoma volumetry after aneurysmal subarachnoid hemorrhage. J Stroke Cerebrovasc Dis. 2023;32(11):107357.
6. Patel TR, Patel A, Veeturi SS, et al. Evaluating a 3D deep learning pipeline for cerebral vessel and intracranial aneurysm segmentation from computed tomography angiography–digital subtraction angiography image pairs. Neurosurg Focus. 2023;54(6):E13.
7. Colombo E, Fick T, Esposito G, Germans M, Regli L, van Doormaal T. Segmentation techniques of brain arteriovenous malformations for 3D visualization: a systematic review. Radiol Med. 2022;127(12):1333–41.
8. van Doormaal JAM, Mensink T, van Doormaal TPC. Augmented reality glasses in the operating room. Ned Tijdschr Geneeskd. 2018;163:D3041.
9. van Doormaal TPC, van Doormaal JAM, Mensink T. Clinical accuracy of holographic navigation using point-based registration on augmented-reality glasses. Oper Neurosurg. 2019;17(6):588–93.
10. Fick T, van Doormaal JAM, Hoving EW, Regli L, van Doormaal TPC. Holographic patient tracking after bed movement for augmented reality neuronavigation using a head-mounted display. Acta Neurochir. 2021;163:879. https://doi.org/10.1007/s00701-021-04707-4.
11. van Doormaal JAM, Fick T, Ali M, Köllen M, van der Kuijp V, van Doormaal TPC. Fully automatic adaptive meshing based segmentation of the ventricular system for augmented reality visualization and navigation. World Neurosurg. 2021;156:e9–e24.
12. Fick T, van Doormaal JAM, Tosic L, van Zoest RJ, Meulstee JW, Hoving EW, van Doormaal TPC. Fully automatic brain tumor segmentation for 3D evaluation in augmented reality. Neurosurg Focus. 2021;51(2):E14.
13. Fick T, Meulstee JW, Köllen MH, Van Doormaal JAM, Van Doormaal TPC, Hoving EW. Comparing the influence of mixed reality, a 3D viewer, and MRI on the spatial understanding of brain tumours. Front Virtual Real. 2023;4:1214520.
14. Colombo E, Bektas D, Regli L, van Doormaal T. Case report: impact of mixed reality on anatomical understanding and surgical planning in a complex fourth ventricular tumor extending to the lamina quadrigemina. Front Surg. 2023;10:1227473.
15. Colombo E, Regli L, Esposito G, Germans M, Fierstra J, Serra C, Van Doormaal T. Mixed reality for cranial neurosurgical planning: a single center usability study with the first 107 subsequent holograms. Oper Neurosurg. 2023;26(5):551–8.
16. Kos T, Colombo E, Bartels W, Robe P, Van Doormaal T. Evaluation metrics for augmented reality in neurosurgical preoperative planning, surgical navigation, and surgical treatment guidance – a systematic review. Oper Neurosurg. 2023;26(5):491–501. https://doi.org/10.1227/ons.0000000000001009.
17. Du G, Cao X, Liang J, Chen X, Zhan Y. Medical image segmentation based on U-net. J Phys Conf Ser. 2020;64(2):020508-1–020508-12.
18. Isensee F, Jaeger PF, Kohl SAA, Petersen J, Maier-Hein KH. nnU-net: a self-configuring method for deep learning-based biomedical image segmentation. Nat Methods. 2021;18(2):203–11.
19. Chen M, Geng C, Wang D, Zhou Z, Di R, Li F, Piao S, Zhang J, Li Y, Dai Y. A coarse-to-fine cascade deep learning neural network for segmenting cerebral aneurysms in time-of-flight magnetic resonance angiography. Biomed Eng Online. 2022;21(1):71.
20. Joo B, Ahn SS, Yoon PH, Bae S, Sohn B, Lee YE, Bae JH, Park MS, Choi HS, Lee S-K. A deep learning algorithm may automate intracranial aneurysm detection on MR angiography with high diagnostic performance. Eur Radiol. 2020;30(11):5785–93.
21. Sichtermann T, Faron A, Sijben R, Teichert N, Freiherr J, Wiesmann M. Deep learning–based detection of intracranial aneurysms in 3D TOF-MRA. AJNR Am J Neuroradiol. 2019;40(1):25–32.
22. Acosta S, Penny DJ, Brady KM, Rusin CG. An effective model of cerebrovascular pressure reactivity and blood flow autoregulation. Microvasc Res. 2018;115:34–43.
23. Helthuis JHG, van Doormaal TPC, Amin-Hanjani S, Du X, Charbel FT, Hillen B, van der Zwan A. A patient-specific cerebral blood flow model. J Biomech. 2020;98:109445.
24. Zhao M, Charbel FT, Alperin N, Loth F, Clark ME. Improved phase-contrast flow quantification by three-dimensional vessel localization. Magn Reson Imaging. 2000;18(6):697–706.

25. Walheim J, Dillinger H, Kozerke S. Multipoint 5D flow cardiovascular magnetic resonance - accelerated cardiac- and respiratory-motion resolved mapping of mean and turbulent velocities. J Cardiovasc Magn Reson. 2019;21(1):42.
26. Helthuis JHG, Bhat S, van Doormaal TPC, Kumar RK, van der Zwan A. Proximal and distal occlusion of complex cerebral aneurysms—implications of flow modeling by fluid–structure interaction analysis. Oper Neurosurg. 2018;15(2):217–30.
27. Müller A, Mould WA, et al. The incidence of catheter tract hemorrhage and catheter placement accuracy in the CLEAR III trial. Neurocrit Care. 2018;29(1):23–32.
28. Woo PYM, Ng BCF, Xiao JX, et al. The importance of aspirin, catheterization accuracy, and catheter design in external ventricular drainage-related hemorrhage: a multicenter study of 1002 procedures. Acta Neurochir. 2019;161(8):1623–32.
29. Ning S, Chautems C, Kim Y, et al. Robotic interventional neuroradiology: progress, challenges, and future prospects. Semin Neurol. 2023;43(03):432–8.

Open Access This chapter is licensed under the terms of the Creative Commons Attribution 4.0 International License (http://creativecommons.org/licenses/by/4.0/), which permits use, sharing, adaptation, distribution and reproduction in any medium or format, as long as you give appropriate credit to the original author(s) and the source, provide a link to the Creative Commons license and indicate if changes were made.

The images or other third party material in this chapter are included in the chapter's Creative Commons license, unless indicated otherwise in a credit line to the material. If material is not included in the chapter's Creative Commons license and your intended use is not permitted by statutory regulation or exceeds the permitted use, you will need to obtain permission directly from the copyright holder.

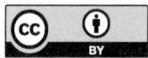

Educational Impact of an Annotation System Integrated with an Exoscope for Cerebral Aneurysm Surgery: Case Description

Yoji Tanaka, Motoki Inaji, Daisu Abe, Kazuhide Shimizu, and Taketoshi Maehara

Introduction

Since the introduction of the three-dimensional (3D) exoscope as a potential alternative to the operative microscope, there have been an increasing number of reports about the advantages of the exoscope in microneurosurgical procedures, including cerebral aneurysm clipping [1–8]. These reports have established the excellent visual clarity, better ergonomics, and educational advantage of the exoscope. They have also drawn attention to an important educational advantage: The exoscope allows the staff attending a surgery to share a high-quality view of the surgical field that realistically replicates the view of the surgeon [4]. However, whether the exoscope can achieve better communication between the main surgeon and the mentor than that achieved by the surgical microscope remains unclear. In addition, in the case of neurosurgical procedures, the mentor may sometimes experience difficult in verbally conveying instructions to the surgeon, especially when the surgical field is narrow and the mentor cannot directly point out the target in the surgical field.

In laparoscopic surgery, the surgeon performs surgery while looking at a surgical monitor, as in exoscope neurosurgery. Research on telementoring during laparoscopic surgery has been conducted; in this case, the telementoring consisted of a mentor in a remote location writing annotations on the monitor to communicate with the surgeon [9]. We have also used this annotation system to improve communication between the surgeon and the mentor during exoscope surgery. This chapter introduces our experience with using an exoscope and annotation system during left middle cerebral aneurysm surgery in a 63-year-old woman.

Case Description

System Details

We used a 3D exoscope (ORBEYE, Olympus, Japan) and an annotation system (ADMENIC ANNOTATOR, Carina Systems, Japan) for aneurysm surgery. Figure 1 shows a schematic of the annotation system and integrated exoscope in the operating room. The images of the surgical field taken with the exoscope camera were displayed on the main monitor and transferred to the annotation system separately. Then the images were sent to a tablet device that was connected to the annotation system via Wi-Fi using a wireless local area network. The mentor added the annotations to the images displayed on the tablet device, and the images with annotations were transferred to a second monitor. The tablet was placed in a sterilized bag when the mentor was scrubbed. The surgeon performed the surgery while confirming both the mentor's verbal instructions and the annotations on the second monitor.

Y. Tanaka (✉) · M. Inaji · D. Abe · K. Shimizu · T. Maehara
Department of Neurosurgery, Tokyo Medical and Dental University, Tokyo, Japan
e-mail: tanaka.nsrg@tmd.ac.jp

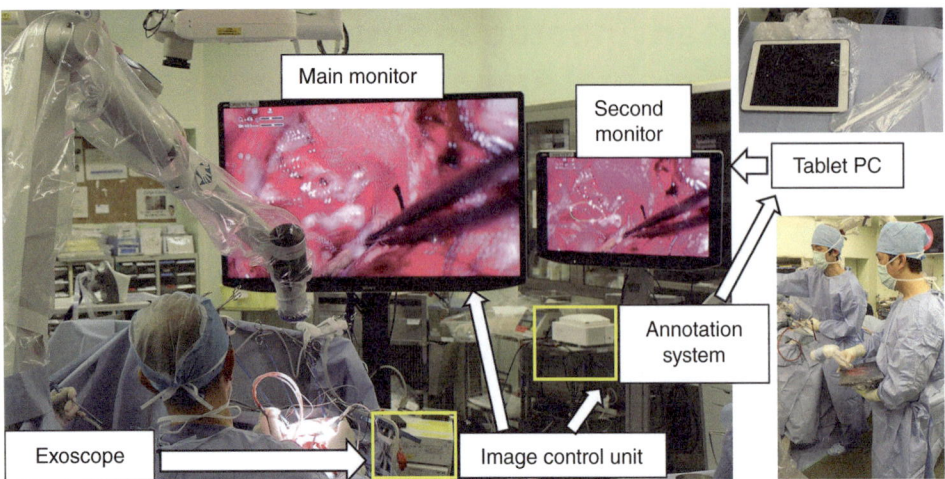

Fig. 1 Schematic of the annotation system with integrated exoscope in the operating room. The images of the surgical field were transferred to the annotation system. The mentor added annotations to the images, and the images with annotations were transferred to a second monitor

Clinical Description

A 63-year-old woman with an incidentally found, unruptured cerebral aneurysm was referred to our hospital. Computed tomography angiography revealed a 7 mm diameter aneurysm located at the bifurcation of the left middle cerebral artery (MCA). The aneurysmal neck was broad and had a daughter's sac (Fig. 2a, b). A left pterional approach was carried out, and a dissection of the Sylvian fissure was performed. The MCA aneurysm was completely exposed from surrounding brain tissue and vessels. The aneurysm had a broad neck, as shown in the preoperative images, and we therefore decided to occlude the aneurysm with two clips. Then the mentor traced the outline of the MCA and the aneurysm and indicated the direction to insert each of the clips on the monitor (Fig. 2c–e). The main surgeon applied the first straight clip as indicated by the annotation (Fig. 2f). As expected, part of the aneurysm remained, so the surgeon closed the remaining part of the aneurysm by applying the mini-clip as indicated by the annotation (Fig. 2g). Finally, the complete occlusion of the aneurysm was confirmed by using indocyanine green (ICG). Postoperatively, the patient did well without neurological deficits and was discharged home.

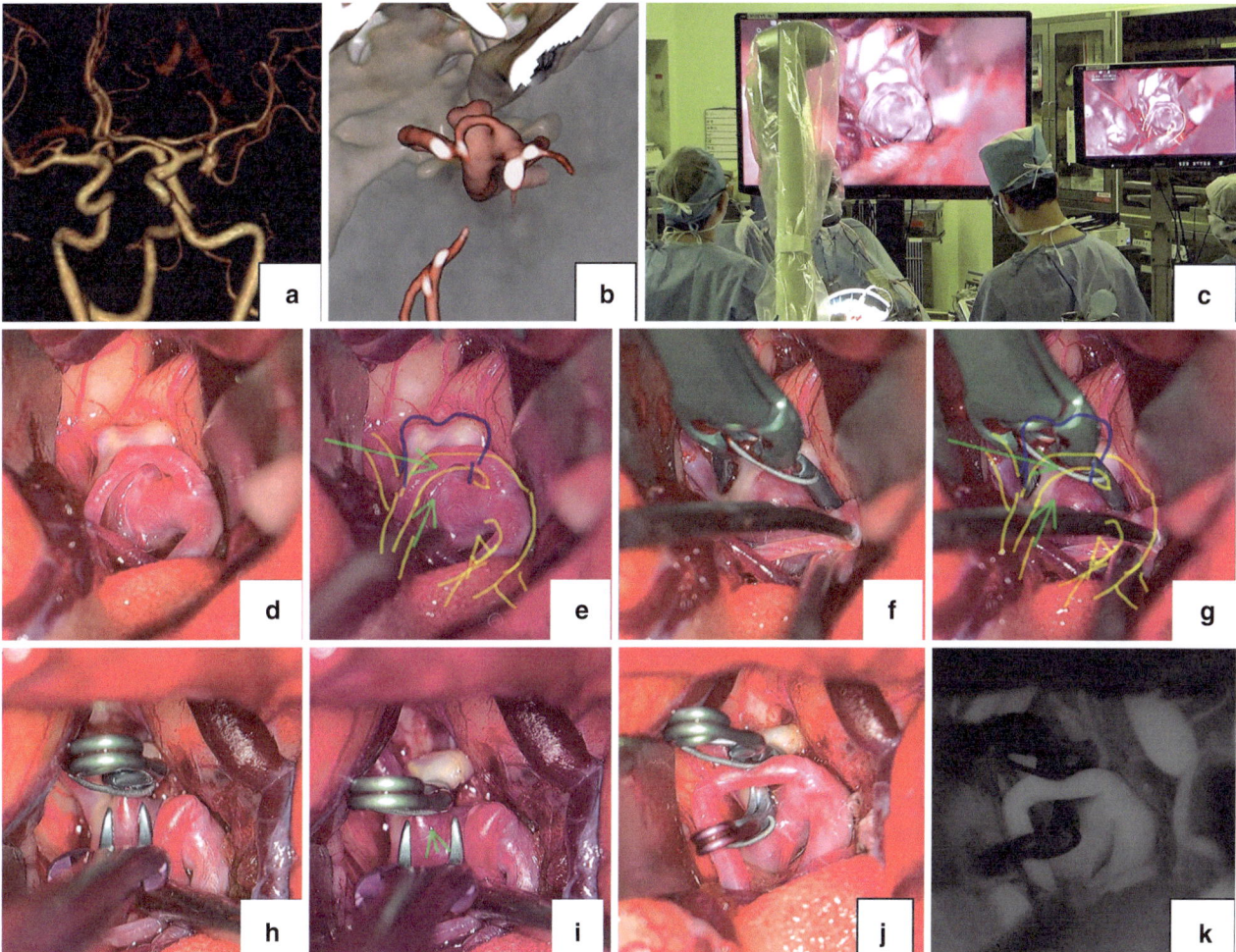

Fig. 2 A 63-year-old woman with left MCA aneurysm. (**a**) A three-dimensional reconstructed image of the computed tomography angiography shows the left MCA aneurysm. (**b**) An operative view image shows that the aneurysm has a broad neck with a daughter sac. (**c**) In the operating room, the surgeon (on the left side) is looking at both the large main monitor and a small second monitor. The mentor (on the right side) draws instructions on the tablet, and the resulting image is displayed on the second monitor. (**d, e**) The aneurysm displayed on the main monitor (**d**) and the second monitor with annotation (**e**). The mentor draws green arrows to indicate the direction of insertion for each clip. (**f, g**) Placing the first clip: The surgeon applies the first clip as the mentor instructed (large green arrow). (**h, i**) Placing the second clip: The mentor redraws the direction of insertion of the clip (**i**), and the surgeon applies the clip as instructed. (**j**) Final view of the clipping. (**k**) An indocyanine green image shows that the aneurysm is completely occluded

Discussion

Our case of aneurysmal surgery demonstrated that the surgeon could accomplish the clipping as the mentor instructed. By adding instructions to the monitor with an annotation system, the mentor was able to clearly convey the instructions to the surgeon. This was shown to be an advantage of heads-up surgery with an exoscope.

Some have reported that the exoscope is equivalent or even superior to a surgical microscope in terms of vision and surgical ergonomics during neurosurgery [1, 2, 4]. Indeed, the surgical results using an exoscope have been reported to be equivalent to those using a surgical microscope [4, 7]. The exoscope also offers an educational advantage: The operator, assistant, and observers can see the same high-resolution 3D image [10, 11]. Moreover, Calloni et al. reported that the exoscope does not obstruct the view of the surgeon's hands, which allows a clear dual perception of the surgical field for the assisting surgeon and consequently a better orientation on the surgical field [12]. However, no reports have examined how the exoscope affects communication between the surgeon and the assistant or instructor. A method of displaying annotations on the surgical monitor has been reported to be useful in the telementoring of other heads-up surgeries using a surgical monitor, including endovascular procedures [13]. Lopes et al. reported that telementoring with augmented reality could reduce the time required for suturing procedures by displaying visual instruction in the field of view of the mentee [14]. Also, in the field of laparoscopic surgery, an annotation system using augmented reality has been reported to shorten the time required for the procedure, reduce failures, and improve the safety of surgery [9]. In the latter two reports, the authors speculated that displaying instructions on the monitor would allow the mentee to clearly and efficiently understand what the mentor is trying to convey, thereby simplifying the process of taking instructions while conducting a surgery and also thereby ultimately shortening the operation time and improving safety. On the other hand, the use of only verbal instructions hampers understanding the contents of the instructions, which may lead to the misidentification of the target or a delay in recognition [15]. Therefore, in aneurysmal clipping surgery via exoscope, the surgeon is expected to perform the procedure safely by indicating the important structures on the monitor and providing explicit directions about where to insert the clip. Because the exoscope surgery is a heads-up surgery using a surgical monitor, it allows for multiple types of information, including the annotations, to be displayed on the monitor along with the surgical field, unlike when using a surgical microscope.

Middle cerebral artery aneurysms may require a combination of clip techniques due to the complicated shape of the aneurysm neck [16]. Also, surgeons must decide how to apply clips for a particular aneurysm to minimize risk of postoperative complications and future recurrence [17]. Although instruction on the number and types of clips can be given outside the surgical field, the mentor cannot easily verbally indicate the direction in which the clips are to be inserted. With the annotation system, however, the mentor can clearly indicate the direction of clip insertion by simply drawing an arrow on the surgical monitor.

Two important limitations of this technique should be mentioned. First, the annotation system that we used was not applicable to 3D images. For this reason, the annotated images were displayed on a second monitor. Second, the added annotations did not follow the camera movement. Therefore, we had to rewrite the annotation each time the viewpoint changed. Future technological advances will likely lead to solutions to both of these problems.

Conclusion

A new method for surgical education using an annotation system integrated with an exoscope was introduced and used during aneurysm clipping surgery. This system is expected to improve communication between surgeons and mentors and improve surgical safety.

Declarations The authors declare that the chapter content was composed in the absence of any commercial or financial relationship that could be construed as a potential conflict of interest.

References

1. Hines K, Hughes LP, Franco D, Sharan AD, Wu C. Exoscope improves visualization and extent of hippocampal resection in temporal lobectomy. Acta Neurochir. 2023;165:259–63. https://doi.org/10.1007/s00701-022-05405-5.
2. Klinger DR, Reinard KA, Ajayi OO, Delashaw JB Jr. Microsurgical clipping of an anterior communicating artery aneurysm using a novel robotic visualization tool in lieu of the binocular operating microscope: operative video. Oper Neurosurg (Hagerstown). 2018;14:26–8. https://doi.org/10.1093/ons/opx081.
3. Li Z, Gui S, Zhao P, Bai J, Cao L, Cheng S, Liu C, Zhu H, Zhang Y, Li C. Combined endoscopic and exoscopic resection of intracranial epidermoid cysts. World Neurosurg. 2022;168:e28–33. https://doi.org/10.1016/j.wneu.2022.08.111.
4. Mamelak AN, Nobuto T, Berci G. Initial clinical experience with a high-definition exoscope system for microneurosurgery. Neurosurgery. 2010;67:476–83. https://doi.org/10.1227/01.NEU.0000372204.85227.BF.
5. Murai Y, Sato S, Yui K, Morimoto D, Ozeki T, Yamaguchi M, Tateyama K, Nozaki T, Tahara S, Yamaguchi F, Morita A. Preliminary clinical microneurosurgical experience with the 4K3-dimensional microvideoscope (ORBEYE) system for microneurological surgery: observation study. Oper Neurosurg (Hagerstown). 2019;16:707–16. https://doi.org/10.1093/ons/opy277.
6. Nossek E, Schneider JR, Kwan K, Kulason KO, Du V, Chakraborty S, Rahme R, Faltings L, Ellis J, Ortiz R, Boockvar JA, Langer DJ. Technical aspects and operative nuances using a high-definition 3-dimensional exoscope for cerebral bypass surgery. Oper Neurosurg (Hagerstown). 2019;17:157–63. https://doi.org/10.1093/ons/opy342.
7. Rossmann T, Veldeman M, Nurminen V, Huhtakangas J, Niemela M, Lehecka M. 3D exoscopes are noninferior to operating microscopes in aneurysm surgery: comparative single-surgeon series of 52 consecutive cases. World Neurosurg. 2023;170:e200–13. https://doi.org/10.1016/j.wneu.2022.10.106.
8. Watanabe T, Iwami K, Kishida Y, Nagatani T, Yatsuya H, Miyachi S. Combined exoscopic and endoscopic two-step keyhole approach for intracranial meningiomas. Curr Oncol. 2022;29:5370–82. https://doi.org/10.3390/curroncol29080426.
9. Wild C, Lang F, Gerhauser AS, Schmidt MW, Kowalewski KF, Petersen J, Kenngott HG, Muller-Stich BP, Nickel F. Telestration with augmented reality for visual presentation of intraoperative target structures in minimally invasive surgery: a randomized controlled study. Surg Endosc. 2022;36:7453. https://doi.org/10.1007/s00464-022-09158-1.
10. Barbagallo GMV, Certo F. Three-dimensional, high-definition exoscopic anterior cervical discectomy and fusion: a valid alternative to microscope-assisted surgery. World Neurosurg. 2019;130:e244–50. https://doi.org/10.1016/j.wneu.2019.06.049.
11. Kwan K, Schneider JR, Du V, Falting L, Boockvar JA, Oren J, Levine M, Langer DJ. Lessons learned using a high-definition 3-dimensional exoscope for spinal surgery. Oper Neurosurg (Hagerstown). 2019;16:619–25. https://doi.org/10.1093/ons/opy196.

12. Calloni T, Roumy LG, Cinalli MA, Rocca A, Held A, Trezza A, Carrabba GG, Giussani CG. Exoscope as a teaching tool: a narrative review of the literature. Front Surg. 2022;9:878293. https://doi.org/10.3389/fsurg.2022.878293.
13. Rai AT, Deib G, Smith D, Boo S. Teleproctoring for neurovascular procedures: demonstration of concept using optical see-through head-mounted display, interactive mixed reality, and virtual space sharing-a critical need highlighted by the COVID-19 pandemic. AJNR Am J Neuroradiol. 2021;42:1109–15. https://doi.org/10.3174/ajnr.A7066.
14. Neves Lopes V, Dantas I, Barbosa JP, Barbosa J. Telestration in the teaching of basic surgical skills: a randomized trial. J Surg Educ. 2022;79:1031–42. https://doi.org/10.1016/j.jsurg.2022.02.013.
15. McKinley SK, Brunt LM, Schwaitzberg SD. Prevention of bile duct injury: the case for incorporating educational theories of expertise. Surg Endosc. 2014;28:3385–91. https://doi.org/10.1007/s00464-014-3605-8.
16. Jeon HJ, Kim SY, Park KY, Lee JW, Huh SK. Ideal clipping methods for unruptured middle cerebral artery bifurcation aneurysms based on aneurysmal neck classification. Neurosurg Rev. 2016;39:215–23; discussion 223–214. https://doi.org/10.1007/s10143-015-0671-x.
17. Ishikawa T, Nakayama N, Moroi J, Kobayashi N, Kawai H, Muto T, Yasui N. Concept of ideal closure line for clipping of middle cerebral artery aneurysms–technical note. Neurol Med Chir (Tokyo). 2009;49:273–7; discussion 277–278. https://doi.org/10.2176/nmc.49.273.

Open Access This chapter is licensed under the terms of the Creative Commons Attribution 4.0 International License (http://creativecommons.org/licenses/by/4.0/), which permits use, sharing, adaptation, distribution and reproduction in any medium or format, as long as you give appropriate credit to the original author(s) and the source, provide a link to the Creative Commons license and indicate if changes were made.

The images or other third party material in this chapter are included in the chapter's Creative Commons license, unless indicated otherwise in a credit line to the material. If material is not included in the chapter's Creative Commons license and your intended use is not permitted by statutory regulation or exceeds the permitted use, you will need to obtain permission directly from the copyright holder.

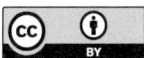

Part VII
Editorials

Microneurosurgical Training on Simulators: The Zurich Microsurgery Lab Experience

Elisa Colombo, Lara Höbner, Martina Sebök, Tristan van Doormaal, Luca Regli, and Giuseppe Esposito

Background and Introduction

Microsurgery is a highly specialized and technically demanding surgical subfield that requires extreme precision, technical skills, and structured and continuous training. Microsurgical techniques play a pivotal role in neurosurgery, enabling surgeons to perform delicate tasks with great precision. Given the critical nature of neurosurgical interventions and the high technical demand of microsurgery, starting microsurgical training during residency becomes of paramount importance. Furthermore, neurosurgical and microsurgical training specifically represent progressive journeys demanding a structured approach for the concrete establishment of skills. Nonetheless, with the increasing complexity of neurosurgical cases, the restrictions of working hours in residency, and legal and ethical factors to consider, a proper training of microneurosurgical skills only in real intraoperative settings becomes difficult to achieve [1].

Therefore, the incorporation of simulation models into neurosurgical training programs is nowadays very useful to provide residents with a safe and nonthreatening environment to develop and refine microsurgical skills [2–4]. In fact, simulation models offer a range of tools that are adaptable to the evolving needs and proficiency levels of neurosurgeons at different levels of training. Simulators not only replicate the complexity of the intraoperative settings but also allow residents at all levels of training to refine their microsurgical techniques and enhance their skill development, muscle memory, and surgical confidence in a risk-free learning space. This allows residents to make and correct mistakes without compromising patient safety [5–7].

Given the importance of progressive training for microsurgical techniques in neurosurgery, we believe that the incorporation of different simulators should be a stepwise process. We describe the progressive training program that uses simulation models implemented at our Zurich Microsurgery Lab of Department of Neurosurgery of University Hospital Zurich.

Training Scheme

The Zurich Microsurgery Lab offers dedicated space and tools for a progressive microneurosurgical training of residents by implementing different simulators. It is equipped with microscopes, microsurgical and surgical instruments, progressive training plans showing the residents which exercises to perform, hardware and software for virtual-reality and augmented-reality training, and simulators made of synthetic or biological material. The microsurgical training is structured according to a precise scheme. Before starting practicing with one simulation model, residents attend a theoretical and visual training session to learn how to properly use and profit from the simulator.

At the beginning of the residency journey, trainees in their first or second year of residency receive a training session on the use of the microscope, the optimal posture to have while working with it, the types of microsurgical instruments, and

E. Colombo (✉) · L. Höbner · M. Sebök · L. Regli · G. Esposito
Department of Neurosurgery, Clinical Neuroscience Center, University Hospital Zurich, University of Zurich, Zurich, Switzerland

Zurich Microsurgery Lab, Department of Neurosurgery, University Hospital Zurich, Zurich, Switzerland
e-mail: elisa.colombo@usz.ch

T. van Doormaal
Department of Neurosurgery, University Medical Center Utrech, Utrecht, Netherlands

Department of Neurosurgery, University Hospital Zurich, Zurich, Switzerland

the correct way to handle them. Then trainees learn microsuturing and microanastomosis techniques on vessel tubes. This first phase of training is performed on 2 mm and 1 mm silicon tubes (Pocket Microvascular Anastomosis Card, Pocket Suture, LLC, Mesa AZ, USA) and hyper-realistic UpSurgeOn three-dimensional models (UpSurgeOn S.r.l. Milano, Italy). Trainees follow a list of microsurgical exercises in a specific sequence (i.e., microsurgical suturing first, microsurgical repair second, and microsurgical anastomoses third: end-to-end, end-to-side, and side-to-side). After the list of exercises has been completed, these exercises are evaluated by a senior attending/lab team member, after which the progress of the residents is charted and graded. If the quality of the performance of the residents is considered sufficient, the second phase of the training can start.

The second phase of the training is offered to neurosurgeons in their second or third year of residency, who participate to the intensive 2-day training at the Zurich Microsurgical Course, where they gain training experience in microdissection, microsuturing, and microanastomosis on a perfused human placenta model. Human placentas have emerged as viable simulators for microsurgical training, mostly for microvascular dissection and anastomoses [6, 8]. The value of the perfused human placenta lies in the possibility of using many human vessels with different diameters to perform the exercises mentioned above as many times as needed. At the Zurich Microsurgery Course, the performed exercises are evaluated and graded by experienced attending team members of the Department of Neurosurgery and Plastic Surgery, and the performance of the participants is charted and analyzed to document any improvement. If the Zurich Microsurgery Course has been attended successfully, residents can have access to regular training on placentas at our lab as a progression in their training. Furthermore, with the placenta model, vessels and aneurysm clipping can also be trained, as can the microsuturing techniques used in carotid endarterectomy surgery, such as primary closure, closure with a patch, and the eversion technique.

In the meantime, residents in their second, third, or fourth year of residency also receive lab craniotomy sessions, where the following craniotomies and approaches are trained by using hyper-realistic 3D UpSurgeOn models: pterional, latero-supraorbital, mini-pterional, subtemporal, parasagittal interhemispheric, suboccipital, retrosigmoidal, endonasal endoscopic transsphenoidal. This is done in a one-to-one or one-to-two training scheme—that is, one or two residents and one junior/senior attending—an approach that is thought to enhance surgical confidence. In this part of the training, other microsurgical techniques, such as dura closure under the microscope, are progressively trained.

Another useful tool in the training pathway of residents is virtual-reality (VR) and mixed-reality (MxR) anatomical reconstructions (Augmedit bv, Aagen, Netherlands) [9, 10]. Augmented-reality simulators offer an immersive and interactive learning environment where trainees can engage with virtual anatomical structures and perform simulated surgical procedures in real time [9]. Sessions of anatomical study and discussions of cases using a dedicated augmented-reality simulator are scheduled during the training. Augmented-reality (AR) sessions allow an enhanced training experience by providing 3D interactive reconstructions of the anatomical structures most relevant to the specific surgical approach, the critical appraisal of the most important intraoperative steps, and a thorough risk assessment. This AR training is offered to residents in their second, third, or fourth year of residency. Indeed, augmented-reality and craniotomy training on 3D models is reinforced by regular attendance in the operating room.

Furthermore, residents in their fourth and fifth year of training who want to focus their career on cerebrovascular surgery then have access to the Zurich Clipping Course. In this course, the following techniques are mastered: the main standard craniotomies on cadavers (pterional, latero-supraorbital, and minipterional; suboccipital, subtemporal, and retrosimoidal, and parasagittal interhemispheric); aneurysm clipping techniques and trapping on perfused cadaver models; and further microsurgical training on perfused human placenta models.

Consideration of the Placenta Model

The entire microsurgical and neurosurgical training at the Zurich Microsurgery Lab is nowadays animal-free. In fact, we have totally replaced the use of animals in our courses and training programs with the use of perfused and pressurized human placenta models. The technique featuring the preparation of the placenta is described elsewhere, as reported by our research group [11]. The placenta model is a very promising and affordable tool for training residents in microsurgical techniques because it resembles the real surgical environment. Each placenta model contains several human vessels of different diameters surrounded by membranes and tissue (stroma), which can be perfused and pressurized to simulate operative conditions and allow very efficient training in techniques such as microdissection, microsuturing, and microanastomoses. Therefore, the placenta model allows trainees to repeat the exercise as many times as needed on vessels of different sizes in a nonthreatening training environment [6, 8]. Dissecting placenta vessels also simulates arachnoid dissection. Further advantages of the placenta models are reported in Table 1. Placenta simulators can be used at all levels of training (beginner, intermediate, or expert trainees). Studies have shown that training on a perfused human placenta may significantly improve surgical skills, particularly in their confidence, technique, and knowledge retention (education outcomes) [12, 13].

Table 1 Advantages of using perfused human placenta

Realistic tissue characteristics: The placenta provides a natural and lifelike simulation of human tissues, including the complexity of the vascular network. This allows surgeons to practice handling delicate blood vessels and soft tissues.

Availability: Placentas are readily available as a byproduct of childbirth, making them accessible resources that lack ethical concerns associated with animal use or the limitations of cadaveric availability.

Cost-effectiveness: The placenta is a cost-effective resource, especially when compared to high-fidelity synthetic models or maintaining animal laboratories. Its availability as a byproduct of childbirth also adds to its cost-effectiveness.

Ethical considerations: The model's affordability and ease of use make it accessible to a wide range of training programs, including those in resource-limited settings. This broadens the scope of high-quality microsurgical training globally. Using the placenta model reduces surgeon's reliance on animal models, aligning with the principles of the 3Rs (replacement, reduction, and refinement) in animal research. It offers an ethical alternative without compromising on the quality of training.

- Increased confidence: By providing a realistic and low-risk environment for practice, the placenta model helps build confidence in trainees. This confidence translates into better performance in the operating room.
- Improved technique: The realistic simulation helps trainees to develop fine motor skills and precision, which are critical in microsurgery (significant improvements in microsuturing, vessel manipulation, and overall surgical skill, including microanastomosis techniques).
- Knowledge retention: The realistic simulation may help trainees to more concretely and stably acquire their skills.

Conclusion

Progressive training in microneurosurgical techniques using simulators in a lab is nowadays an important component of neurosurgical residency. Neurosurgical residents at all levels of training can benefit from training in a lab with the realistic replication of surgical scenarios, the development of muscle memory, the enhancement of surgical confidence, and the mitigation of risks associated with delicate procedures. A progressive training approach in neurosurgical residency that uses simulation models at different training stages is important in the comprehensive development of neurosurgeon residents.

Silicon tubes serve as initial tools, providing exposure to basic skills and a 3D spatial reconstruction of the intraoperative settings. Placental simulators are great tools to train microsurgical techniques, can be used at all levels of training (beginner, intermediate, or expert trainees), and represent a milestone in our lab training programs. Hyper-realistic 3D skull models allow good-quality craniotomy training sessions. Mixed reality allows for teaching surgical anatomy with 3D interactive reconstructions of the most relevant anatomical structures. Cadaver models offer a realistic anatomical setting for advanced specialistic training.

We think that a well-designed resident curriculum integrating simulators to ensure a seamless and effective progression in neurosurgical and specifically microsurgical skill acquisition is nowadays of great importance for residents.

References

1. Weber M, Backhaus J, Lutz R, et al. A novel approach to microsurgical teaching in head and neck surgery leveraging modern 3D technologies. Sci Rep. 2023;13(1):20341. https://doi.org/10.1038/s41598-023-47225-2.
2. Mishra R, Narayanan MDK, Umana GE, Montemurro N, Chaurasia B, Deora H. Virtual reality in neurosurgery: beyond neurosurgical planning. Int J Environ Res Public Health. 2022;19(3):1719. https://doi.org/10.3390/ijerph19031719.
3. Belykh E, Abramov I, Bardonova L, et al. Seven bypasses simulation set: description and validity assessment of novel models for microneurosurgical training. J Neurosurg. 2023;138(3):732–9. https://doi.org/10.3171/2022.5.JNS22465.
4. Oliveira LM, Figueiredo EG. Simulation training methods in neurological surgery. Asian J Neurosurg. 2019;14(2):364–70. https://doi.org/10.4103/ajns.AJNS_269_18.
5. Chawla S, Devi S, Calvachi P, Gormley WB, Rueda-Esteban R. Evaluation of simulation models in neurosurgical training according to face, content, and construct validity: a systematic review. Acta Neurochir. 2022;164(4):947–66. https://doi.org/10.1007/s00701-021-05003-x.
6. de Oliveira MMR, Ferrarez CE, Ramos TM, et al. Learning brain aneurysm microsurgical skills in a human placenta model: predictive validity. J Neurosurg. 2018;128(3):846–52. https://doi.org/10.3171/2016.10.JNS162083.
7. Gmeiner M, Dirnberger J, Fenz W, et al. Virtual cerebral aneurysm clipping with real-time haptic force feedback in neurosurgical education. World Neurosurg. 2018;112:e313–23. https://doi.org/10.1016/j.wneu.2018.01.042.
8. Oliveira MM, Wendling L, Malheiros JA, et al. Human placenta simulator for intracranial-intracranial bypass: vascular anatomy and 5 bypass techniques. World Neurosurg. 2018;119:e694–702. https://doi.org/10.1016/j.wneu.2018.07.246.
9. Colombo E, Regli L, Esposito G, et al. Mixed reality for cranial neurosurgical planning: a single-center applicability study with the first 107 subsequent holograms. Oper Neurosurg (Hagerstown). 2023;26:551. https://doi.org/10.1227/ons.0000000000001033.
10. Efe IE, Cinkaya E, Kuhrt LD, Bruesseler MMT, Muhrer-Osmanagic A. Neurosurgical education using cadaver-free brain models and augmented reality: first experiences from a hands-on simulation course for medical students. Medicina (Kaunas). 2023;59(10):1791. https://doi.org/10.3390/medicina59101791.
11. Hobner LM, Staartjes VE, Colombo E, Sebok M, Regli L, Esposito G. How we do it: the Zurich microsurgery lab technique for pla-

centa preparation. Acta Neurochir. 2023;165(12):3821–4. https://doi.org/10.1007/s00701-023-05847-5.

12. Oliveira MM, Ferrarez CE, Lovato R, et al. Quality assurance during brain aneurysm microsurgery-operative error teaching. World Neurosurg. 2019;130:e112–6. https://doi.org/10.1016/j.wneu.2019.05.262.

13. Apaza-Tintaya RA, Canache Jimenez LA, Salvagni Pereira F, et al. Topographical systematization of human placenta model for training in microneurosurgery. World Neurosurg. 2024;182:e471–7. https://doi.org/10.1016/j.wneu.2023.11.123.

Open Access This chapter is licensed under the terms of the Creative Commons Attribution 4.0 International License (http://creativecommons.org/licenses/by/4.0/), which permits use, sharing, adaptation, distribution and reproduction in any medium or format, as long as you give appropriate credit to the original author(s) and the source, provide a link to the Creative Commons license and indicate if changes were made.

The images or other third party material in this chapter are included in the chapter's Creative Commons license, unless indicated otherwise in a credit line to the material. If material is not included in the chapter's Creative Commons license and your intended use is not permitted by statutory regulation or exceeds the permitted use, you will need to obtain permission directly from the copyright holder.

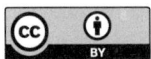

Index

A

Acute ischemic stroke, 115, 132
Akaike Information Criterion (AIC), 39
Analysis of variance (ANOVA), 123, 125
Aneurysm, 154, 166
Aneurysmal subarachnoid hemorrhage (aSAH), 19, 20, 23
Angiographic effects, 27
Angiographic factor, 89
Angiography, 75, 85
Antiplatelet management, 27, 29
Apparent diffusion coefficient (ADC), 129, 130, 132
    limitations, 132
    methods, 129, 130
    reduction, 132
Arterial spin labeling (ASL), 121–123, 125, 126, 135
Arterial transit artifacts (ATA), 85, 121, 122, 125
Arteriovenous malformations (AVMs), 37, 47, 65, 154
Artificial intelligence (AI), 157, 158
    5D by adding flow and pulsatility, 160
    integration of AR, 159, 160
    methods, 158
    treatment guidance, 161
    treatment planning, 160
Asymmetry index (AI), 37, 39
Atherosclerotic occlusive disease, 114, 115
Augmented reality (AR), 157, 158, 174
    5D by adding flow and pulsatility, 160
    integration of AI, 159, 160
    methods, 158
    treatment guidance, 161
    treatment planning, 160

B

Balloon assist technique, 27
Balloon neck-plasty technique, 27
Bayesian network (BN), 23
Bayes' theorem, 20, 22
Bias, 20, 96
Bifrontal hypoperfusion, 114
Blood blister-like aneurysm (BBA), 29, 30
BOLD-CVR, 115, 116
Bone flap, 101
Brain, 37
Brain hemodynamic and collaterals, 115
Bypass surgery, 93, 94

C

Carotid cavernous aneurysms (CCAs), 29
Carotid Occlusion Surgery Study (COSS), 121
Carotid stenosis/occlusion, 154
Cerebral blood flow (CBF), 85, 121–123, 125, 126, 139
Cerebral cavernous malformations (CCMs), 143
    and developmental venous anomalies, 146
    epidemiology, 143
    genetic mutations, 144, 145
    genotype–phenotype correlations, 145
    GJA4, a novel cavernous malformation-associated gene, 147
    molecular pathogenesis, 145, 146
    natural history of, 143
Cerebral embolism, 31
Cerebral hyperperfusion syndrome, 99, 100, 103
Cerebral ischemic complications of surgical treatment with Moyamoya disease, 85–87, 89, 90
Cerebral perfusion, 121
Cerebrovascular insufficiency (CVI), 85, 121, 126
    compensation group, 125
    decompensation, 125, 126
    materials and methods, 122, 123, 125
    MR perfusion methods, 125
    subcompensation, 125, 126
Choroidal channel, 101
Cilostazol, 14
Circle of Willis, 19, 89, 115
Clinical factor, 89
Clopidogrel, 95
Cognitive biases, 19, 20
Combined revascularization surgery for Moyamoya disease, 103
    inclusion criteria of patients and surgical procedure, 99, 100
    outcome, 100
    postoperative CBF measurement and peri-operative management protocol, 100
    representative case, 101
Complementary metal oxide semiconductor (CMOS), 110
Computed tomography (CT), 69
Cone beam computed tomography (CBCT), 73, 74
    conjunction with superselective angiography, 77
    contrast from microcatheter, 74
    deposition of platinum coils, 75
    disadvantage, 80
    protocol for, 74
    selective injection, 75
    vs. traditional computed tomography (CT), 80
Contrast agents, 121
CorPath GRX vascular robotic system, 31
Cortical venous drainage (CVD), 61
Corticospinal tract (CST), 37
Craniotomy, 101
Craniovertebral junction (CVJ), 65

D

Decision-making process, 19, 20
Definite MMD (dMMD), 94
Dehydration, 90
Delayed cerebral ischemia (DCI), 3, 11, 13, 14
De novo PHTSs, 71
Developmental venous anomalies, 146
Diagnostic perfusion techniques, 126
Diffusion tensor tractography (DTT), 37
Diffusion weighted imaging (DWI), 129
Digital subtraction angiography (DSA), 48
Digital zoom, 110
Direct angiography, 123
Directed acyclic graph (DAG), 23
Doppler sonography, 62
Dual ASL perfusion imaging, 139
    background, 135
    hemodynamic parameters, 136
    incomplete filling-up in the MMD group, 138
    methods, 135, 136
    of mild ischemia, 136, 137
    of moderate ischemia, 136, 137
    for normal control, 138
Dural arteriovenous fistula (DAVF), 73
Dyna CT, 153

E

Early brain injury (EBI), 11
Early slow-in, 135
Early stagnation, 135
Elective secondary surgery, 69
Endovascular embolization, 27
Endovascular thrombectomy (EVT), 129
Endovascular treatment (EVT)
    BBA, challenges for, 29, 30
    dAVF, 61, 63
    and GKRS, 49
    large/giant aneurysms, challenges for, 29
    remote telesurgery, 31, 32
    robotics, challenges for, 30, 31
    structure, 31
    transition in, 27–28
Ethmoidal dAVF, 65
Euvolemia, 3
Exoscopes, 105, 168
    advantages, 110
    annotation system, 165–168
    disadvantages, 110
    educational advantage, 167
    in microneurosurgical procedures, 165
    vision and surgical ergonomics, 167
Exoscopic STA-MCA bypass
    clinical outcomes, 108
    limitations, 111
    methods, 105
        questionnaire, 106
        setup and setting of exoscope, 107
        statistical analysis, 108
        surgical procedure, 106
    patient characteristics, 108
Extracranial-intracranial (EC-IC) bypass surgery, 113

F

Familial cerebral cavernous malformations, 144, 145
Fasudil hydrochloride, 14
Fiber assignment by the continuous tracking (FACT) method, 39
Fibronectin type III (FNIII), 11
Fisher's exact test, 39
Flow-augmentation bypass surgery, 113
    atherosclerotic occlusive disease of ICA and MCA, 114, 115
    intra- and post-operative measurements, 116
    Moyamoya vasculopathy, 113, 114
    studying brain hemodynamic and collaterals, 115
Flow-augmentation revascularization, 116
Flow disruptor, 27
Flow diverters (FD), 27–29
Fluoroscopy, 31
Fractional anisotropy (FA), 37, 39
Fragile moyamoya collateral vessels, 114
Functional disability, 6

G

Galectin-3, 14
Gamma knife radiosurgery (GKRS), 47
    basic radiosurgical techniques, 48
    history, 47
    limitations, 58
    radiosurgical advancement
        endovascular treatment, 49
        integration of tractography, 48
        rotational angiography (RA), integration of, 48, 49
    radiosurgical outcomes
        baseline characteristics, 52
        haemorrhagic events and survival, 52
        obliteration, 52, 57
        post-GKRS early signal change and neurological outcomes, 53, 57
    study population, 47, 48
Germline mutations, 69–71
Giant symptomatic paraclinoid aneurysms, 29
GJA4, a novel cavernous malformation-associated gene, 147

H

Head mounted display (HMD), 157
Hemispheric VFR (hVFR), 116
Hemodilution, 3
Hemodynamic cerebral ischemia, 138, 139
HiRes-XperCT, 48
Houkin classification, 123
Hybrid operating room, 153
    advantage, 153, 154
    AVM/fistula, 154
    carotid stenosis/occlusion, 154
    hybrid interventions, 154
    intraoperative angiography, 154
    methods and materials, 153
    in neurosurgery, 153
    surgical strategy, 154
Hyperdynamic therapy, 3, 7
Hyper-realistic UpSurgeOn three-dimensional models, 174
Hypertension, 6
Hyperventilation, 90
Hypervolemia, 3
Hypervolemia, hypertension, hemodilution (HHH) therapy, 6

Hypotension, 90
Hypovolemia, 90

I
Inadequate collateral pathways, 114
Indirect brain revascularization, 90
Indirect revascularization, 86
Indocyanine green (ICG), 101, 153, 166
Informed consent, 61
Integrated parallel acquisition technique (iPAT), 38
Internal carotid artery (ICA) stenosis, 105
Intra-arterial spasmolysis, 4
Intracerebral hemorrhage, 101, 114
Intracranial aneurysms (IAs), 19
    Bayes' theorem, 20
    complexity with Bayesian networks, 23
    decision-making for, 19
    management, 19
    recruitment population and at-risk demographics
        risk estimations for, 21
        rupture cases, 20, 21
        sex-associated risks in diagnosis and rupture, 21–23
    risk factors, 19
Intracranial dural arteriovenous fistulas (dAVF), 61
    CVJ and tentorial, 65
    ethmoidal, 65
    factors for selecting surgery and endovascular attempts, 63
    limitation, 65
    massive ICH presentation, 65
    methods
        data collection and outcome evaluation, 61, 62
        direct surgical procedure, 62
        indication and selection of treatment modality, 62
        patient, 61
    patient characteristics, 62, 63
    pial arterial supply, 65
    surgical outcomes, 63, 64
    surgical procedural details, 63
Intracranial hemorrhage (ICH), 61
Intradural reflux, 70
Intraoperative angiography, 154, 155
Intravenous fasudil, 6
Ischemic cerebrovascular disease, 114
Ischemic penumbra, 132
Ischemic region, 130
Ischemic stroke, 86, 89

J
Japan Adult Moyamoya (JAM) trial, 99, 113

K
Knowledge gaps, 20

L
Lacosamide, 100
LactoSorb®, 101
Laminectomy, 69
Laparoscopic surgery, 165
Large artery atherosclerosis (LAA), 135
Large/giant aneurysms, 29
Late complete filling-up, 136
Late filling-up, 135, 136

Late stagnation/over-stagnation, 136
Leksell Gamma Knife, 48
Leksell GammaPlan, 48
Leptomeningeal collaterals, 123, 125
Lhermitte-Duclos disease, 70
Lipiodol, 74
Logistic regression model, 86
LumiNE software, 158

M
Machine learning, 157
Magnetic resonance imaging (MRI), 37, 69
Magnetization-prepared rapid acquisition gradient-echo sequences (MPRAGE), 38
Mann-Whitney U-test, 39
Manual muscle test (MMT), 39
Massive ICH presentation, 65
Matrix metalloproteinases (MMPs), 11
MDAC, 43, 44
Mechanical thrombectomy, 155
Microanastomosis, 174
Microcatheterization, 31
Microdissection, 174
Microsurgery, 62, 173
    placenta model, 174, 175
    scheme, 173, 174
Microsuturing, 174
Middle cerebral artery aneurysms, 168
Milrinone, 3
    published controlled studies, 4–7
    vasospasm and DCI, 5
Minimal targeting embolization (MTE), 49
Mitogen-activated protein kinase (MAPK), 12, 13
Mixed reality (MxR), 157, 159, 174
MMA, *see* Moyamoya angiopathy
Modified Rankin Scale (mRS), 61, 94–96, 129
Motor function, 39
Motor weakness, 39
Moyamoya angiopathy (MMA), 85, 121, 122, 125
Moyamoya disease (MMD), 85, 89, 93, 126, 135, 136, 138
    cerebral ischemic complications of surgical treatment, 85–87, 89, 90
    combined revascularization surgery for, 103
        inclusion criteria of patients and surgical procedure, 99, 100
        outcome, 100
        postoperative CBF measurement and peri-operative management protocol, 100
        representative case, 101
    dual ASL perfusion imaging (*see* Dual ASL perfusion imaging, hemodynamic cerebral ischemia)
    etiology, 85
    long-term outcome of, 94, 96
        academic level in pediatric patients, 95
        characteristics of the cohort, 94
        cohort population, 93
        data availability statement, 94
        income source, 95
        medical and surgical management, 94, 95
        revascularisation surgery, 94
        statistical analysis, 94
        strengths and limitations, 96, 97
        structured telephone interviews, 95
        study timeline, 94
        subgroup analyses, 95
    systemic risk factors, 85

Moyamoya syndrome, 122
Moyamoya vasculopathy, 113, 114
mRS, see Modified Rankin Scale
Multiple primary cancers, 69, 71

N
N-butyl cyanoacrylate (NBCA), 74
NeuroRegistration program, 122
Nimodipine, 3, 4
N-isopropyl-p-[123I] iodpamphetamine single-photon emission computed tomography, 102
nnUNet framework, 159
Non-contrast ASL perfusion, 121
Non-invasive optimal vessel analysis (NOVA), 115
NOVA-qMRA, 115
Nuclear factor-kappa B (NF-κB), 12, 13

O
Optic radiation (OR), 37
ORBEYE, 110, 111
Orbital cavernous venous malformations (OCVMs), 147
Orthostatic hypoperfusion syndrome, 115
Osteopontin, 14
Oxygen extraction fraction (OEF) ratio, 114

P
Paraspinal arteriovenous shunt (PAVS), 69, 70
Pearson's chi-square test, 39, 123
Penumbra evaluation, 132
Perampanel, 14
Perfused human placenta models, 174, 175
Perfusion factor, 89
Pericallosal artery, 154
Periostin, 14
Permanent symptoms, 39
Phosphatase and tensin homolog (PTEN), 69
Phosphodiesterase-3 inhibitors, 4
Pial arterial supply, 65
Placenta simulators, 174
Post-labeling delay (PLD), 135
Pressurized human placenta models, 174
Probable MMD (pMMD), 94
Prospect theory, 19
Pseudoaneurysm, 101
Pseudo-continuous ASL perfusion (3D pCASL), 122
PTEN hamartoma tumor syndrome (PHTS), 69, 71
Pulsed continuous ASL (pCASL), 135

Q
Q-ball based tractography, 48
Quantitative analysis, 125
Quantitative magnetic resonance angiography (qMRA), 115

R
Radiofrequency (RF), 135
Radiosurgical planning, 48
Randomized controlled trials (RCTs), 114
Randomized Trial of Unruptured Brain Arteriovenous Malformations (ARUBA) study, 47
ReadyView program, 122
Red-color shift, 110

Regions of interest (ROI), 39, 122, 126
Remote telesurgery, 31, 32
Revascularization procedures, 89
Revascularization surgery, Moyamoya disease, 114
Revised PHTS clinical diagnostic criteria, 70
Robotic intelligence, 32
Robotics, 30, 31
Receiver operating characteristic (ROC) analysis, 39, 130
ROIs, see Regions of interest
Rotational angiography (RA), 48, 49

S
SAH, see Subarachnoid hemorrhage
Sensor system, 31
Simulation models, 173
Slave manipulator, 31
Spetzler-Martin Grading (SMG), 44
Sporadic cerebral cavernous malformations (CCMs), 144, 145, 147
Stabilization, 111
Staged revascularization, 86
STA-MCA anastomosis, 99, 103
Steno-occlusive cerebrovascular pathology, 121, 125, 126
Steno-occlusive disease, 113–116
Stent-assisted coiling, 29
Stereotactic radiosurgery (SRS), 47
Subacute stroke, 115
Subarachnoid hemorrhage (SAH), 4, 11–13
Superficial temporal artery (STA), 99, 102, 105, 113
  See also Exoscopic STA-MCA bypass
Superselective angiography, 75, 77
Surgical deconstructive techniques, 30
Surgical revascularization, 99
Suzuki classification, 123
Symptomatic ischemia, 136
Symptomatic vasospasm, 6
Symptom-disease relationships, 20
Systemic therapy, 3

T
Target Registration Error (TRE), 161
Telementoring, 165, 167
Telesurgery, 31
Tenascin-C (TNC), 11
  active form, 11
  DCI
    biomarker for, 13
    development, 13, 14
  drugs antagonizing functions, 14
  intact monomer of, 11
  isoforms, 12
  perspective, 14
  post-SAH upregulation of, 12
Tentorial dAVFs, 65
Therapeutic vessel occlusion, 155
Three-dimensional (3D) exoscope, 165
3D holograms, 160
3D rotational angiography, 78, 153
3D TOF magnetic resonance angiography, 123
3-tesla magnetic resonance tractography (MRT), 37
  estimation of CST by visual inspection, 41
  materials and methods
    characteristics of patients, 37, 38
    evaluation of tract injury on, 39
    imaging protocol, 38

    minimal distance vs. nidus and CST measurement, 39
    motor disfunctions evaluation, 39
    size of the nidus measurement, 39
    statistical analysis, 39
  multivariate analysis, 43, 44
  permanent motor dysfunction and findings, 42
  preoperative motor dysfunction and findings, 41
  receiver operating character analysis of MDAC, 43
  SMG, 44
  transient motor dysfunction and findings, 41
Time to peak (TTP), 4
Toll-like receptor 4 (TLR4), 12, 13
Traditional computed tomography (CT) scans, 80
Transarterial embolization (TAE), 61, 70
Transdural collaterals, 123, 125
Transient symptoms, 39
Transitory ischemic attack (TIA), 114
Transvenous approach, 74, 77
Transvenous embolization (TVE), 61

Transverse-sigmoid junction, 74
2D angiography, 155

U
Unruptured aneurysms, 27

V
Virtual reality (VR), 174

W
Watershed shift phenomenon, 100, 103
Wilcoxon rank-sum test, 129

X
Xper CT system, 74

If you have any concerns about our products,
you can contact us on
ProductSafety@springernature.com

In case Publisher is established outside the EU,
the EU authorized representative is:
**Springer Nature Customer Service Center GmbH
Europaplatz 3, 69115 Heidelberg, Germany**

Printed by Libri Plureos GmbH
in Hamburg, Germany